S0-BET-896

SEXUALLY TRANSMITTED DISEASES

Epidemiology, Pathology, Diagnosis, and Treatment

Edited by

Kenneth A. Borchardt, Ph.D.
Center for Biomedical Laboratory Science
San Francisco State University

Michael A. Noble, M.D., F.R.C.P.C.
Department of Pathology and
Laboratory Medicine
The University of British Columbia

CRC Press
Boca Raton   New York

Senior Editor: Paul Petralia
Editorial Assistant: Norina Frabotta
Project Editor: Debbie Didier
Cover design: Dawn Boyd
PrePress: Kevin Luong

Library of Congress Cataloging-in-Publication Data

Sexually transmitted diseases : epidemiology, pathology, diagnosis,
    and treatment / edited by Kenneth A. Borchardt, Michael A. Noble.
        p.   cm.
    Includes bibliographical references and index.
    ISBN 0-8493-9476-7
    1. Sexually transmitted diseases.   I. Borchardt, Kenneth A.
II. Noble, Michael A.
    [DNLM: 1. Sexually Transmitted Diseases.   WC 140 S5174 1997]
    RC200.S499   1997
    616.95'1--dc21
    DNLM/DLC
    for Library of Congress   96-39561
                                                                        CIP

No claim to original U.S. Government works
International Standard Book Number 0-8493-9476-7
Library of Congress Card Number 96-39561
Printed in the United States of America 1 2 3 4 5 6 7 8 9 0
Printed on acid-free paper

Introduction

Since the 1950s, sexually transmitted diseases (STDs) have become an important medical challenge worldwide. The ubiquitousness of STDs affects all nations and races. This is particularly evident in developing countries, such as those in Africa. Some regions have a significant incidence of gonorrhea, chlamydia, syphilis, and the human immunodeficiency virus (HIV). Insufficient health care centers, inadequate laboratory capabilities, and the unavailability of appropriate treatment perpetuates the prevalence of these STDs. However, it is important to appreciate that underservicing of areas and regions is not found exclusively in developing countries, but is evident in developed regions as well.

The identification of new infectious agents such as HIV have presented the medical and scientific communities with some of its most significant therapuetic challenges. Subsequent infections in these patients have created additional diagnostic and treatment dilemmas.

Antimicrobial resistance has become important in treating various STDs. *Neisseria gonorrhoeae* which initially was sensitive to penicillin G has developed resistance requiring different treatment regimens. The successful treatment of patients with HIV and cryptosporidiosis infections remains a vexing problem. As we near the end of this millenia, it is important to realize that while the medical community has effectively eliminated smallpox and is successful in controlling many bacterial and viral infections, the worldwide prevalence of STDs remains a major infectious disease conundrum.

This textbook presents contributors from Brazil, Canada, China, and the U.S. They have graciously extended their clinical expertise and scientific knowledge in their respective chapters. We respectively appreciate each author's contribution.

The editors appreciate the contributions of Axel W. Hoke, M.D., for the clinical photographs he provided.

K.A.B.
M.A.N.

Editors

Kenneth A. Borchardt, Ph.D., is a Professor of Clinical Science at the Center for Biomedical Laboratory Science, San Francisco State University. He received his doctorate from Tulane University School of Medicine and Graduate School. He completed a Fellowship in Tropical Medicine at Louisiana State University School of Medicine, New Orleans. Presently he is a Fellow, Royal Society of Tropical Medicine and Hygiene; Fellow, American Academy of Microbiology; and Affiliate, American Academy of Dermatology. He is a former Chief of Clinical Microbiology at Letterman Army Medical Center, San Francisco, and former Chief of Clinical Microbiology at the United States Public Health Services Hospital, San Francisco. He retired as a Captain in the United States Public Health Service.

Michael A. Noble, M.D., F.R.C.P.(C), is an Associate Professor in the Department of Pathology and Laboratory Medicine, University of British Columbia, and a Consultant Microbiologist at the Vancouver Hospital and Health Sciences Centre, Vancouver, British Columbia. He received his M.D. from the University of Western Ontario and earned Fellowships in Internal Medicine and Medical Microbiology. He is a member of the American Society for Microbiology, Royal College of Physicians and Surgeons of Canada, the past-chair of the Infectious Diseases Committee for the Council on Health Promotion, British Columbia Medical Association, past-president of the Canadian Association for Clinical Microbiology and Infectious Diseases, and presently the chair of the Clinical Microbiology Proficiency Testing program for Western and Eastern Canada.

Contributors

Nero Araújo Barreto, Professor, Master, Department of Microbiology and Parasitology, Universidade Federal Fluminense, and Coordinator, Course of Postgraduation (Especialization) In STD, Universidade Federal Fluminense, Brazil.

Barbara A. Body, Ph.D., is National Director of Microbiology for Laboratory Corporation of America. She received her doctoral degree from the University of Kentucky and completed a postdoctoral fellowship in Clinical and Public Health Microbiology in the Department of Pathology at the Medical College of Virginia, Virginia Commonwealth University. She is a Diplomat of the American Board of Medical Microbiology and has served on the editorial boards of the *Journal of Clinical Microbiology, Diagnostic Testing Alert,* and *Clinical Microbiology Reports.*

Brian P. Currie, M.D., M.P.H., is an Assistant Professor of Medicine and Epidemiology and Social Medicine, Albert Einstein College of Medicine, Bronx, New York. He is attending physician in Infectious Diseases and Director of Infection Control, Montefiore Medical Center, Bronx, New York.

Gerald J. Domingue, Sr., Ph.D., received his doctorate from Tulane University School of Medicine and Graduate School, New Orleans, Louisiana, and completed a postdoctoral fellowship at Children's Hospital and the University of Buffalo School of Medicine, Buffalo, New York. He is a Professor of Urology and Professor of Microbiology and Immunology at Tulane University School of Medicine and Graduate School. He is Director of Research in Urology and Chief of the Laboratory of Microbiology and Immunology in the Urology Department.

José Trindade Filho, M.D., Professor, Master, Discipline of Dermatology, Faculty of Medicine, Universidade Federal Fluminense, and Professor, Course of Post Graduation In STD, Universidade Federal Fluminense, Brazil.

Janice I. French, C.N.M., M.S., is a graduate of Lycoming College and the University of Colorado. She is a Ph.D. student in Epidemiology at the University of North Carolina, Chapel Hill. She is a Senior Instructor-Research Associate in the Department of Obstetrics and Gynecology at the University of Colorado Health Sciences Center, Denver, Colorado.

Lynne S. Garcia, M.S., M.T., F(AAM), obtained her M.S. in Health Care Administration from the University of La Verne, La Verne, California. She is Manager of the Clinical Microbiology Division of the Clinical Laboratories in the Department of Pathology and Laboratory Medicine at the University of California at Los Angeles. She is a member of the editorial board of several journals, one of the senior editors of *Clinical Microbiology Reviews,* and Chair of the Parsitology Committee of the National Committee for Clinical Laboratory Standards.

Robert F. Garry, Ph.D., is Professor of Microbiology and Immunology at Tulane University School of Medicine and obtained his doctorate from the University of Texas at Austin. He is an investigator on both the Adult and Pediatric AIDS Clinical Trials Units at Tulane University. He was a charter member of the AIDS Molecular Biology Study Section (AIDS and Related Research Section C) for NIH.

Axel W. Hoke, M.D., is a Clinical Professor of Dermatology at the University of California, San Francisco.

Michael H. Levi, Sc.D., is an Assistant Professor of Pathology, Albert Einstein School of Medicine, and an Associate Director of Microbiology and Immunology, Montefiore Medical Center, Bronx, New York. He received his Sc.D. from the Graduate School of Public Health at the University of Pittsburgh, and then completed a two-year Fellowship in Clinical Public Health Microbiology at the Montefiore Medical Center.

Zhijian Li, M.D., M.S., is an Associate Professor of Laboratory Medicine in the School of Laboratory Medicine at Hunan Medical University, Changsha, Hunan, the People's Republic of China. He recieved his M.D. from the Department of Human Parasitology of Hunan Medical University and the M.S. degree in Clinical Science from the Center for Advanced Medical Technology, San Francisco State University, San Francisco, California.

Nino Maida, M.S., received his degree at San Francisco State University and presently is performing research in cell and molecular biology at the University of California, San Francisco.

James A. McGregor, M.D., C.M., is a graduate of McGill University, Faculty of Medicine. He is Professor and Vice Chairman of Academic Affairs for the Department of Obstetrics and Gynecology at the University of Colorado Health Sciences Center, Denver.

Julio S.G. Montaner, M.D., received his M.D. with honors at the University of Buenos Aires and completed his residency in Internal and Respiratory Medicine at the University of British Columbia. He is the Director, Clinical Activities of the B.C. Centre for Excellence in HIV/AIDS and a founding Co-Director of the Canadian HIV Trials Network. He is an Associate Professor in the Department of Medicine at the University of British Columbia and in 1996 was appointed to the Endowed Chair on AIDS at St. Paul's Hospital, University of British Columbia, Canada.

Rene Garrido Neves, M.D., Ph.D., is a Titular Professor at the Universidade Federal do Rio de Janeiro, Brazil; Curso de Pos-Graducao em Medicina-Dermatologia.

Michael V. O'Shaughnessy, Ph.D., is Director, Canadian HIV Trials Network, Vancouver, British Columbia, and the Director, B.C. Centre for Excellence in HIV/AIDS, St. Paul's Hospital, Vancouver, British Columbia. He received his doctorate at Dalhousie University, Halifax, Nova Scotia, Canada.

Mauro Romero Leal Passos, M.D., Ph.D., is a Professor in the Department of Microbiology and Parasitology, Universidade Federal Fluminense. He is Coordinator for the Health Ministry Course of Postgraduation in Sexually Transmitted Diseases, and Chief, Sector of Sexually Transmitted Diseases, Universidade Federal Fluminse; and the STD National Reference Center-STD/AIDS Program National Health Ministry. He is President of the Brazilian STD Society.

Omar Lupi Da Rosa Santos, M.D., Ph.D., M.Sc., is a Professor at the Universidade Federal do Rio de Janerio, Brazil; Curso de Pos-Graduacao em Medicina-Dermatologia.

Martin T. Schecter, M.D., Ph.D., M.Sc., is Professor and Chair, Division of Epidemiology and Biostatistics, in the Department of Health Care at the University of British Columbia, Faculty of Medicine, Canada. He received his Ph.D. in mathematics at the Polytechnic Institute of New York, his M.D. at McMaster University, and his M.Sc. in Epidemiology at the University of Toronto. He is a Fellow of the Royal College of Physicians and Surgeons of Canada and currently holds the National Health Research Scientist Award of Health in Canada from 1991–98.

Walter F. Schlech III, M.D., is a Professor of Medicine and Head of the Division of Infectious Diseases at Dalhousie University, Halifax, Nova Scotia, Canada. He received his M.D. degree from Cornell University and completed an Internal Medicine residency at Dartmouth. He studied the pathogenicity of *Neisseria gonorrhoeae* with a fellowship from the American Venereal Diseases Association and subsequently joined the Epidemic Intelligence Service at CDC prior to taking his current position. Presently he is a member of the CDC Advisory Committee on the Prevention of STD, HIV, and TB infection.

Dawn M. Sokol, M.D., is an Assistant Professor of Pediatrics in the Section of Infectious Diseases at the Tulane University School of Medicine. She obtained her M.D. degree from the University of Missouri in Kansas City and served an Internship, Residency, and Fellowship at Baylor College of Medicine, Houston, Texas. Her research has resulted in development of polymerase chain reaction (PCR) staining techniques for diagnosis of herpesvirus infections. She is a co-investigator with the Tulane-LSU Pediatric Clinical Trials Units and is active in basic and clinical research designed to prevent and treat HIV infection in infants.

Nancy G. Warren, Ph.D., is Science Advisor for the Association of State and Territorial Public Health Laboratory Directors and is a Research Professor of Dermatology in the George Washington University's Department of Dermatology. She obtained her Ph.D. from the Department of Pathology, Medical College of Virginia, Virginia Commonwealth University. She serves on the editorial board of the *Journal of Clinical Microbiology.*

Michael Z. Zhang, M.D., received his M.D. from Hubei Medical University, China. After completing his residency in surgery, he was an Assistant Professor in the Department of Surgery. He received his M.S. in Biomedical Laboratory Science, at San Francisco State University, San Francisco, California.

Contents

Bacterial

Chapter 1 Bacterial Vaginosis: History, Epidemiology, Microbiology, Sequelae, Diagnosis, and Treatment..3
Janice I. French and James A. McGregor

Chapter 2 Sexually Transmitted Infections Associated with *Chlamydia trachomatis*..41
Michael A. Noble

Chapter 3 Chancroid..59
Brian P. Currie

Chapter 4 Current Concepts in the Laboratory Diagnosis of Gonorrhea..75
Michael H. Levi

Chapter 5 Donovanosis..103
Mauro Romero Leal Passos, José Trindade Filho, and Nero Araújo Barreto

Chapter 6 Lymphogranuloma Venereum..117
Rene Garrido Neves and Omar Lupi da Rosa Santos

Spirochete

Chapter 7 Syphilis..131
Gerald J. Domingue

Fungal

Chapter 8 Candidiasis..149
Nancy G. Warren and Barbara A. Body

Protozoan

Chapter 9 Amebiasis..167
Lynne S. Garcia

Chapter 10   Cryptosporidiosis 189
Lynne S. Garcia

Chapter 11   Trichomoniasis 205
Kenneth A. Borchardt

Viral

Chapter 12   Herpesviruses..217
Dawn M. Sokol and Robert F. Garry

**Chapter 13   Infection with the Human Immunodeficiency Virus and the
                Acquired Immunodeficiency Syndrome** 245
Julio S.G. Montaner, Michael V. O'Shaughnessy, and Martin T. Schechter

Chapter 14   Condyloma Acuminatum 271
Michael Z. Zhang, Kenneth A. Borchardt, and Zhijian Li

Chapter 15   Molluscum Contagiosum 283
Zhijian Li, Kenneth A. Borchardt, and Michael Z. Zhang

The Gay Bowel Syndrome

Chapter 16   The Gay Bowel Syndrome: A 20-Year Retrospective 295
Walter F. Schlech III

Ectoparasites

Chapter 17   Scabies 315
Kenneth A. Borchardt, Axel W. Hoke, Nino Maida, and Michael Z. Zhang

Chapter 18   Lice 323
Kenneth A. Borchardt, Axel W. Hoke, Nino Maida, and Michael Z. Zhang

Index 333

Dedication

This textbook is dedicated in the memory of Morris F. Shaffer, Ph.D., former Chairman of the Department of Medical Microbiology and Immunology at the Tulane University School of Medicine and Graduate School. Dr. Shaffer was a distinguished research scientist, teacher, and humanitarian. His persona was an inspiration to all of his students. Any success achieved by them was a result of his efforts.

SEXUALLY TRANSMITTED DISEASES

Epidemiology, Pathology, Diagnosis, and Treatment

Bacterial

chapter one

Bacterial vaginosis: history, epidemiology, microbiology, sequelae, diagnosis, and treatment

Janice I. French and James A. McGregor

1.1	Introduction	4
1.2	History of bacterial vaginosis	4
1.3	Microbiology and pathology of BV	5
1.4	Epidemiology of BV	7
	1.4.1 Natural history of BV	10
1.5	Gynecologic complications associated with BV	11
	1.5.1 Pelvic inflammatory disease	11
	1.5.2 Abnormal bleeding and endometritis	12
	1.5.3 Postoperative infections following gynecologic surgery	13
	1.5.4 Cervical cancer	13
	1.5.5 Transmission of HIV infection	14
1.6	Obstetrical complications associated with BV	15
	1.6.1 Preterm birth	15
	1.6.2 Antimicrobial treatment trials for the prevention of preterm birth	18
	1.6.3 Intrapartum and post partum infections	19
1.7	Diagnosis of BV	19
	1.7.1 Clinical diagnosis	20
	1.7.2 Papanicolaou smear diagnosis	21
	1.7.3 Gram stain diagnosis	22
	1.7.4 Bacterial metabolic by-products	24
	1.7.5 Microbial culture	24
	1.7.6 New diagnostic techniques	25
1.8	Treatments for BV	25
	1.8.1 Treatment during pregnancy	27
	1.8.2 Adverse effects from treatment	28
	1.8.3 Probiotic treatments	28
1.9	Conclusions	29
	References	30

> " the Excrementitious Humors are somtimes white and flegmatick,
> very like to Whey, or Barley Cream...; Somtimes they are pale, or
> yellow, or green...; somtimes watery...; somtimes they are of a strong
> and beastly smel, and other whiles again, not at all offensive in that
> kind."
>
> "leukorrhoea" as described by Riverius, 1655[1]

1.1   Introduction

Bacterial vaginosis (BV) is a common abnormal vaginal condition which is the leading cause of abnormal vaginal discharge and other symptoms world wide.[2] Over the past 40 years researchers have sought to define and describe the pathobiology, etiologic factors, clinical characteristics, diagnostic methods, pathologic sequelae, and effective treatments for bacterial vaginosis. Prior to the early 1980s, bacterial vaginosis was commonly regarded as a "nuisance" infection, and either not recognized or ignored by clinicians. Considerable work over the past decade has focused national and international attention on this common condition. Bacterial vaginosis is increasingly recognized as directly related to a number of serious obstetrical and gynecologic complications.[3-20] Importantly, a number of these complications including some instances of preterm birth can be prevented by identification and effective treatment of bacterial vaginosis.[23-27]

1.2   History of bacterial vaginosis

Clinical signs consistent with BV have been recognized as abnormal throughout recorded history. Prior to the late 19th century BV was included in the discussion of the global condition of "leukorrhoea" or commonly "the whites." The predominant Döderlein's lactobacillus characteristic in normal vaginal flora was first described by Döderlein in 1892.[28] Others subsequently identified facultative and anaerobic bacteria from vaginal fluid obtained from healthy women.[29] As early as 1894, the entity subsequently called BV was accurately described. Because a single causative microorganism had not been identified, the condition was referred to as "nonspecific" vaginitis.[29] In their classic work, Gardner and Dukes further described the clinical characteristics of this condition, described the characteristic "clue" cell, and suggested that these findings represented a specific clinical entity.[30] Gardner and Dukes proposed that this condition was caused by a single agent, the facultative bacterium *Haemophilus vaginalis*, and proposed the name "*Haemophilus vaginalis* vaginitis."[30] Further study of the bacillus determined that the microorganism was not appropriately classified as *Haemophilus* and it was reclassified and renamed *Corynebacterium vaginalis* in 1963.[31] Again, testing of the organism determined that it was not characteristic of the *Corynebacterium* genus and in 1980 it was named *Gardnerella vaginalis* to honor Gardner eponymously.[32,33] Subsequently, many North American clinicians inappropriately termed this condition "Gardnerella vaginitis."

In the early 1980s, the integral role of anaerobic bacteria in the pathobiology of the condition was acknowledged and other names for the clinical condition were suggested including: anaerobic vaginitis, anaerobic colpitis, and anaerobic vaginosis.[34,35] The term bacterial vaginosis was proposed and became generally accepted in 1984.[36] The name bacterial vaginosis was selected to reflect the characteristic vaginal discharge and the polymicrobial nature of the condition as well as the relative absence of an inflammatory response.[36] Concurrently, Amsel's diagnostic criteria based upon aggregate clinical findings were evaluated and accepted as the "gold standard" for detecting the condition.[36,37]

Although disagreement concerning nomenclature has subsided, recently a new name, vaginal bacteriosis, has been suggested to reinforce the concept of excessive bacteria in the vagina.[38] Doubtlessly disputes over identification of a single bacterial etiologic factor and repeated name changes have handicapped our understanding of this condition and hindered effective clinical care.

1.3 Microbiology and pathogenesis of BV

BV is distinguished as a polymicrobial condition in which a characteristic set of bacterial species appear to synergistically overgrow and cause local genital symptoms as well as upper reproductive tract pathology.[3,34,37] Current understanding best defines BV as a massive microbiologic change in the vaginal ecosystem, rather than an infection caused by a single microorganism.[39] In addition to dynamic ecological shifts in the vaginal microflora, there are important alterations in the biochemical properties of BV-associated vaginal fluid.[34,37] Indeed, BV may be considered similar to a "red tide" resulting from blooming of various oceanic bacteria. Current understanding of factors which initiate and perpetuate such microbiologic and biochemical shifts remains incomplete.

In the healthy vagina, between 5 and 15 principle microbial species are recovered.[39-41] The predominant microorganisms detected are acidophilic facultative lactobacilli.[39-41] Recent advances in microbiologic identification techniques indicate that hydrogen peroxide (H_2O_2) producing *Lactobacillus crispatus, L. jensenii, L. fermentum,* and *L. gasseri* represent the predominant species rather than *L. acidophilus* as traditionally accepted.[42] Other bacteria account for approximately 10% of the bacteria recovered from the healthy vagina.[40] Facultative aerobes including *Staphylococcus epidermidis, Streptococcus* spp. and *G. vaginalis* also are common among women without evidence of vaginal discharge.[37,40] Characteristically low concentrations (10^2 to 10^5 per gram of vaginal fluid) of BV-associated anaerobic microorganisms including *Bacteroides* spp., *Prevotella* spp., and *Peptostreptococcus* spp. as well as *G. vaginalis*, genital mycoplasmas, *Mycoplasma hominis,* and *Ureaplasma urealyticum* may also be commonly present in the healthy vaginal flora of sexually active women.[34,40,41,43,44]

BV is characterized by high concentrations (10^8 to 10^{11} CFU/g of fluid or greater) of *G. vaginalis* and a set of potentially pathogenic BV-associated microorganisms, most notably *Prevotella* spp. (formerly *Bacteroides* spp.), *Peptostreptococcus* spp., *Porphomonas* spp., and *Mobiluncus* spp., along with *M. hominis*.[34,41,45] These microorganisms are present in concentration which are 100- to 1000-fold higher than found in the healthy vagina.[40,44] *Lactobacillus* spp., which are normally present in high numbers (10^5 to 10^6 per gram of fluid), are decreased in number or absent in bacterial vaginosis.[40,41,44]

A number of potentially important vaginal fluid biochemical components are altered with BV. Biochemical changes include elevated pH, increased vaginal fluid concentrations of diamines, polyamines, and organic acids, as well as enzymes such as mucinases, sialidase, IgA proteases, collagenases, nonspecific proteases, and phospholipase A_2 and C.[34,37,46,47-55] Endotoxin and the cytokine interleukin-1-α and the prostaglandins E_2 and $F_2\alpha$ are also increased in the presence of BV.[54,55] These enzymes and organic compounds likely serve to overcome host defense mechanisms, facilitate entrance of cervicovaginal microorganisms into the upper reproductive tract, and contribute to the initiation of a number of BV-associated obstetric or gynecologic complications.[49,56]

Knowledge of the biology of the vagina in health and disease continues to be fragmentary. The role of lactobacilli in maintaining a healthy vaginal ecosystem is increasingly recognized. Lactobacilli likely contribute to the acidic environment characteristic of the healthy vagina through metabolism of glucose, produced by vaginal epithelial cells from glycogen, to lactic acid.[57] *In vitro* experiments demonstrate that lactobacilli inhibit growth of other bacterial species and also produce antimicrobial factors including acidolin, lactacin B, and H_2O_2.[58-64] H_2O_2-producing *Lactobacillus* spp. are predominant in the vaginal fluid of healthy women.[65] The microbicidal action of H_2O_2 is further enhanced in the presence of a halide ion, such as chloride from cervical mucus, and peroxidase enzymes such as myeloperoxidase produced by neutrophils and macrophages.[66] Each of these factors is present in the vaginal fluid of healthy women in sufficient concentrations to produce *in vitro* bactericidal effects.[66] It remains to be determined, however, whether BV-associated bacteria become established in the vagina because of the absence of H_2O_2-producing lactobacilli, or if invasion of abnormal bacteria or other factors such as phages or antibiotic use cause declines in the numbers of normally "protective" lactobacilli. In any case, absence of H_2O_2-producing lactobacillus appear important for establishment or perturbation of BV. In a longitudinal study, Hillier and Eschenbach found that women without H_2O_2-producing lactobacillus more often developed BV and more frequently relapsed after successful treatment.[67,68] These findings support the hypothesis that an absence of H_2O_2-producing lactobacillus precedes the development of BV.[67]

Increased vaginal pH may also contribute to the initiation of BV.[69] An acidic vaginal pH (3.8 to 4.2) favors attachment and growth of lactobacilli and limits attachment of *G. vaginalis* and other BV-associated microorganisms.[69-71] Increased pH tends to displace lactobacilli from receptor sites on vaginal epithelial cells and maximizes adherence of *G. vaginalis*.[70] Elevations in vaginal pH following intercourse or douching with basic solutions have been suggested as mechanisms contributing to the initiation of BV. Vaginal pH may remain elevated for up to 8 h following coitus.[72] Other factors must be required to establish BV; however, since elevations in vaginal fluid pH are also noted during menstruation, among postmenopausal women, and in women suffering trichomoniasis, as well as following intercourse.[39,57] Young black women are also reputed to have relatively increased vaginal pH.[99] Whether or not pH contributes to the initiation of BV or becomes elevated as the condition becomes established remains to be determined.

Currently, there is little understanding of the interrelationships between the constituent flora of BV and biochemical changes in vaginal fluid and cervical mucin. Amines, primarily trimethalamine, putrescine, and cadaverine, are produced during amino acid metabolism by BV-associated anerobic bacteria.[47,73] These volatile amines are released as pH increases and are responsible for the characteristically "sharp" or "fishy" odor noticed in the presence of BV.[47,73] Several vaginal fluid short chain fatty acids are also increased in BV.[34] These include succinate, acetate, propionate, isobutyrate, butyrate, and isovalerate.[34] Of these, acetate is also present among women with healthy vaginal fluid, although at considerably lower concentrations.[34] Chen postulates that release of acid insoluble carbon dioxide gas from amino acid decarboxylase activity may account for the "frothy" appearing discharge noted among up to 27% of women with BV.[46,47]

Chen suggests that symbiotic relationships exist between *G. vaginalis* and the anaerobic components of BV flora.[46,47] *In vitro* studies demonstrate release of high concentrations of pyruvic acid and amino acids during *G. vaginalis* growth.[47] These metabolic byproducts were further metabolized to putrescine and cadaverine and short chain fatty acids when anaerobic bacteria recovered from women with BV (nonspecific vaginitis) were added to *in vitro* cultures.[47] Although symbiotic relationships between bacteria are increasingly recognized in a number of clinical diseases including peritonitis, gingivitis, and peridontal disease, further work is required to explore such bacterial interdependencies in BV.[74,75]

Effects of the altered biochemical milieu characteristic of BV fluid on vaginal and cervical tissues appear important for understanding sequelae of BV. *In vitro* studies demonstrate that succinic acid in concentrations similar to those found in clinical abscesses with high pH (5.5), dramatically impair neutrophil phagocytic killing, response to chemotactic stimuli, and generation of the respiratory burst.[76] Butyrate inhibits lymphocyte activation by endotoxin and is toxic to human fibroblast and mouse neuroblastoma cells in culture.[76-78] Whether or not these bacterial virulence factors contribute to the relative paucity of inflammatory cells noted in the vaginal fluid of women suffering from BV remains to be determined.

The potential role of BV-associated virulence factors in both gynecologic and obstetrical sequelae of BV is of keen interest. Elevated vaginal pH has been implicated in heterosexual HIV transmission and susceptibility, as well as in preterm premature rupture of fetal membranes and preterm birth.[79,80] Studies in pregnant women with BV demonstrated elevated vaginal fluid levels of sialidase, mucinase, phospholipase A_2, phospholipase C, IgA protease, and nonspecific proteolytic enzymes.[48-51,81,82]

Mucinases and sialidases are established bacterial virulence factors. These enzymes can effectively lyse components of protective mucin layers and promote bacterial attachment, allowing invasion and subsequent spread to underlying epithelial cells. These enzymes may play roles in disruption of cervical mucus and other host defenses, leading to upper genital tract invasion of BV-associated microflora.[49] During pregnancy, phospholipase A_2 and C as well as nonspecific proteases may act on cervical and amniochorion connective tissue and promote cervical ripening and focal amniochorion weakening. In addition, phospholipase A_2 and C may promote the release of prostaglandins and further the processes leading to preterm birth. Whether or not such potential virulence factors may be useful in identifying infected women more likely to experience recurrent infection or adverse gynecologic or obstetrical complications remains to be determined.

Further understanding of the pathogenesis of BV requires elucidation of bacterial interdependencies and determination of the types and minimum number of species required to produce the disease. Knowledge of the factors which facilitate the development and course of infection should aid in development and implementation of strategies for long-term cure and prevention of adverse sequela.

1.4   Epidemiology of BV

Our understanding of the distribution of BV within populations and risk factors for developing the condition has accumulated largely through convenience samples of women in selected clinical settings rather than from population based studies. Vaginal infections are not reportable and surveillance data is not available. Reported prevalences and risk factors obtained by examination of self-selected women, i.e., those seeking healthcare are likely biased. As many as 50 to 60% of women with BV do not report symptoms. Therefore, unless specific screening strategies are used, asymptomatic women are less likely to be included in many clinical studies.[37,83] Each study's methods must be reviewed carefully to ascertain if the results are generalizable to other populations.

Elucidation of the epidemiology of BV is further complicated by the use of varying diagnostic criteria. The misclassification that may arise with differing diagnostic methods for BV is best illustrated in a study by Krohn, Hillier, and Eschenbach.[84] Three methods used to detect BV were compared with the standard clinical diagnosis proposed by Amsel.[37] Among the 593 pregnant women studied, the prevalence of BV was 21% by clinical criteria, 12% by Gram stain, 28% by gas-liquid chromatography, and 41% by heavy growth of *G. vaginalis* on culture.[84] Clearly, very different numbers of women would be deemed as having BV depending on which diagnostic criteria were used.

Despite these limitations, review of current information about BV is informative. BV has been generally detected among 10 to 41% of women from studies around the world.[3,9,12,14-18,25,37,83-108] The prevalence of BV varies widely between the different populations studied (Table 1). BV has been most widely studied among women attending publicly supported sexually transmitted infection clinics, family planning clinics, and obstetrical clinics.

Women seen in sexually transmitted disease (STD) clinics have the highest prevalence of BV ranging up to 64%.[3,85-92,94] Several studies of unselected women from the Seattle-King County, WA, STD clinic report BV prevalences of 33 to 37%.[3,44] Similar findings of from 26 to 37% are reported from STD clinics in Sweden and Halifax, Nova Scotia.[83,91,92]

Table 1 Prevalence of BV in Selected Clinic Populations

Population	Location	Symptomatic/ asymptomatic	Number studied	Prevalence BV
STD clinics	U.S.[85]	Not described	11,264	12.3%
	Boston, Massachusetts[86]	Symptomatic	33	64%
	Columbus, Ohio[87]	Not described	10,500	17.7%
	Denver, Colorado[88]	Symptomatic	4162	10.7%
	Seattle, Washington[3]	Symptomatic	640	33%
	Seattle, Washington	Both	633	32.4%
	Halifax, Nova Scotia, Canada[83]	Not described	40	37%
	Australia[89]	Both	5365	13.7%
	Oslo, Norway[90]	Not described	3500	30%
	Uppsala, Sweden[91]	Both	455	24%
	Orebro, Sweden[92]	Not described	3800	26.2%
Juvenile detention center commercial sex workers	Seattle, Washington[93]	Both	57	26%
			35	23%
Abortion clinics	Halifax, Nova Scotia,Canada[94]	Not described	22	29%
	Stockholm, Sweden[6]	Both	1300	26.9%
Family planning clinics	Halifax, Nova Scotia[83]	Not described	75	23%
	France[95]	Symptomatic	392	27.2%
	U.K.[96]	Both	114	11%
	Manchester, England[97]	Symptomatic	226	26.8%
		Asymptomatic	138	5.6%
	Sköude/Göteborg, Sweden[98]	Both	235	22.6%
	Los Angeles, California[85]	Not described	5742	9.5%
Adolescents	Denver, Colorado[99]	Both	719	15.5%
Gynecology clinics	Columbus, Ohio[100]	Asymptomatic	270	5.6%
	Houston, Texas[101]	Both	1204	12.2%
	Ålborg, Denmark[102]	Symptomatic	188	41%
		Asymptomatic	407	13%
	New Delhi, India[103]	Both	248	32.2%

Nonreportable STDs and vaginal infections were examined in six STD clinics throughout the U.S. between 1976 and 1977.[85] Prevalence of "nonspecific vaginitis" ranged from 3% in New Haven, CT, to 31.5% in DeKalb County, GA, with an average prevalence of 12.3% overall.[85] Use of more consistent diagnostic criteria recommended since the early 1980s could explain the differences in prevalence noted between this study and more recently evaluated populations.

Among women attending family planning clinics in studies from the U.K., the prevalence of BV is 11% among unselected women, and ranges from 5.6% among women who deny symptoms on direct questioning to 27% among symptomatic women.[96,97] Work from France and Sweden report similar prevalences of 23 to 27% among symptomatic women.[95,98] Among university students attending clinics for routine gynecologic or contraceptive care, Amsel identified BV among 15% of asymptomatic women and 29% of women with complaints of vaginitis.[37] Little information is available from private gynecologic practices in the U.S.; studies by Bump and Gardner reported BV among 5.6 and 12% of women in their practices.[100,101]

Studies of pregnant women demonstrate prevalences for BV similar to those found among nonpregnant populations. Numerous studies have prospectively examined BV among populations of pregnant women and demonstrated prevalences ranging from 6 to 32% (Table 2).[9,12,14-18,104-110] Studies from Sweden and Denmark report BV among 14% of pregnant women.[109,110] Among pregnant research volunteers in U.S. studies the prevalence

Table 2 Prevalence of BV in Pregnant Women Followed Prospectively

Study population	Diagnostic method	Prevalence
U.S.		
Seattle, Washington[9,84,104,105]	GLC	14–28%
	Clinical	6–21%
	Gram stain	12–21%
New York, New York[106]	Clinical	20.1%
Denver, Colorado[12,25,107]	Gram stain	18.7–23%
	Clinical	32%
Vaginal Infections and Prematurity Study[18]	Gram stain and pH>4.5	16%
Maternal Fetal Medicine Network Centers[108]	Gram stain and pH>4.5	23.4%
Halifax, Nova Scotia, Canada[83]	Clinical	23%
Finland[15]	Quantitative cultures	21.4%
Göteborg, Sweden[109]	Pap smear and pH>4.5	14.3%
Odense, Denmark[110]	Clinical	14%
Harrow,U.K.[16,96]	Gram stain	12–14%
Adelaide, Australia[14]	*G. vaginalis* culture (heavy growth)	28%
Jakarta, Indonesia[17]	Gram stain	17%

of BV varies from 16 to 23%.[9,12,18,84,106-107] In comparison, in a survey of all pregnant women attending an inner city clinic, McGregor identified BV among 32% of clinic attendees.[25] Importantly, fully 43% of poor African-American women studied had BV.[25]

When groups of U.S. women are examined in greater detail, the prevalence of BV is highest among African-American women and lowest among Asian-American women and highest among women with multiple sexual partners and lowest among women with no history of heterosexual contact.[9,25,44,100,101,111,112] BV has been detected more often among women not using any method of contraception and among contracepting women using an intrauterine contraceptive device.[37,113,114] BV has not been related to oral contraceptive use. Importantly, the incidence of BV is reduced somewhat among women using the spermicide nonoxynol-9 (RR,0.86, 95% CI 0.69-1.12).[115]

As noted, exactly how BV occurs remains elusive, but information indicates that acquisition of BV often is related to sexual behavior.[44,111] Whether BV is sexually transmitted continues to be debated. There are a number of factors which link BV to sexual activity. BV most often occurs among sexually active women and may be related to acquiring a new male sexual partner.[115,116] In general, BV occurs more frequently among women who have initiated sexual activity at earlier ages, among women reporting more sexual partners, and among women with concurrent or prior sexually transmitted infections.[37,94,115,116] BV is also noted among sexually abused children.[117] Microbiologic examination of male partners of women with BV demonstrates that BV-associated microorganisms including *M. hominis*, *G. vaginalis*, *Peptostreptococcus* spp., *Mobiluncus* spp., and *Bacteroides* spp. are recovered from 17 to 52% of urethral cultures.[44,118] Furthermore, the same *G. vaginalis* biotypes are isolated within couples.[119] Holst suggests that BV-associated microorganisms recovered from men may originate in the vagina; however, carriage by men may be transient. Microorganisms were no longer recovered from male partners following two weeks of condom use.[118] Holst suggests further that the anaerobic component of BV microflora is derived from the gastrointestinal tract.[118]

Recent examination of a series of lesbian couples identified BV among eight partners of women with BV (73%) and in one partner of ten women without BV.[120] This suggests that among women who have sex with women BV may indeed be sexually transmitted possibly by direct genital contact, fingers, or sharing of sexual devices. Additional work is required to further examine aspects of both male and female sexual behavior which may influence acquisition or recurrence of BV.

Conversely, detection of BV among virginal women and children, even though the occurrence is low, weighs against sexual transmission as the exclusive means for acquisition of BV.[112,117] Twelve percent of adolescent study volunteers who denied sexual contact were found by Bump and colleagues to have BV.[112] In clinical studies of the university students examined by Amsel, BV was not detected among the 18 students who denied sexual experience.[37] In addition, BV has been detected among 4% (1/23) of nonabused children ages 2.5 to 13 years who served as a comparison group for the study of STD transmission among sexually abused children.[117] Strong evidence contradicting exclusive heterosexual transmission of BV comes from a number of randomized controlled trials demonstrating the recurrence of BV among women despite treatment of male contacts.[121-123] Today BV is best thought of as a massive microecologic change in the vagina involving greatly increased numbers of specific microflora along with characteristic patterns of biochemicals including increased pH.

1.4.1   *Natural history of bacterial vaginosis*

Despite the frequency of BV among women, its natural history remains poorly studied. BV may be acute, chronic, resolve spontaneously, or be recurrent.[109,124] Prospective studies of both pregnant and nonpregnant women show shifts in carriage of BV over time. Among pregnant women participating in the National Institutes of Health sponsored Vaginal Infections and Prematurity Study, BV developed among 12% of women examined between 23 to 26 weeks gestation and again at 31 to 36 weeks gestation.[111] In addition, 31% of untreated positive women resolved the condition during this interval.[111] A similar incidence (13%) was noted by Hauth and colleagues among women without BV between 22 to 24 weeks gestation and re-examined at approximately 28 weeks gestation.[26] Among Indonesian women without BV between 16 to 20 weeks gestation, 7.3% developed BV by re-examination at 28 to 32 weeks gestation and 50% of initially positive women had resolved their infection during this interval.[17] Studies from the U.K. and Sweden provide information on the most consistently followed pregnant women.[109,125] Between the initial first trimester examinations and follow-up examinations at 28 weeks gestation only 47 to 55% of initially positive women continued to have findings of BV.[109,125] Additionally, none of the 102 initially negative Swedish women developed clue cells with elevated pH during the study interval and 2.9% of British women developed Gram stain findings of BV by 28 weeks gestation.[109] A further 2.4% of women without BV in the first trimester had developed BV by term.[109,125] Women who may have had BV and delivered before either follow-up examination and those who may have developed BV and delivered prematurely would not be included in these assessments of persisting or incident infection. Therefore these findings likely represent low estimates of the actual incidence of BV and numbers of women with persisting infection.

Studies among nonpregnant women also suggest that BV may resolve spontaneously among large numbers of women. Bump et al. reported that only 36% of untreated women continued to have clue cells upon examination at a six-month follow-up visit.[100] Subsequently, these authors reported that only one of eight virginal adolescents with BV diagnosed by clinical criteria continued to have BV at a three-month follow-up visit.[112] Longitudinal studies among nonpregnant women and children demonstrate development of BV among 13% of sexually assaulted children within one week of assault, 7% of adolescents followed for 3 months, and among 13.6 and 25% of women attending STD clinics and followed for 5 to 6 months.[112,115-117]

Prospective treatment studies show that BV regularly recurs over time regardless of initial successful treatment.[124] Well-controlled treatment trials document BV recurrences among 30 to 40% of women within 3 months of oral metronidazole therapy.[126] McGregor and colleagues examined the effectiveness of 2% vaginal clindamycin cream for BV during

Table 3   Gynecologic Complications Associated with Presence of BV

Gynecologic complications	Risk ratio	95% Confidence intervals[a]	Ref.
PID	7.5	ND[b]	Paavonen, 1987[4]
	9.2	ND[c]	Eschenbach, 1988[3]
Post abortion PID	3.7	(1.1–12.1)	Larsson, 1989[6]
Post hysterectomy cuff cellulitis	3.2	(1.5–6.7)	Soper, 1990[5]
	6.2	(1.3–30.7)	Larsson, 1991[146]
Abnormal uterine bleeding	3.8	(1.8–8.2)	Wolner-Hanssen,1990[139]
Cervical intraepithelial neoplasia	7.2	(3.7–14.0)	Platz-Christensen, 1994[153]

[a] Risk ratio and 95% confidence intervals calculated from data provided.

[b] Case Control Study BV was present among 25.5% of cases and none of the controls.

[c] 3% of women (8/311) with BV and none of 350 women without BV had a clinical diagnosis of PID.

pregnancy.[49] One week post-treatment, 4% of women continued to have findings of BV; however, it gradually recurred during the pregnancy with approximately 10% of women having findings of BV 8 weeks post-treatment and approximately 20% having BV by 36 weeks gestation.[49] Other authorities report recurrence of BV in up to 80% of women within 9 months of initially effective treatment.[44,127] Heterogeneity of BV, differing susceptibilities between women, misclassification due to differing diagnostic criteria, and other methodologic issues may contribute to differences in studies examining the natural history of BV. Understanding of how BV recurs after initially effective treatment may give us important clues to its biology.

Eschenbach and colleagues determined that the absence of H_2O_2-producing lactobacillus predisposes one to developing BV after treatment.[65] Cook identified that persistence of at least one abnormal BV-associated microbiologic or vaginal fluid biochemical factor was a predictor for frequent recurrence of BV among nonpregnant women.[124] Cook suggests that a number of individuals with BV appear to be unable to re-establish a normal vaginal ecosystem following treatment.[124]

1.5   Gynecologic complications associated with BV

Increasing information over the past decade demonstrates that BV is related to a number of morbid and costly gynecologic complications. These include endometritis, pelvic inflammatory disease (PID), postsurgical abortion infections, post-hysterectomy infection, and perhaps cervical intraepithelial neoplasia and facilitation of heterosexual HIV transmission (Table 3).

1.5.1   Pelvic inflammatory disease

Elucidation of the causes of nonchlamydial, nongonococcal PID (endometritis, salpingitis, peritonitis) is increasingly important as chlamydial and gonorrheal infections have become increasingly amenable to effective diagnosis and treatment. While anaerobic bacteria and *M. hominis* have been associated with PID, the direct link between PID and BV is less well studied.[4,128-131] In the absence of *Neisseria gonorrhoeae* and *Chlamydia trachomatis*, the bacterial species most commonly isolated from the upper genital tracts of women with laparoscopically confirmed PID represent the constituent flora of BV.[4,130-131] These sets of upper tract microflora include: *Bacteroides* spp., *Prevotella* spp., *Peptostreptococcus* spp., *G. vaginalis*, and *M. hominis*. In a uniquely detailed cross-sectional study of the microbiology of acute salpingitis, Soper and colleagues identified vaginal fluid Gram stain findings of BV among 61.8% of women with laparoscopically confirmed PID.[130] Paavonen examined vaginal wash specimens for volatile fatty acids and identified a profile consistent with BV among 9 of 35 (25.5%) women with acute salpingitis or histologic endometritis.[4] Importantly, women with PID were 7.5 times more likely to have BV than comparison women without PID.[4] Subsequently, in a cross-sectional study of 661 women attending an STD clinic, clinical signs of upper genital tract infection were present among approximately 4% of women with Gram stain findings of BV and 1% of women without BV.[3] Controlling for co-infection with *N. gonorrhoeae* and *C. trachomatis*, women with BV were 9.2 times more likely to have adnexal tenderness compared to women without BV.[3]

Conversely, using the standard composite clinical diagnosis of PID and semi-quantitative vaginal cultures to identify BV, Faro studied 41 women with clinical PID and concluded that BV is not associated with the development of PID.[132] As would be expected, the vast majority of the cases in Faro's series could be associated with *N. gonorrhoeae* and/or *C. trachomatis*. However, endometrial cultures yielded *M. hominis* from 63.4% of women, *G. vaginalis* from 36.6%, *U. urealyticum* from 31.7%, and *Bacteroides bivius* from 21.9% of studied women.[132] These microbiologic findings from the upper reproductive tract are similar to findings reported by others and represent prominent constituents of BV.[4,128-131] Further work, which utilizes appropriately selected women as controls, is being conducted to explore relationships between BV and PID. These studies could lead to strategies to further reduce risks of salpingitis by screening and treating BV as well as chlamydia and gonorrhea.

1.5.2   Abnormal bleeding and endometritis

Abnormal reproductive tract bleeding, metrorrhagia or menometrorrhagia, is a common finding among 40 to 60% of women with clinically recognized PID and is considered indicative of endometrial infection.[133-136] Abnormal reproductive tract bleeding frequently is the only symptom of endometritis noted by women.[137] The actual incidence of abnormal reproductive tract bleeding associated with endometritis is not well defined, but histologic findings of endometritis have been reported among 3 to 10% of women being evaluated for irregular bleeding.[138] Recently, use of standardized criteria identified endometrial inflammatory changes among 48% of women being evaluated for abnormal menstrual bleeding.[139] Abnormal bleeding due to endometritis is thought to result from abnormal responsiveness of the infected endometrium to ovarian hormones or from direct physical disruption of the endometrium from infection and inflammation.[136,140]

An initial link between BV and abnormal bleeding was provided by a case series in which *G. vaginalis* was recovered in pure culture from the uterine cavity of three patients who underwent hysterectomy for persistent irregular bleeding.[141] Similarly, two studies by Larsson have demonstrated prompt resolution of metrorrhagia following successful treatment of BV and *Mobiluncus* spp. infection with oral metronidazole.[7,142] Resolution of bleeding following treatment of the infection suggests that the two conditions are related; however, endometrial infection or inflammation was not directly evaluated by the authors. Subsequently, Wolner-Hanssen, Kiviat, and Holmes reported that BV was 3.8 times more common among women not using oral contraceptives who were examined for menorrhagia compared with women without this complaint.[139] Most recently, work by Korn directly supports the association between BV and upper genital tract infection.[143] Women attending an urban STD clinic for complaints of vaginal discharge were examined for histologic plasma cell endometritis using endometrial biopsy. Among the 60 women with symptomatic vaginal complaints, 36.7% (N=22) were found to have Gram stain finding of BV without microbiologic findings of *N. gonorrhoeae*, *C. trachomatis*, or clinical evidence of upper genital tract tenderness. Pipelle biopsy detected plasma cell endometritis among 45% of BV-positive women vs. 5% of control women without BV.[143]

1.5.3 Postoperative infections following gynecologic surgery

Among women undergoing therapeutic pregnancy terminations, Larsson reported the incidence of PID as increased 3.7 times (95% CI, 1.1-12.1) for women with BV (11.8%) compared with the incidence among women without BV (3.2%).[6] Larsson further substantiated this important association between BV and post-termination endometritis by eliminating the increased risk for infection through effective treatment for BV.[23] In this double-blind, randomized, placebo-controlled treatment trial among the women undergoing surgical abortions oral metronidazole treatment (500 mg 3 times daily for 10 days) reduced the risk of postoperative PID by 70% (metronidazole: 3.6% vs. placebo 12.2%; RR 0.3, 95% CI 0.08-1.0).[23] This is similar to the risk of infection noted among women without BV (3.2%).

The occurrence of postoperative infection following hysterectomy ranges from 9 to 50%.[144,145] Important reductions in postoperative infections following vaginal and frequently abdominal hysterectomy are achieved with perioperative administration of prophylactic antibiotics which provide antibiotic coverage for vaginal flora.[144] How chemoprophylaxis works and how to best select candidates for prophylaxis is of continuing interest. BV has been associated with increased risk for infection following abdominal hysterectomy in two clinical studies.[5,146] Soper and colleagues examined 161 women undergoing abdominal hysterectomy to identify potential microbiological risk factors for postoperative infection.[5] Clinical findings of BV were present among 19.9% of studied women.[5] Risk of postoperative cuff cellulitis, cuff abscess, or both was significantly increased among women with BV (RR, 3.2, 95% CI 1.5-6.7).[5] Similar results are reported for 70 premenopausal, Swedish women by Larsson and colleagues.[146] BV was detected among 28.6% of women. Vaginal cuff and wound infections occurred among 35% of women with BV and among 8% of women without BV (calculated from data provided, RR 6.2, 95% confidence intervals 1.3-30.7).[146] The association between BV and postoperative hysterectomy infection was independent of other traditional risk factors of postoperative infection such as age, estimated blood loss, and the duration of the operation.[146] Calculations of attributable risk suggest that BV accounted for the majority of post-hysterectomy infectious morbidity in these studies. Preoperative diagnosis and treatment of BV should effectively reduce the occurrence of these postoperative infections.

1.5.4 Cervical cancer

BV has been suggested as a potential co-factor in the pathogenesis and progression of cervical intraepithelial neoplasia. A number of observations support these suggestions. BV and cervical intraepithelial neoplasia, as well as genital human papilloma virus infection, share several epidemiologic associated risk factors, i.e., younger age at onset of intercourse, increased numbers of sexual partners, and history of STDs. Several older studies which examined women with invasive cervical cancer identified a predominance of anaerobic bacteria and *M. hominis* within the vaginal flora of these women.[147-150] Whether or not the vaginal flora was altered as a result of the patient's condition or the altered vaginal flora preceded the cancer is unclear. Subsequently, Pavic hypothesized that anaerobic bacteria present in BV may metabolize vaginal fluid amines to potentially oncogenic nitrosamines.[150,151] Similar processes are thought to occur in the pathogenesis of colonic neoplasia. Increased vaginal fluid concentrations of phospholipase C and A_2 characteristic of BV may play roles in facilitating human papilloma virus infection and/or transformations of cervical epithelial cells.

Despite these intriguing putative molecular mechanisms, clear proof of an association between cervical neoplasia and BV is not available. Guijon and colleagues examined the cervico/vaginal flora of 106 women with and 79 women without colposcopic findings of cervical intraepithelial neoplasia.[152] *M. hominis, N. gonorrhoeae*, yeast, and koilocytotic atypia were identified more often and vaginal fluid Gram stains were more often abnormal among case-women with cervical intraepithelial neoplasia (grades I-III).[152] BV occurred among 48% of the women with cervical intraepithelial neoplasia and among 22% of control women.[152] Presence of other studied microorganisms did not differ significantly between cases and controls.[152] However, the identification methods used for a number of studied microorganisms lacked sensitivity (i.e., koilocytosis for human papilloma virus and microscopic examination for *Trichomonas vaginalis*), therefore large numbers of infected women may have been misclassified as negative.

Additional information linking BV with cervical intraepithelial neoplasia comes from a large study from Sweden which re-examined 6150 archived Pap smear slides for clue cells.[153] Clue cells were 7.2 times (calculated from data provided, 95% CI 3.7-14.0) more common among specimens with cervical intraepithelial neoplasia II-III.[153] Unfortunately, other potential co-factors for cervical intraepithelial neoplasia were not evaluated in this study including smoking and human papilloma virus infection; therefore whether or not BV is a co-factor or a marker of increased risk for sexually transmitted infection could not be reliably determined. Most recently, a group of 280 women with dyskaryotic cervical smears participated in a cross-sectional study to examine the relationships between BV, human papilloma virus, and cervical histological changes.[154] Human papilloma virus (any viral type) was detected equally among women with and without BV. In this study, BV was not related to cervical intraepithelial neoplasia.[154]

Considerable further work is required to determine if a link between BV and cervical intraepithelial neoplasia exists. Study design issues must be carefully addressed to provide meaningful results. Sensitive methods for assessing potential confounding factors must be employed in order to examine an independent role for BV or a potential synergist role for BV with human papilloma virus infection. In addition, due to the relatively long latency for development of neoplastic cervical lesions, consideration of the most appropriate time to assess for the proposed risk factors must be addressed. Cross-sectional assessment for risk factors at the time of the disease diagnosis may be inappropriate for factors which may change over time such as presence of BV, other STDs, contraceptive use, and smoking.

1.5.5   *Transmission of HIV infection*

A number of genital tract infections which alter the integrity of the reproductive tract mucosa (i.e., syphilis, chancroid, herpes simplex virus infections) have been shown to increase risks of heterosexual HIV transmission. Theoretical reasons and empirical findings suggest that BV may also increase risk of heterosexual HIV transmission. Elevated vaginal fluid pH is a primary means by which BV may increase risk for HIV transmission. Free and lymphocyte-associated HIV virus are both inactivated and less likely to adhere at low pH levels (≤ 4.5) such as those found in the healthy vagina.[155] Conversely, as pH increases both viability and adherence of HIV virus increases and transmission may be favored.[155]

As previously discussed, a number of other biochemical properties are altered in the vaginal fluid of women with BV; these also may serve to perturb host defense mechanisms and facilitate HIV infection. BV fluid has increased levels of IgA protease, nonspecific proteases, sialidase, and decreased levels of hydrogen peroxide.[48-50,65,81] Presence of these substances may increase access of HIV to reproductive tract epithelium in men and women.

Most prior clinical studies did not evaluate BV as a potential risk factor for heterosexual HIV transmission. In a longitudinal study of seroconversion among 343 partners of HIV-infected men, Saracco reported a 30% (95%CI 0.3-5.8) increase in risk for HIV seroconversion among women with a history of prior "vaginitis."[156] However, BV was not separated from other causes of "discharge."[156] Most recently, among a group of commercial sex workers in Thailand, BV was significantly associated with HIV seropositivity (OR, 2.7, 95% CI 1.3-5.0).[157] Whether or not BV directly effects transmission and acquisition or is merely a marker for women at risk for HIV infection requires urgent study.

1.6 Obstetrical complications associated with BV

Considerable information from around the world links BV directly to a number of serious obstetrical complications including spontaneous abortion, preterm birth, preterm labor, preterm premature rupture of membranes, amniotic fluid infection, post partum endometritis, and post-cesarean wound infections (Table 4). Most importantly, BV represents a potentially preventable risk factor for these common and costly complications of pregnancy.

1.6.1 Preterm birth

Associations between BV and increased risk for preterm birth are well documented. The influence of BV on adverse pregnancy outcomes has been investigated through case-control, cross-sectional, prospective cohort studies and randomized controlled treatment trials (Tables 4 and 5).[8-18,24-26,49,158-161] Direct comparison of studies must consider methodologic differences in study design, definitions of preterm birth, and the techniques used to identify BV. Despite study differences, research repeatedly supports the association between BV and increased risk of preterm labor, preterm premature rupture of membranes, and preterm birth.[9-18,25,26,49,158] Of great importance, BV and associated microorganisms appear to increase risk of preterm birth at the lowest gestational ages.[13] Two published studies report an association between pre-viable pregnancy loss and BV, suggesting that pathophysiologic processes which disrupt pregnancy may occur throughout gestation.[16,25]

Multiple prospective cohort studies indicate that BV may be detected a number of weeks to months prior to the onset of preterm labor or preterm birth.[9,12,15-18] Eschenbach, Gravett, and colleagues were the first to implicate BV as a risk factor for preterm labor and low birthweight.[8-11] BV was identified using gas-liquid chromatography among 19% of 534 pregnant women studied.[9] The presence of BV in the mid-third trimester (mean 32.6 weeks) was associated with increased risk for preterm labor (OR, 2.0; 95% CI, 1.1-3.5) and preterm premature rupture of membranes (OR, 2.0; 95% CI, 1.1-3.7).[9] McDonald and colleagues examined BV (culture for high colonization with *G. vaginalis*) earlier in gestation (22–28 weeks) and demonstrated similar risks for preterm birth following labor (OR 1.8) and preterm premature rupture of membranes (OR 2.7).[14] Subsequent work by McGregor and colleagues identified 22% of preterm births in their inner city, indigent population in Denver, CO, as attributable to BV.[25] Most recently, results of a large prospective cohort study from the National Institute of Child Health and Human Development sponsored, Vaginal Infections and Prematurity Study Group demonstrated a 40% increase in risk of delivering a preterm low birthweight infant (born less than 37 weeks gestation and weighing less than 2500 g) among women with BV and a 10% increase in risk of preterm premature rupture of membranes.[18]

Of interest, studies which examine for BV at the earliest gestations and carefully control for intervening antimicrobial treatment demonstrate the strongest association between BV and preterm birth and rupture of membranes. Kurki examined women between 8 to 17 weeks gestation and identified significantly increased risks for preterm birth (OR=6.9), preterm premature rupture of membranes (OR=7.3), and preterm labor (OR=2.6) among women with BV as defined by quantitative vaginal cultures.[15] None of these women received treatment, and re-evaluation for BV at later gestational ages was

Table 4 Obstetrical Complications Associated with Presence of BV

Obstetric complications	Risk ratio	95% Confidence intervals	Ref.
Preterm birth	3.1	1.6–6.0	Eschenbach, 1984[8]
	2.3	0.96–5.5[a]	Minkoff, 1984[106]
	2.3	1.1–5.0	Martius, 1988[11]
	3.3	1.2–9.2[a]	Hillier, 1988[13]
	3.2	1.1–9.6	McGregor, 1991[158]
	1.8	1.0–3.2	McDonald, 1992[14]
	6.9	2.5–18.8	Kurki, 1992[15]
	2.0	1.0–3.9	Joesoef, 1993[17]
	2.1	1.2–3.7	Holst, 1994[160]
	3.3	1.2–9.1	McGregor, 1994[49]
	5.2	2.0–13.5[a]	Hay,1994[16]
	1.9	1.2–3.0	McGregor, 1995[25]
	1.8	1.2–3.0	Meis, 1995[108]
	1.6	1.3–2.0	Hauth, 1995[26]
	1.4	1.2–1.7	Hillier, 1995[18]
pPROM	1.5	0.9–2.6[a]	Minkoff, 1984[106]
	2.4	1.4–4.3	Gravett, 1986[9]
	2.7	0.7–2.7	McDonald, 1991[158]
	7.3	1.8–29.4	Kurki,1992[15]
	5.7	0.9–36	McGregor, 1994[49]
	3.5	1.4–8.9	McGregor, 1995[25]
	1.1	0.8–1.6	Hillier, 1995[18]
Preterm labor	1.5	0.8–2.8[a]	Minkoff, 1984[106]
	2.2	1.3–3.8	Gravett, 1986[9]
	3.8	1.2–11.6	Gravett, 1986[10]
	2.6	1.1–6.5	McGregor, 1990[12]
	1.8	1.1–3.1	McDonald, 1991[158]
	2.6	1.3–4.9	Kurki, 1992[15]
	2.0	0.9–9.4	Holst, 1994[160]
	1.5	0.8–2.6	McGregor, 1994[49]
	1.8	0.9–3.5	McGregor, 1995[25]
Spontaneous abortion	5.4	1.5–19.5	Hay, 1994[16]
	3.1	1.4–6.9	McGregor, 1995[25]
Amniotic fluid infection	1.5	1.1–2.0[a]	Silver, 1989[20]
	1.5	1.2–2.2	Krohn, 1995[163]
Post partum endometritis	5.8	3.0–10.9[a]	Watts, 1990[19]
Post-cesarean section wound infection	3.1	0.9–11.8[a]	Watts, 1989[164]

[a] Risk ratio and 95% confidence limits calculated from data provided.

not reported.[15] Convincingly similar results were reported by Hay for women with Gram stain findings of BV prior to 16 weeks gestation and preterm birth (calculated from data provided, RR 5.2, 95 % CI. 2.0-13.5).[16]

In an innovative analysis, Joesoef examined risk of preterm birth for women found to have BV between 16 and 20 weeks gestation and/or between 28 and 32 weeks gestation.[17] Women with BV in early second trimester experienced a two-fold increase in premature birth compared with women without BV.[17] Women with BV at 28 to 32 weeks gestation experienced somewhat less increased risk for premature birth (O.R. 1.5, 95% C.I. 0.7-3.0). The authors note that women who developed BV between the screening intervals (i.e., those negative at 16 to 20 weeks gestation and positive at 28 to 32 weeks gestation)

Table 5 Summary of Controlled Treatment Trials to Prevent BV-Associated Complications

Outcome	Relative risk (95% confidence interval)	Outcome among treated	Outcome among control	Ref.
		Metronidazole 500 mg b.i.d. × 7 days	Placebo	
Preterm birth[a]	0.4 (0.2–0.85)	18%	39%	Morales, 1993[24]
pPROM	0.14 (0.03–0.57)	5%	33%	
		Clindamycin 300 mg t.i.d. × 7	Observational control	
Preterm birth	0.52 (0.3–0.9)	9.8%	18.8%	McGregor, 1995[25]
pPROM	0.5 (0.2–1.4)	3.5%	6.9%	
Preterm labor with PTB	0.2 (0.1–0.7)	1.8%	8.8%	
		Metronidazole and erythromycin	Placebos	
Preterm birth[b]	0.6 (0.48–0.9)	31%	49%	Hauth, 1995[26]
		2% Clindamycin vaginal cream	Placebo cream	
Preterm birth	2.0 (0.7–5.8)	15.0%	7.2%	McGregor, 1994[49]
pPROM	1.1 (0.2–5.4)	5.0%	4.4%	
PTL	1.5 (0.7–3.2)	21.7%	14.5%	
Preterm birth	1.1 (0.7–1.7)	15.0%	13.5%	Joesoef, 1995[161]
		Metronidazole 500 mg t.i.d. × 10 days	Placebo	
Post abortion PID	0.3 (0.1–1.0)	3.6%	12.2%	Larsson, 1992[23]

[a] All women with prior preterm birth.

[b] All women with prior preterm birth or maternal pre-pregnant weight <50 kg.

were not at increased risk for preterm birth (10.7% preterm birth among women developing BV vs. 11.8% among women never positive for BV; calculated OR 0.9).[17] Cross-sectional screening at 28 to 32 weeks gestation in essence created an exposed group of women which was comprised of those at low risk for preterm birth (42% without BV between 16 to 20 weeks gestation) and women with elevated risk (58% with early and continuing BV). Therefore, the association between BV and preterm birth was reduced and not statistically significant when screening occurred later in pregnancy.

Importantly, women with findings of BV at 16 to 20 weeks gestation were at increased risk for preterm birth even if they no longer had findings of BV at the later follow-up visit (20.5% preterm birth among women with BV at both visits and 20.5% preterm birth among women with BV only at the first visit vs. 11.8% preterm birth among women without BV).[17] These findings suggest that physiologic processes present or initiated at, or prior to, 16 to 20 weeks gestation are important for the subsequent development of preterm birth. These authors concluded that "only BV in early pregnancy plays a major role as a risk factor for preterm delivery."[17]

Recent results reported from a National Institute of Child Health and Human Development sponsored Maternal-Fetal Medicine Network Study appear to contradict the results of Joesoef.[17,108] Women with BV between 22 and 24 weeks gestation (OR, 1.38, 95% CI 0.94-2.05) and 26 to 29 weeks gestation (OR,1.84, 95% CI 1.15-2.95) experienced increased risk for preterm birth. However, the greatest increase in risk for preterm birth (defined as birth <35 weeks gestation) occurred among women who developed BV between screenings at 22 to 24 weeks gestation and 26 to 29 weeks gestation (OR, 2.53,

95% CI 1.3–4.8).[108] Although these authors discussed the information that women who received "antibiotics" between the first and second screening visit tended to have lower risk of preterm birth (OR, 0.44, 95% CI 0.11–1.9); the risk for preterm birth among untreated women with BV is not presented separately.[108] The "exposure group" (women with BV) appears to be comprised of both untreated and treated women for much of the data presented. Failure to separate results for women who have received intervening, nonstudy, effective antimicrobial treatment and results for untreated women will yield an inaccurate assessment of risk and may account for conflicting results.

1.6.2   Antimicrobial treatment trials for the prevention of preterm birth

Most importantly, several recent, well-controlled, treatment trials to prevent preterm birth demonstrate reductions in the rate of preterm birth among women with both symptomatic and asymptomatic BV during pregnancy (Table 5).[24,25] McGregor and colleagues identified BV using standard clinical criteria among 32% of pregnant women.[25] Risk of preterm birth was reduced by 50% among women with BV who received oral clindamycin treatment compared with untreated observational controls.[25] Risks of otherwise unexplained "idiopathic" preterm birth and rupture of membranes were also reduced by systematic treatment of BV.[25] Morales randomized pregnant women with both BV and a prior preterm birth to receive either oral metronidazole or placebo.[24] This protocol also demonstrated a 50% reduction in the rate of preterm births among treated women compared with those who received placebo.[24] Finally, Hauth presented results from an antenatal trial of prophylactic metronidazole and erythromycin vs. dual placebos among women considered at increased risk for preterm birth because of a prior preterm birth or because of low maternal weight.[26] Subset analyses of these data indicate that only the subgroup of women with BV achieved important reductions in the rates of preterm birth compared with women given placebos (Table 5).[26]

In contrast, two randomized, placebo-controlled trials to prevent preterm birth by treatment of BV with 2% intravaginal clindamycin cream failed to demonstrate reduced incidence of preterm birth despite apparently adequate treatment for BV.[49,161] Indeed, data suggest that the outcomes of women treated with active intravaginal drug tended to have arithmetically higher rates of preterm births (15%) than women receiving placebo (7.2% to 13.5%).[49,161] Just why intravaginal treatment might not be effective in preventing preterm birth is unclear. McGregor and colleagues suggest that BV-associated susceptible microorganisms may be present within the decidual tissues and systemic treatment (oral or intravenous) is required for effective eradication and reduction in the risk of preterm birth.[25,49] Alternately, women receiving placebo are more likely to continue to have BV and have this condition detected by their care providers. Use of nonstudy, effective, oral antimicrobial therapy among the placebo recipients would likely reduce the incidence of preterm birth, similar to the decreases noted in the treatment arms of clinical trials using oral medications. Finally, Hillier and colleagues demonstrated a transient increase in recovery of *E. coli* and *Enterococcus* spp. for up to one month following intravaginal clindamycin cream treatment.[162] *E. coli* has also been associated with increased risk for preterm birth especially when acquired mid-pregnancy.[159] Joesoef and colleagues speculate that presence of this change in the vaginal flora (to *E. coli*, *Enterococcus* spp. predominant) may have further increased the risk for preterm birth among studied women who received clindamycin vaginal cream.[161]

Overall the information from these treatment trials supports the idea that screening and standard oral treatments for BV is beneficial in preventing potentially large portions of preterm births. Conversely, mid-gestational antenatal intravaginal treatment does not appear to prevent BV-associated preterm birth.

A number of questions remain to further our understanding of associations between BV and preterm birth and allow further reductions in risks of preterm birth. Studies are ongoing which address optimal timing of screening and treatment of BV during pregnancy. Unpublished work shows maximum benefit if women are screened and orally treated for BV at the time of the initial antenatal visit in early pregnancy. Similarly our studies as well as the studies of Hauth, Hillier, and Morales show that both symptomatic and asymptomatically infected women receive benefit from treatment. Decisions of whether to screen and treat women at "high risk" for preterm birth because of a prior preterm birth or low body mass appear unnecessary. In the study by McGregor all women benefited from screening and treatment for BV and other common reproductive tract infections.

1.6.3 *Intrapartum and post partum infections*

BV has been linked with clinical amniotic fluid infection as well as postoperative endometritis and post partum endometritis in several studies. These associations were first suggested by observations that the microorganisms frequently recovered from women with these complications often include the common constituents of BV, i.e., *Prevotella bivius*, *G. vaginalis*, *M. hominis*, and *Peptostreptococcus* spp.[163,164] Clinical studies have examined BV, identified by either Gram stain or gas-liquid chromatography and shown that women with clinical amniotic fluid infection more commonly have findings of BV compared with women without clinical infection.[10,20,21] Among the 286 (2.4%) women from the Vaginal Infections and Prematurity Study who developed amniotic fluid infection, antenatal carriage (23 to 26 weeks gestation) of BV (RR=1.5, 95% CI 1.2–2.2) and BV-associated microorganisms were significantly associated with amniotic fluid infection.[163] This increase in risk for amniotic fluid infection associated with BV was independent of duration of labor, duration of rupture of membranes, concurrent infection with *N. gonorrhoeae*, *C. trachomatis*, *T. vaginalis*, group B streptococcus, and effective antimicrobial treatment.[163] Future large studies are required to determine if antenatal treatment for BV or intrapartal screening and treatment for BV are of benefit in reducing rates of amniotic fluid infection.

Post partum endometritis occurs following 2 to 5% of vaginal births and 10 to 20% of cesarean deliveries.[165] Among over 80% of affected women this infection is polymicrobial in nature.[164] In a series of 161 women with post partum endometritis described by Watts, the common sets of BV constituents (i.e., *G. vaginalis*, *P. bivius*, *Peptostreptococcus* spp., and *Bacteroides* spp.) were recovered from endometrial cultures in up to 60% of women.[164] Wound infections developed among 18% (16/79) of women with endometrial BV-associated flora and among 8% (4/53) of women with other bacteria recovered from the endometrium.[164] Subsequent work by Watts demonstrated a 5.8-fold increased risk for post-cesarean section endometritis among women with BV.[19] Reduction of post partum endometritis associated with BV is being examined. However, it seems reasonable that treatment of BV aimed at reducing risks of preterm birth and premature rupture of membranes could also reduce risks of both chorioamnionitis and post partum infection.

1.7 *Diagnosis of BV*

Diagnosis of BV is complicated by the polymicrobial nature of the condition. Culture for single microorganisms such as *G. vaginalis* does not provide an accurate diagnosis for the clinical condition BV.[3,37] The current, recognized gold standard, examined in 1984 by Amsel and colleagues, is based upon a combination of clinical criteria.[3,37] These clinical criteria can be criticized because each criterion is subject to interpretation by untrained care providers. A variety of other diagnostic techniques have been developed and explored in the attempt to decrease the subjectivity of the diagnosis and improve consistency between examiners including: identification of clue cells on Pap smear sampled from the posterior fornix, often in combination with elevated vaginal fluid pH;[92,166] Gram stains of vaginal fluid interpreted using one of several systems;[96,167,168] identification of several different vaginal fluid biochemicals (amines and proline aminopeptidase);[47,169] ratio of normal biochemicals to abnormal biochemicals;[34] culture or DNA probes for a predominant microorganism (i.e., *G. vaginalis*);[170] and quantitative microbiologic cultures.[14,15]

1.7.1   Clinical diagnosis

Accurate clinical diagnosis is based on the presence of 3 of 4 clinical criteria (Amsel's criteria):

1. Homogeneous, thin vaginal fluid that adheres to the vaginal walls
2. Vaginal fluid pH >4.5
3. Release of amine odor with alkalinization of vaginal fluid, the "whiff test"
4. Presence of vaginal epithelial cells with borders obscured with adherent, small bacteria called "clue" cells.

Microscopic examination of a saline "wet" mount preparation of vaginal fluid is essential for the accurate assessment of BV. Clue cells may be distinguished from normal vaginal epithelial cells by their characteristic stippled and ragged appearance (Figure 1). The cell borders are obscured by adherent small coccobacilli-type bacteria, as compared to normal vaginal epithelial cells where the cell borders are distinct and clearly seen (Figure 2). In addition to the presence of clue cells, the bacterial flora appears grossly altered on microscopic examination when BV is present. The characteristic long rods, or normal *Lactobacillus* morphotypes, are absent or rare. Background bacterial flora appear greatly increased in number and short rods and coccobacillary forms predominate. *Mobiluncus* spp. may be identified by their characteristic spiral or serpent-like motility.[171] Identification of clue cells may be hindered by adherence of normal bacteria, cellular debris and availability and quality of the microscopy.[170]

Of these four clinical criteria, presence of clue cells on saline wet mount examination is the single most specific and sensitive indicator of BV.[172] Identification of clue cells accurately predicts 85 to 90% of women with clinical BV (positive predictive value).[172]

Alkalinization of vaginal fluid releases volatile amines, putrescine, cadaverine, and trimethylamine which give off the characteristic unpleasant "fishy" or sharp odor, distinctive of BV.[46,47,73] This odor may be released spontaneously by other agents which raise the vaginal pH, such as sexual intercourse and menses. Presence of an amine odor is highly predictive of BV. However, putrescine is also present in semen, and other anaerobic infections may result in positive amine tests.[46] In addition, release of odor is the least sensitive of the criteria, therefore absence of odor does not negate the presence of BV.[3]

Normal vaginal pH from menarche through menopause ranges between 3.8 and 4.2.[37] Amsel and colleagues determined that vaginal fluid pH over 4.5 best discriminated between BV and normal vaginal fluid.[37] Identification of pH over 4.5 is highly sensitive for the diagnosis of BV but it is not specific.[3,37,172] Other factors present in the vagina may provide an elevated pH measurement. These include semen, cervical mucus, menses, trichomoniasis, and possibly residue from recent douching. Samples for examination of vaginal fluid pH must be obtained from the lateral vaginal side wall or posterior fornices in order to accurately reflect vaginal and not cervical pH. Similarly, the pH indicator paper must allow distinction between the normal vaginal pH (3.8 to 4.2) from pH over 4.5.

The characteristic thin, homogeneous, and adherent vaginal fluid is the most subjective indicator of BV. BV fluid is described as if "milk or cream" had been poured into the

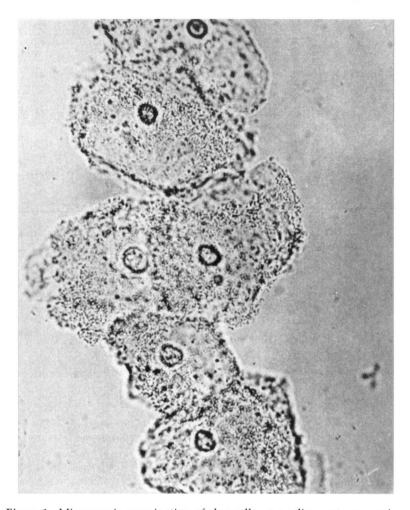

Figure 1 Microscopic examination of clue cells on a saline wet preparation.

vagina. Vaginal fluid may appear "frothy" in up to 27% of women with BV.[30] Although increased discharge is a common presenting complaint for women with BV, the quantity often differs and may range from scant, moderate, or profuse. Due to low sensitivity and specificity, the characteristics of vaginal fluid should be used in conjunction with other diagnostic criteria and not as the only indicator of BV. Especially, leukorrhea, which is characteristic of normal pregnancy, may interfere with recognition of the discharge characteristic of BV.

1.7.2 *Papanicolaou smear diagnosis*

The sensitivity, specificity, and positive predictive value of Pap smear findings suggestive of BV compared with the standard clinical criteria have not been completely studied. Schnadig and colleagues examined 149 women attending a dysplasia clinic and compared identification of clue cells from endocervical Pap smears with vaginal fluid wet prep detected clue cells and found poor correlation (phi coefficient=0.22).[173] These authors further explored associations between three bacterial patterns identified on the Pap smears (large lactobacillus, anaerobic predominant, and scant growth pattern), Gram stains of cervical smears and culture results for *G. vaginalis* and *Mobiluncus* spp. Although interesting positive associations were found between culture results and the anaerobic pattern

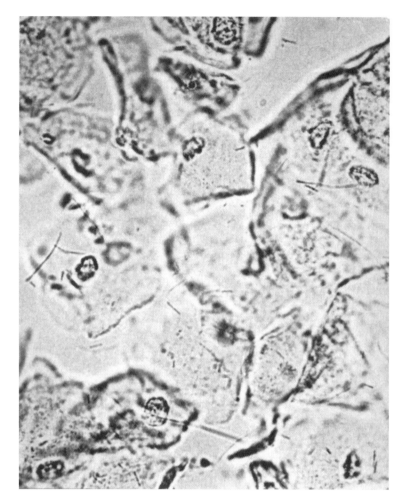

Figure 2   Microscopic examination of normal vaginal epithelial cells on a saline wet preparation.

and negative associations with the lactobacillus predominant pattern, standard diagnostic criteria for BV were not used, therefore, the results are difficult to interpret.[173]

A further study reported excellent agreement between Pap smear detection of clue cells and the standard clinical diagnosis of BV.[153,166] The sensitivity, specificity, and positive predictive value were 90, 97, and 94%, respectively, for the study.[153,166] However, a vaginal sample from the posterior vaginal fornix is part of routine cytological screening in this setting and the vaginal sample was reviewed for clue cells.[153,166] Current practice in the U.S. of collecting cervical and endocervical samples for cytologic cervical smear screening does not provide an ideal test for identification of vaginal fluid clue cells.

1.7.3   Gram stain diagnosis

Dunkelberg first examined vaginal fluid Gram stains for the presence of clue cells and adjacent dense bacteria.[174] Subsequent examinations of vaginal fluid Gram stains to diagnose BV are not based upon examination for clue cells, rather quantitative estimations of the types of bacteria in the vaginal fluid are evaluated.[96,167,168] BV is characterized by a shift from predominance of lactobacillus morphotypes to predominance of coccobacillary morphotypes and Gram-negative rods.

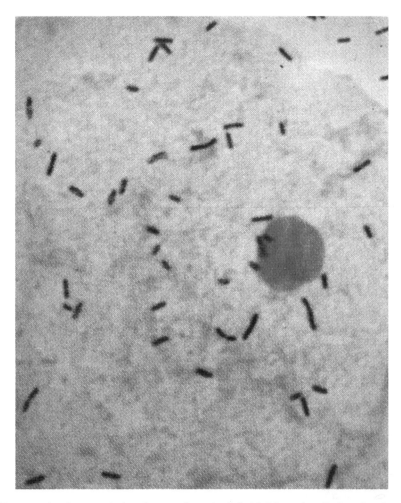

Figure 3   Gram stain characteristic of normal vaginal fluid. Note the distinct borders of the epithelial cells and predominance of long, Gram-positive rods, morphotypically characteristic of *Lactobacillus* spp.

Spiegel re-introduced the idea of Gram stain detection for BV in 1983, and further characterized the vaginal fluid Gram stain findings of BV.[167] Normal fluid is described by a predominance of large Gram-positive rods considered *Lactobacillus* morphotypes, with or without smaller Gram-variable bacilli considered *Gardnerella* morphotypes (Figure 3).[167] A pattern of mixed vaginal flora which includes *Gardnerella* morphotypes, Gram-negative rods, fusiform curved rods and Gram-positive cocci and absent or reduced numbers of *Lactobacillus* morphotypes (less than 5 per high power field) is consistent with BV (Figure 4).[167] Subsequent work by Nugent, Krohn, and Hillier provides a method to further standardized Gram stain interpretation for BV.[168] This technique specifically examines four bacterial morphotypes and assigns a summary score to the vaginal specimen based on the semi-quantitative assessment for *Lactobacillus* morphotypes, *G. vaginalis* and *Prevotella* spp. morphotypes and *Mobiluncus* spp. morphotypes (Table 6).[168] A score of 7 to 10 is considered BV.[168] Compared with other diagnostic methods, this standardized scheme has demonstrated superior reproduciblity comparing examinations by separate individuals and duplicate examinations by the same individual.[175,176] Gram stain interpretation for BV is being made increasingly available in microbiologic laboratories.

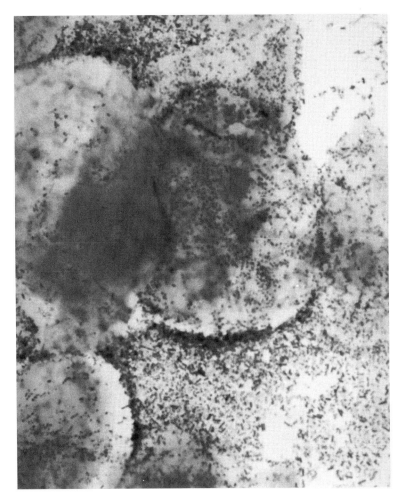

Figure 4 Gram stain characteristic of BV. Note the overall increase in number of bacteria present with predominance of small, Gram-variable coccobacilliary morphotypes, Gram-negative rods, and the general absence of lactobacillus morphotype bacteria.

1.7.4   Bacterial metabolic by-products

Detection of proline amniopeptidase activity, diamine concentration, and organic acid metabolites was examined to characterize BV among older research studies.[34,46,169] These methods are being adapted to allow for paper based "dip stick" diagnostic tests.

1.7.5   Microbial culture

For nearly 20 years, culture for *G. vaginalis* was promoted as the method for diagnosis of the clinical condition now called BV. Research in the early 1980s re-introduced the importance of anaerobic bacteria in this condition and brought forth our current understanding of the polymicrobial nature of BV. Subsequent comparison of the recommended composite clinical criteria for BV with *G. vaginalis* culture results demonstrate presence of this microorganism in up to 60% of women without BV.[3,84] Therefore, single culture for *G. vaginalis* would categorize up to 60% of healthy women as having BV.[3,37,84] Even semi-quantitative examination for heavy colony growth, suggesting presence of high concentrations of *G. vaginalis* accurately predicts as few as 41 to 49% women with the composite clinical criteria

Table 6   Gram Stain Scoring for BV

Quantitation per oil immersion field Quantity	*Lactobacillus* morphotypes Score	*G. vaginalis/Prevotella* spp. morphotypes Score	*Mobiluncus* morphotypes Score
4+	0	4	2
3+	1	3	2
2+	2	2	1
1+	3	1	1
0	4	0	0

Note: The average number of each bacterial morphotype seen in 10 oil immersion fields is counted and assigned a score. The total score for slide is the sum of scores for *Lactobacillus, G. vaginalis, Prevotella,* and *Mobiluncus* morphotypes.

Quantitation per oil immersion field is derived as follows:

Count	Quantitation
0	0
<1	1+
1–5	2+
6–30	3+
>30	4+

From Nugent, RP, Krohn MA, Hillier SL. Reliability of diagnosing bacterial vaginosis is improved by a standardized method of gram stain interpretation. *J. Clin. Microbiol.* 1991;29:297-301. With permission.

for BV among populations with low prevalence.[3,84] More than one half of women with clinical BV would remain undetected using this method. Therefore, culture for *G. vaginalis* without other adjunctive information is not helpful, is misleading, and should be avoided.

Quantitative aerobic and anaerobic vaginal cultures have been used in clinical research studies to evaluate BV, but this technique is costly and impractical for clinical use.[14,15]

1.7.6   New diagnostic techniques

New techniques which include nucleic acid probes for high concentrations of *G. vaginalis* have recently become available.[170,177] Other methodologies are in the developmental stage. Development of "easy to use," reliable and reproducible diagnostic techniques for BV would benefit care providers and women. The Affirm VP III Microbial Identification Test (Becton Dickinson and Company, Sparks, MD) may provide a less subjective test for BV than other current methods. Briselden and Sheiness report accurate detection of 95 to 97% of women with clinical criteria for BV (sensitivity) using the Affirm VP III test.[170,177] Specificity for this test ranged from 71 to 98%.[170,177] Briselden and Hillier note that the false-positive tests (compared with clinical criteria) occurred most often among women with Gram stain findings consistent with BV. This highlights an important difficulty encountered in the development of new tests which must be compared with an imprecise standard for diagnostic method such as with BV.

1.8   Treatments for BV

Several effective treatments for BV are currently available. Variations in reported treatment efficacies often can be attributed to a number of methodologic differences such as different populations studied, diagnostic criteria for BV, inclusion criteria, length of followup, criteria for "cure" and analyses procedures. Duration of followup is probably the most important variable in determining effectiveness. Women examined within one to two weeks post treatment generally show successful resolution rates of 85 to 95%. Women

Table 7   Treatment Regimens for BV and Wholesale Costs

		Cost	
Drug	Dosage	Trade	Generic
Metronidazole	2 g	$14.90	$1.36
	500 mg oral b.i.d. × 7 days	$33.97	$4.46
Clindamycin capsules	300 mg orally b.i.d. × 7 days	$32.95	None
Metro-Gel Vaginal (Curatek)	5 g intravaginally b.i.d. × 5 days	$24.00	None
Cleocin Vaginal Cream (Upjohn)	5 g intravaginally once daily × 7 days	$28.03	None

who are followed for 4 to 5 weeks post treatment show recurrence rates as high as 25 to 35%. Few studies have followed women for longer intervals. Importantly, despite evidence which suggests that BV is linked to sexual activity, a number of randomized controlled trials which examined co-treatment of male partners have failed to demonstrate reduced recurrence rates of BV for women.[121,122]

With their classic study in 1978, Pheifer and colleagues demonstrated the superiority of oral metronidazole for treatment of what was then called nonspecific vaginitis.[178] Oral metronidazole, 500 mg twice daily for seven days, continues to be the standard therapy recommended by the Centers for Disease Control in the U.S. for treatment of BV (Table 7).[179] Follow-up examination of women approximately one week following completion of oral metronidazole treatment demonstrates resolution of BV among 85 to 100% of studied women.[180-185] The percentage of women without BV 4 to 5 weeks following completion of treatment, ranges from 60 to 95% and averages approximately 80%.[180-195]

A number of different regimens of oral metronidazole have been examined in clinical trials and observational reports. Among three randomized, blinded studies, cure rates at 4 weeks post dosing with a single 2 g dose of metronidazole were 45, 47, and 69%.[181-183] However, a number of open treatment trials reported 4-week cure rates of approximately 80% (range 68 to 90%) with the single-dose regimen.[126,184-194] A few authors have examined the efficacy of a 2-g dose of oral metronidazole given on days 1 and 3.[121,122,184] Cure rates are similar with this regimen and single-dose regimens (range 73 to 94%).[121,122,126,184,188-190] In general, when the single-dose regimens are compared with the standard 7-day regimen in the same populations, cure rates with a single 2-g dose of metronidazole are lower.[44,126]

Clindamycin also is active against anaerobic bacteria, *M. hominis* and *G. vaginalis*. Greaves examined 49 women 7 to 10 days following completion of a 7-day course of oral clindamycin 300 mg twice daily and demonstrated a 94% cure rate.[189] McGregor examined 194 pregnant women and found a 92% cure rate 2 to 4 weeks post treatment.[25] Importantly, among a subgroup of women who received treatment early in pregnancy and were followed for the remainder of the pregnancy, 90% remained cured for up to 11 weeks (McGregor, unpublished data).

Intravaginal treatment for BV may have considerable appeal. Local therapy provides high medication levels at the site of the infection and should reduce systemic side effects. Two effective regimens have been developed to meet this need. Clindamycin vaginal cream (2%) used once daily for 7 days provides a cure for BV among 72 to 94% of women at 4 to 10 days following treatment and 50 to 75% of women examined at one month post treatment.[162,190-193] Microorganisms associated with BV, i.e., *G. vaginalis*, *M. hominis*, *Prevotella* spp., and *Peptostreptococcus* spp. are greatly reduced in numbers and *Lactobacillus* spp. colonization is greatly increased following treatment with clindamycin vaginal cream.[162] As previously mentioned, recovery of *E. coli* increased from 13 to 66% of women and *Enterococcus* spp. from 0 to 62% of women at one week after completing treatment. Although *E. coli* colonization did not persist to the one month follow-up visit, recovery of *Enterococcus* spp. continued in up to 50% of women at one month following treatment.[162] The clinical importance of these findings are unclear.

Several forms of metronidazole have been derived for intravaginal administration. Intravaginal metronidazole gel (0.75%) formulated at a pH of 4 is approved within the U.S. for BV treatment. Intravaginal metronidazole treatment has been achieved with vaginal tablets (400 or 500 mg tablets), pessaries, and metronidazole-containing vaginal sponges.[194-197] These preparations are not currently available in the U.S.

Bistoletti examined the effectiveness of intravaginal tablets (500 mg at bedtime for 7 days) vs. oral metronidazole and demonstrated similar efficacies — resolution of BV among 79% of women using intravaginal medication and 74% of women who were randomized to receive oral metronidazole.[194] In a randomized, double-blind, placebo-controlled study, Bro compared 500 mg metronidazole pessaries daily for 7 days with placebo. All 41 women studied using the metronidazole pessaries were cured at one week following treatment. None of the women reported systemic side effects; however, 17% reported vaginal itching and burning.[195] Similarly, Edelman and North examined use of intravaginal sponges containing 1000 mg of metronidazole, for 24 h on 3 consecutive days, in an open trial and identified 88% of studied women as cured 4 weeks after treatment.[197]

Several small randomized, controlled trials demonstrate equivalent efficacy rates for metronidazole vaginal gel and both oral metronidazole and clindamycin vaginal cream.[162,198-201] Hillier examined 60 symptomatic women randomized to either metronidazole vaginal gel or placebo gel, twice daily for 5 days, in a double-blind randomized trial.[198] Initially at 1 to 2 weeks post treatment, 87% of treated women were without findings of BV. Subsequent followup at approximately 4 weeks post treatment yielded an overall cure rate of 73% for women who received metronidazole gel.[198] Similar results were reported by Livengood with 78% of treated women "cured" at the initial followup and an overall cure rate of 69% at one month post treatment.[199] Hanson compared metronidazole vaginal gel with oral metronidazole and again demonstrated equivalent efficacies for the two treatments.[200] BV was eliminated by one week post treatment among 83.7% (36/43) of women randomized to metronidazole vaginal gel and 85.1% (40/47) of women randomized to oral metronidazole.[200] Similarly, BV was absent at 4 weeks post treatment among 70.7 and 71% of women who received intravaginal and oral metronidazole, respectively.[200]

Other treatments for BV have been used. These included ampicillin, Augmentin, ofloxacin, erythromycin, triple sulfa cream, and vaginal acidification.[105,178,202,203] These treatments are less effective than either oral or vaginal preparations of metronidazole or clindamycin and are not recommended.

1.8.1 Treatment during pregnancy

Treatment trials of BV during pregnancy show that cure rates are similar to those obtained among nonpregnant women. McDonald reported 76% of women were cured of BV findings 4 weeks following treatment with oral metronidazole.[204] This is similar to the 70% resolution of BV approximately 4 weeks post treatment reported by Hauth for women who received metronidazole and erythromycin.[26] Oral treatment with clindamycin may be used throughout pregnancy, including the first trimester and provides resolution of BV equivalent to oral metronidazole. Two studies which examined 2% clindamycin vaginal cream demonstrated cure rates of 85 to 95% at examinations 1 to 2 weeks after treatment.[49,161] Metronidazole vaginal gel has not been systematically examined among pregnant women, but is effective anecdotally.

Traditionally metronidazole has been avoided during early pregnancy due to laboratory evidence of mutagenicity in several bacterial and cellular systems and oncogenicity in prolonged high dose exposures in selected animal models. Despite these concerns, after 30 years of clinical use carcinogenic effects in humans have not been detected. Similarly several retrospective studies and a recent meta-analysis have examined the pregnancy

Table 8   Adverse Effects of Standard BV Treatment Regimens

Adverse event	Metronidazole 500 mg b.i.d. × 7	2 g × 1	0.75% Metro-Gel Vaginal b.i.d. × 5	Clindamycin 300 mg b.i.d. × 7	2% Clindamycin Vaginal Cream q.h.s. × 7
Unpleasant taste	35–46%	52%	1.7%	ND	0
Nausea	12–23%	29%	2.0%	12%	1–4%
Vomiting	8–23%	8.8%	<1%	6%	1–4%
Abdominal cramping	1.4–16.7%	11.8%	3.4%	1.6%	1–16%
Decreased appetite	4–23%	14.7%	<1%	ND	ND
Dark urine	33%	17.6%	ND	ND	ND
Diarrhea	1.4–13.3%	8.8%	<1%	6.3%	<1%
Constipation	4–10%	2.9%	<1%	ND	<1%
Headache	8.7%	ND	<1%	ND	<1%
Dizziness	20%	11.8%	<1%	ND	<1%
Yeast vaginitis	4.7–22%	ND	4–6%	8.5 to 24%	12.5–15%

Note: ND = Not described.

outcomes for women who received metronidazole during each trimester of pregnancy. No evidence of increased birth defects has been detected.[205,206] First trimester use of metronidazole is not associated with adverse pregnancy or neonatal outcomes.

1.8.2   Adverse effects from treatment

Side effects with metronidazole treatment are well recognized. An unpleasant taste is the most common complaint occurring to between 35 and 50% of patients.[191] Nausea, vomiting, abdominal pain, headache, and dizziness are also noted (Table 8). Incidence of yeast vaginitis following oral metronidazole treatment varies from 5 to 22%.[191,192]

Among studied women receiving oral treatment with clindamycin, nausea (12%) and yeast vaginitis (8.5 to 24%) were the most common adverse effects.[25,189] Complaints of loose stools or diarrhea occur similarly in numbers of women receiving oral clindamycin (6.3%) and among women given a single 2-g dose of oral metronidazole (8.8%).[25,182] Systemic side effects from intravaginal treatments occur less often than among orally treated women, with the exception of yeast vaginitis.[198-200]

1.8.3   Probiotic treatments

Interest in vaginal infection treatment and vaginal recolonization with *Lactobacillus* sp. preparations originated in the 1890s and has continued throughout this century. Attempts to re-establish normal vaginal "Döderlein Bacillus" with bacteriotherapy have been described in the medical literature since 1917.[207] Metchnikoff's work promoting ingestion of lactobacillus-containing foods for relief of gastrointestinal problems is credited as the first use of probiotic lactobacillus to restore or maintain health.[208] Reports from the early 1900s examined treatment for "leukorrhea" (which included infection with gonorrhea, trichomonas, and monilia as well as likely BV) with bacteria derived from milk fermentation as well as cultured from healthy women.[207,209-211] Differences between milk product acidophilus bacteria and vaginal preparations of Döderlein Bacillus were noted as early as 1933 by Mohler and Brown.[210] Following this Mohler discontinued use of "Bacillus acidophilus" for leukorrhea treatment and established a preparation of Döderlein Bacillus from a healthy volunteer. Daily treatment with this preparation demonstrated resolution of symptoms and recovery of implanted organisms among 6 of 21 women treated.[210] In a recent randomized, controlled clinical trial Hallen examined twice daily treatment with H_2O_2-producing *Lactobacillus acidophilus* intravaginal suppositories vs. placebo among 57 Danish women with BV.[212] Initially, 57% (16/28) of treated women no longer had findings for BV one week after treatment; however, for most of the patients who had received active treatment BV recurred after their next menstrual period.[212]

Commercial lactobacillus powders and capsules as well as yogurt and acidophilus milk continue to be used by women in attempts to restore or continue vaginal health. Most have either not been systematically examined for their effectiveness or have not been shown to provide long-term relief from BV. Importantly, Wood examined bacterial attachment to vaginal epithelial cells by vaginal *Lactobacillus* isolates, several commercial strains of human *Lactobacillus* isolates, yogurt, and other commercial isolates.[213] Isolates derived from human sources demonstrated adherence to vaginal epithelial cells, whereas isolates from yogurt demonstrated low adherence. Importantly, many of the nondairy products have been shown to be contaminated with other potentially harmful bacteria such as *Clostridium sporogenes* and *Enterococcus* spp.[214]

Work continues in multiple centers to develop strains of lactobacillus which will (1) adhere to vaginal epithelial cells, (2) establish mucosal colonization, and (3) provide ecologic regulation for the new host. Such probiotics used following or in conjunction with traditional antimicrobial agents for the treatment of BV will potentially provide long-term cure and reduce recurrences for women with BV.

1.9 Conclusions

BV is defined as replacement of normal healthy vaginal lactobacillus by a characteristic set of genital anaerobes, mycoplasmas, and *G. vaginalis*. This massive microecologic perturbation is similar to a red tide with blooming characteristic sets of bacteria and dramatic increases in microbial products within the vaginal fluid including endotoxins, proteases, and phospholipases. Epidemiologic studies show that this condition is common (10 to 41%) among reproductive age women and although associated with intercourse, it can occur in the absence of sexual contact.

Morbidity associated with BV is now well documented. BV is the most common cause of vaginal discharge and "vaginitis" in the U.S. BV is a direct antecedent if not the direct cause of upper reproductive tract infection including non-gonococcal, non-chlamydial endometritis and salpingitis. BV is directly and consistently linked with post-termination and hysterectomy infectious morbidity.

BV in pregnancy is consistently and causally associated with important numbers of second trimester losses, premature labor, preterm premature rupture of membranes, and preterm birth. Controlled trials conducted among "high" and "low" risk pregnant women with both symptomatic and asymptomatic BV now demonstrate dramatic reductions of prematurity through systematic diagnosis, screening, treatment with oral agents (clindamycin or metronidazole), and "test of cure" followup.

New research imperatives include elucidation of the pathobiology and natural history of BV; refinement of diagnostic techniques and treatments; and further demonstration of benefits of screening and treatment for BV in more recently recognized risk settings such as prior to elective pelvic operation, prior to cesarean section at the initial antenatal visit, and possibly during preconceptional counseling and preparation for pregnancy.

"BV is a disease that has finally been recognized."[215]

References

1. Riverius. *The Practice of Physick.* 1655, p.413. as cited in Eccles A. *Obstetrics and Gynecology in Tudor and Stuart England.* The Kent State University Press. Ohio.1982.
2. Eschenbach DA. Vaginal infection. *Clin. Obstet. Gynecol.* 1983;26(1):186-202.
3. Eschenbach DA, Hillier SL, Critchlow C, Stevens C, DeRousen T, Holmes KK. Diagnosis and clinical manifestations of bacterial vaginosis. *Am. J. Obstet. Gynecol.* 1988;158:819.
4. Paavonen J, Teisala K, Heinonen PK, Aine R, Laine S, Lehtinen M, Miettinen A, Punnonen R, Gronroos P. Microbiological and histopathological findings in acute pelvic inflammatory disease. *Br. J. Obstet. Gynaecol.* 1987;94:454-60.
5. Soper, DE, Bump RC, Hurt WG. Bacterial vaginosis and trichomoniasis vaginitis are risk factors for cuff cellulitis after abdominal hysterectomy. *Am. J. Obstet. Gynecol.* 1990;163;1016-23.
6. Larsson P-G, Bergman B, Försum U, Platz-Christensen J-J, Påhlson C. Mobiluncus and clue cells as predictors of pelvic inflammatory disease after first trimester abortion. *Acta Obstet. Gynecol. Scand.* 1989;68:217-20.
7. Larsson P-G, Bergman B, Försum U, Påhlson C. Treatment of bacterial vaginosis in women with vaginal bleeding complications of discharge and harboring *Mobiluncus. Gynecol. Obstet. Invest.* 1990;29:296-300.
8. Eschenbach DA, Gravett MG, Chen KCS, Hoyme UB, Holmes KK. Bacterial vaginosis during pregnancy. An association with prematurity and post partum complications. In Mårdh PA, Taylor-Robinson D. (Eds) *Bacterial Vaginosis.* Almqvist and Wiksill Stockholm. 1984; 213-22.
9. Gravett MG, Nelson HP, DeRouen T, et al. Independent associations of bacterial vaginosis and *Chlamydia trachomatis* infection with adverse pregnancy outcome. *JAMA* 1986;256: 1899-1903.
10. Gravett MG, Hummel D, Eschenbach DA, Holmes KK. Preterm labor associated with sub-clinical amniotic fluid infection and with bacterial vaginosis. *Obstet. Gynecol.* 1986;67:229-37.
11. Martius J, Krohn MA, Hillier SL, et al. Relationships of vaginal *Lactobacillus* species, cervical *Chlamydia trachomatis,* and bacterial vaginosis to preterm birth. *Obstet. Gynecol.* 1988;71:89-95.
12. McGregor JA, French JI, Richter R, et al. Antenatal microbiologic and maternal risk factors associated with prematurity. *Am. J. Obstet. Gynecol.* 1990;163:1465-77.
13. Hillier SL, Martius J, Krohn MA et al. A case-control study of chorioamnionic infection and histologic chorioamnionitis in prematurity. *N. Engl. J. Med.* 1988;319:972-8.
14. McDonald HM, O'Loughlin JA, Jolley P, et al. Prenatal microbiological risk factors associated with preterm birth. *Br. J. Obstet. Gynaecol.* 1992;99:190-6.
15. Kurki T, Sivonen A, Renkonen O-V, et al. Bacterial vaginosis in early pregnancy and pregnancy outcome. *Obstet. Gynecol.* 1992;80:173-7.
16. Hay PE, Lamont RF, Taylor-Robinson D, Morgan DJ, Ison CA, Pearson J. Abnormal bacterial colonization of the genital tract and subsequent preterm delivery and late miscarriage. *Br. Med. J.* 1994;308:295-8.
17. Joesoef MR, Hillier SL, Utomon B, Wiknjosastro G, Linnan M, Kandun N. Bacterial vaginosis and prematurity in Indonesia: Association in early and late pregnancy. *Am. J. Obstet. Gynecol.* 1993;169:175-8.
18. Hillier SL, Nugent RP, Eschenbach DA, Krohn MA, Gibbs RS, Martin DH, Cotch MF, Edelman R, Pastorek JG II, Rao AV, McNellis D, Regan JA, Carey JC, Klebanoff MA, for the Vaginal Infections and Prematurity Study Group. Association between bacterial vaginosis and pre-term delivery of a low-birth-weight infant. *N. Engl. J. Med.* 1995;333:1737-42.
19. Watts DH, Krohn MA, Hillier SL, Eschenbach DA. Bacterial vaginosis as a risk factor for post cesarean endometritis. *Obstet. Gynecol.* 1990;75:52-58.
20. Silver HM, Sperling RS, St. Clair P, Gibbs RS. Evidence relating bacterial vaginosis to intramniotic infection. *Am. J. Obstet. Gynecol.* 1989;161:808:12.
21. Hillier SL, Krohn MA, Cassen E, Easterling TR, Rabe LK, Eschenbach DA. The role of bacterial vaginosis and vaginal bacteria in amniotic fluid infection in women in preterm labor with intact fetal membranes. *Clin. Infect. Dis.* 1995;20(Suppl. 2):S276-8.
22. McGregor JA, French JI, Seo K. Premature rupture of membranes and bacterial vaginosis. *Am. J. Obstet. Gynecol.* 1993;169:463-6.

23. Larsson P-G, Platz-Christensen J-J, Thejls H, Försum U, Påhlson C. Incidence of pelvic inflammatory disease after first-trimester legal abortion in women with bacterial vaginosis after treatment with metronidazole: A double-blind, randomized study. *Am. J. Obstet. Gynecol.* 1992;166:100-3.

24. Morales WJ, Schorr S, Albritton J. Effects of metronidazole in patients with preterm birth in preceding pregnancy and bacterial vaginosis: A placebo-controlled, double-blind study. *Am. J. Obstet. Gynecol.* 1994;171:345-9.

25. McGregor JA, French JI, Parker R, Draper D, Patterson E, Jones W, Thorsgard K, McFee J. Prevention of premature birth by screening and treatment for common genital tract infections: Results of a prospective controlled evaluation. *Am. J. Obstet. Gynecol.* 1995;173:157-67.

26. Hauth JC, Goldenberg RL, Andrews WW, DuBard MB, Cooper RL. Reduced incidence of preterm delivery with metronidazole and erythromycin in women with bacterial vaginosis. *N. Engl. J. Med.* 1995;333:1732-6.

27. McDonald HM, O'Loughlin JA, Vigneswaran R et al. Metronidazole treatment of bacterial vaginosis in pregnancy and preterm birth: a randomized, placebo-controlled trial. Abstract presented at Infectious Diseases Society for Obstetrics and Gynecology. August 14–17, 1996; Beaver Creek, CO.

28. Döderlein A. Das Scheidensekret und seine bedeutung fur das puerperalfieber. Leipzig, O. Durr. 1892.

29. Thomason JL, Gelbart SM, Broekhuizen FF. Advances in the understanding of bacterial vaginosis. *J. Reprod. Med.* 1989;34:581-7.

30. Gardner HL, Dukes CD. *Haemophilus vaginalis* vaginitis. *Am. J. Obstet. Gynecol.* 1955;69:962-76.

31. Zinneman K, Turner GC. The taxonomic position of *Haemophilus vaginalis* (*Corynebacterium vaginale*). *J. Pathol. Bacteriol.* 1963;85:213-9.

32. Dunkelburg WE Jr., Skaggs R, Kellogg DS Jr. A study and new description of *Corynebacterium vaginale* (*Haemophilus vaginalis*). *Am. J. Clin. Pathol.* 1970;53:370-7.

33. Greenwood JR, Pickett MJ. Transfer of *Haemophilus vaginalis* Gardner and Dukes to a new genus *Gardnerella*: *G. vaginalis* (Gardner and Dukes) comb. nov. *Int. J. Syst. Bacteriol.* 1980;30:170-8.

34. Spiegel CA, Amsel R, Eschenbach D, Schoenknecht F, Holmes KK. Anaerobic bacteria in nonspecific vaginitis. *N. Engl. J. Med.* 1980;303:601-7.

35. Blackwell AL, Phillips I, Fox AR, Barlow D. Anaerobic vaginosis (non-specific vaginitis): Clinical, microbiological, and therapeutic findings. *Lancet* 1983;1379-82.

36. Weström L, Evaldson G, Holmes KK, van der Meijden W, Rylander E, Fredriksson B. Taxonomy of vaginosis: Bacterial vaginosis — a definition. In Mårdh P-A, Taylor-Robinson D. (Eds) *Bacterial Vaginosis.* Uppsala, Sweden: Almqvist and Wiksell, Stockholm. 1984;259-60.

37. Amsel R, Totten PA, Spiegel CA, Chen KCS, Eschenbach DA, Holmes KK. Nonspecific vaginitis. Diagnostic criteria and microbial and epidemiologic associations. *Am. J. Med.* 1983;74:14.

38. Sobel JD. Bacterial vaginosis — an ecologic mystery. *Ann. Int. Med.* 1989;111:551-3.

39. Mårdh P-A. The vaginal ecosystem. *Am. J. Obstet. Gynecol.* 1991;165:1163-8.

40. Eschenbach DA. Bacterial Vaginosis: Emphasis on upper genital tract complications. *Obstet. Gynecol. Clin. N. Am.* 1989;16(3):593-610.

41. Spiegel CA. Bacterial vaginosis. *Clin. Microbiol. Rev.* 1991;4(4):485-502.

42. Giorgi A, Torriani S, Dellaglio F, Bo G, Stola E, Bernuzzi L. Identification of vaginal lactobacilli from asymptomatic women. *Microbiologica* 1987;10:377-84.

43. Paavonen J, Miettinen A, Stevens CE, Chen KCS, Holmes KK. *Mycoplasma hominis* in non-specific vaginitis. *Sex. Trans. Dis.* 1983;10(Suppl):271-5.

44. Hillier SL, Holmes KK. Bacterial vaginosis. Chapter 47 in Holmes KK, Mårdh P-A, Sparling PF, Wiesner PJ, Cates W Jr, Lemon SM, Stamm WE. (Eds) *Sexually Transmitted Diseases.* Second Edition. McGraw-Hill Information Services Company. New York, NY. 1990;547-59.

45. Piot P, VanDyke E, Godts P, Vanderheyden J. The vaginal microbial flora in non-specific vaginitis. *Eur. J. Clin. Microbiol.* 1982;1:301-6.

46. Chen KCS, Amsel R, Eschenbach DA, Holmes KK. Biochemical diagnosis of vaginitis: Determination of diamines in vaginal fluid. *J. Inf. Dis.* 1982;145:337-47.

47. Chen KCS, Amsel R, Eschenbach DA, Holmes KK. Amine content of vaginal fluid from untreated patients with nonspecific vaginitis. *J. Clin. Invest.* 1979;63:828-35.

48. Briselden AM, Moncla BJ, Stevens CE, Hillier SL. Sialidases (neuraminidases) in bacterial vaginosis and bacterial-vaginosis-associated microflora. *J. Clin. Microbiol.* 1992;30:663-6.

49. McGregor JA, French JI, Jones W, Milligan K, McKinney PJ, Patterson E, Parker R. Bacterial vaginosis is associated with prematurity and vaginal fluid sialidase: Results of a controlled trial of topical clindamycin cream. *Am. J. Obstet. Gynecol.* 1994;170:1048-60.

50. Glasson JH, Woods WH. Immunoglobulin proteases in bacteria associated with bacterial vaginosis. *Austr. J. Med. Lab. Sci.* 1988;9:63-5.

51. McGregor JA, French JI, Jones W, Parker R, Patterson E, Draper D. Association of cervico/vaginal infections with increased vaginal fluid phospholipase A_2 activity. *Am. J. Obstet. Gynecol.* 1992;167:1588-94.

52. McGregor JA, Lawellin D, Franco-Buff, Todd JK. Phospholipase C activity in microorganisms associated with reproductive tract infection. *Am. J. Obstet. Gynecol.* 1991;164:682-6.

53. McGregor JA, Lawellin D, Franco-Buff A, et al. Protease production by microorganisms associated with reproductive tract infection. *Am. J. Obstet. Gynecol.* 1986;154:109.

54. Platz-Christensen JJ, Brandberg A, Wiqvist N. Increased prostaglandin concentrations in the cervical mucus of pregnant women with bacterial vaginosis. *Prostaglandins.* 1992;43(2):133-41.

55. Platz-Christensen JJ, Mattsby-Baltzer I, Thomsen P, Wiqvist N. Endotoxin and interleukin-1-α in the cervical mucus and vaginal fluid of pregnant women with bacterial vaginosis. *Am. J. Obstet. Gynecol.* 1993;169:1161-6.

56. McGregor JA. Prevention of preterm birth: New initiatives based on microbial-host interactions. *Obstet. Gynecol. Survey.* 1988;43:1-14.

57. Redondo-Lopez V, Cook RL, Sobel JD. Emerging role of lactobacilli in the control and maintenance of vaginal bacterial microflora. *Rev. Infect. Dis.* 1990;12(5):856-72.

58. Mårdh P-A, Soltesz LV. *In vitro* interactions between lactobacilli and other microorganisms occurring in the vaginal flora. *Scand. J. Infect. Dis.* 1983;40(Suppl.):47-51.

59. Hamdan IY, Mikolajcik EM, Acidolin: An antibiotic produced by *Lactobacillus acidophilus. J. Antibiot. (Tokyo)* 1974;27:632-6.

60. Barefoot SF, Klaenhammer TR. Detection and activity of lactacin-β, a bacteriocin produced by *Lactobacillus acidophilus. Appl. Environ. Microbiol.* 1983;45:1808-15.

61. Wheater DM, Hirsh AM, Mattick ATR. Possible identity of lactobacilli with hydrogen peroxide produced by lactobacilli. *Nature* 1952;170:623-24.

62. Chan RCY, Reid G, Irvin RT, Bruce AW, Costerton JW. Competitive exclusion of uropathogens from human uroepithelial cells by lactobacillus whole cells and cell wall fragments. *Infect. Immun.* 1985;47:84-9.

63. Mårdh P-A, Weström L. Adherence of bacteria to vaginal epithelial cells. *Infect. Immun.* 1976;13:661-6.

64. West CA, Warner PJ, Plantacin β, a bacteriocin produced by *Lactobacillus plantarium* NCDO 1193. *Microbiol. Lett.* 1988;49:163-5.

65. Eschenbach DA, Davick PR, Williams BL, Klebanoff SJ, Young-Smith K, Critchlow CM, Holmes KK. Prevalence of hydrogen peroxide-producing *Lactobacillus* species in normal women and women with bacterial vaginosis. *J. Clin. Microbiol.* 1989;27:251-6.

66. Klebanoff SJ, Hillier SL, Eschenbach DA, Waltersdorph AM. Control of the microbial flora of the vagina by H_2O_2-generating lactobacilli. *J. Infect. Dis.* 1991;164:94-100.

67. Hillier SL, Krohn MA, Rabe LK, Klebanoff SJ, Eschenbach DA. The normal vaginal flora, H_2O_2-producing lactobacilli, and bacterial vaginosis in pregnant women. *Clin. Infect. Dis.* 1993;16(Suppl. 4):S273-81.

68. Hillier SL, Krohn MA, Klebanoff SJ, Eschenbach DA. The relationship of hydrogen peroxide-producing lactobacilli to bacterial vaginosis and genital microflora in pregnant women. *Obstet. Gynecol.* 1992;79:369-73.

69. Paavonen J. Physiology and ecology of the vagina. *Scand. J. Infect. Dis.* 1983;40:31-35.

70. Peeters M, Piot P. Adhesion of *Gardnerella vaginalis* to vaginal epithelial cells: variables affecting adhesion and inhibition by metronidazole. *Genitourin. Med.* 1985;61:391-5.

71. Nagy E, Froman G, Mårdh P-A. Fibronectin binding of Lactobacillus species isolated from women with and without bacterial vaginosis. *J. Med. Microbiol.* 1992;37:38-42.
72. Freidrich EA JR. The vagina: an ecologic challenge. *Ariz. Med.* 1979;36:443-5.
73. Brand JM, Galask RP. Trimethylamine: the substance mainly responsible for the fishy odor often associated with bacterial vaginosis. *Obstet. Gynecol.* 1986;68:682-5.
74. MacDonald, JB, Socranshy SS, Gibbons RJ. Aspects of the pathogenesis of mixed anaerobic infections of mucous membranes. *J. Dent. Res.* 1963;42:529-44.
75. Mayrand D, McBride BC. Ecological relationships of bacteria involved in a simple, mixed anaerobic infection. *Infect. Immun.* 1980;27:44-50.
76. Rotstein OD, Pruett TL, Fiegel VD, Nelson RD, Simmons RL. Succinic acid, a metabolic by product of *Bacteroides* species, inhibits polymorphonuclear leukocyte function. *Infect. Immun.* 1985;48:402-8.
77. Kyner D, Zabos P, Christman J, Acs G. Effects of sodium butyrate on lymphocyte activation. *J. Exp. Med.* 1976;144:1674-8.
78. Singer RE, Buckner BA. Butyrate and propionate: Important components of toxic dental plaque extracts. *Infect. Immun.* 1981;32:458-63.
79. Voeller B, Anderson D. Heterosexual transmission of HIV. JAMA 1992;267:1917-1919.
80. Ernest JM, Meis PJ, Moore ML, Swain M. Vaginal pH: a marker of preterm premature rupture of the membranes. *Obstet. Gynecol.* 1989;74:734-8.
81. Heine RP, Draper D, Jones W, French JI, McGregor JA. Vaginal fluid enzymes correlate with wet mount positivity but not symptomatology in pregnant patients with *Trichomonas vaginalis*. Presented at the annual meeting of the Infectious Disease Society for Obstetrics and Gynecology. Stowe, VT. August 4–7, 1993.
82. McGregor JA, French JI, Parker R, Draper D, Jones W, Heine P, Patterson E, Hastings C, Thorsgard K. Vaginal fluid enzymes in pregnancy: Correlation with cervico-vaginal infections. Presented at the annual meeting of the Infectious Disease Society for Obstetrics and Gynecology. Stowe, VT. August 4–7, 1993.
83. Hill LH, Ruparelia H, Embil JA. Nonspecific vaginitis and other genital infections in three clinic populations. *Sex. Trans. Dis.* 1983;10:114-8.
84. Krohn MA, Hillier SL, Eschenbach DA. Comparison of methods for diagnosing bacterial vaginosis among pregnant women. *J. Clin. Microbiol.* 1989;27:1266-71.
85. Centers for Disease Control. Nonreported sexually transmissible diseases — United States. *MMWR* 1979;28(6):61-3.
86. Embree J, Caliando JJ, McCormack WM. Nonspecific vaginitis among women attending a sexually transmitted diseases clinic. *Sex. Trans. Dis.* 1984;11:81-4.
87. Lossick JG. The descriptive epidemiology of vaginal trichomoniasis and bacterial vaginosis. Horowitz BJ, Mårdh P-A (Eds) In *Vaginitis and Vaginosis*. Wiley-Liss, New York, NY. 1991, pp.77-84.
88. Rosenberg MJ, Davidson AJ, Chen J-H, Judson FN, Douglas JM. Barrier contraceptives and sexually transmitted diseases. A comparison of female dependent methods and condoms. *Am. J. Public Health.* 1992;82:669-74.
89. Hart G. Factors associated with trichomoniasis, candidiasis, and bacterial vaginosis. *Int. J. STD AIDS* 1993;4:21-5.
90. Moi H. Epidemiologic aspects of vaginitis and vaginosis in Scandinavia. Horowitz BJ, Mårdh P-A (Eds) In *Vaginitis and Vaginosis*. Wiley-Liss, New York, NY. 1991, pp.85-91.
91. Hallén A. Påhlsson C. Försum U. Bacterial vaginosis in women attending STD Clinic: diagnostic criteria and prevalence of *Mobiluncus* spp. *Genitourin. Med.* 1987;63:386-9.
92. Moi H. Prevalence of bacterial vaginosis and its association with genital infections, inflammation, and contraceptive methods in women attending sexually transmitted disease and primary health clinics. *Int. J. STD AIDS* 1990;1(2):86-94.
93. Bell TA, Farrow JA, Stamm WE, et al. Sexually transmitted diseases in females in a juvenile detention center. *Sex. Trans. Dis.* 1985;12:140-4.
94. Hill LVH, Luther ER, Young D, Pereira L, Embil JA. Prevalence of lower genital tract infections in pregnancy. *Sex. Trans. Dis.* 1988;15:5-10.

95. Lefevre JC, Averous S, Bauriaud R, Blanc C, Bertrand MA, Lareng MB. Lower genital tract infections in women: Comparison of clinical and epidemiologic findings with microbiology. *Sex. Trans. Dis.* 1988;15:110-3.
96. Hay PE, Taylor-Robinson D, Lamont RF. Diagnosis of bacterial vaginosis in a gynaecology clinic. *Br. J. Obstet. Gynecol.* 1992;99:63-6.
97. Riordan T, Macaulay ME, James JM, Leventhall PA, Morris EM, Neal BR, Rowland J, Evans BM. A prospective study of genital infections in a family planning clinic. *Epidemiol. Infect.* 1990;104:47-53.
98. Larsson P-G, Platz-Christensen JJ, Enumeration of clue cells in rehydrated air-dried vaginal wet smears for the diagnosis of bacterial vaginosis. *Obstet. Gynecol.* 1990;76:727-30.
99. Stevens-Simon C, Jamison J, McGregor JA, Douglas JM. Racial variations in vaginal pH among healthy sexually active adolescents. *Sex. Trans. Dis.* 1994;21(3):168-72.
100. Bump RC, Zuspan FP, Buesching WJ, Ayers LW, Stephens TJ. The prevalence, six-month persistence and predictive values of laboratory indicators of bacterial vaginosis (nonspecific vaginitis) in asymptomatic women. *Am. J. Obstet. Gynecol.* 1984;150:917-24.
101. Gardner HL, Damper TK, Dukes CD. The prevalence of vaginitis. A study in incidence. *Am. J. Obstet. Gynecol.* 1957;73:1080-7.
102. Schmidt H, Hansen JG. A wet smear criterion for bacterial vaginosis. *Scand. J. Prim. Health Care* 1994;12:233-8.
103. Singh V, Gupta MM, Satyanarayana L, Parashari A, Sehgal A, Chattopadhya D, Sodhani P. Association between reproductive tract infections and cervical inflammatory epithelial changes. *Sex. Trans. Dis.* 1995;22:25-30.
104. Paavonen J, Hienonen PK, Aine R, Laine S, Grönroos P. Prevalence of nonspecfiic vaginitis and other cervicovaginal infections during the third trimester of pregnancy. *Sex. Trans. Dis.* 1986;13:5-8.
105. Duff P, Lee ML, Hillier SL, Herd LM, Krohn A, Eschenbach DA. Amoxicillin treatment of bacterial vaginosis during pregnancy. *Obstet. Gynecol.* 1991;77:431-5.
106. Minkoff H, Grunebaum AN, Schwarz RH, Feldman J, Cummings M, Cromblehome W, Clark L, Pringle G, McCormack WM. Risk factors for prematurity and premature rupture of membranes: A prospective study of the vaginal flora in pregnancy. *Am. J. Obstet. Gynecol.* 1984;150:965-72.
107. McGregor JA, French JI, Richter R, Vuchetich M, Bachus V, Hillier S, Judson FN, McFee J, Schoonmaker J, Todd JK. Cervicovaginal microflora and pregnancy outcome: Results of a double-blind, placebo-controlled trial of erythromycin treatment. *Am. J. Obstet. Gynecol.* 1990;163:1580-91.
108. Meis PJ, Goldenberg RL, Mercer B, Moawad A, and the National Institute of Child Health and Human Development Maternal-Fetal Medicine Units Network. The preterm prediction study: Significance of vaginal infections. *Am. J. Obstet. Gynecol.* 1995;173:1231-5.
109. Platz-Chritensen JJ, Pernevi P, Hagmar B, Andersson E, Brandberg A, Wiqvist N. A longitu-dinal follow-up of bacterial vaginosis during pregnancy. *Acta Obstet. Gynecol. Scand.* 1993;72:99-102.
110. Thorsen P, Jensen IP, Molsted K, Arpi M, Bremmelgaard A, Moller BR. An epidemiologic study of bacterial vaginosis in a population of 3600 pregnant women: First antenatal visit. Abstract #204 Presented at 11th Annual meeting of the International Society for STD Re-search. New Orleans. LA, August 27–30, 1995.
111. Hillier SL, Krohn MA, Nugent RP, Gibbs RS, for the Vaginal Infections and Prematurity Study Group. Characteristics of three vaginal flora patterns assessed by Gram stain among pregnant women. *Am. J. Obstet. Gynecol.* 1992;166:938-44.
112. Bump RC, Buesching WJ III. Bacterial vaginosis in virginal and sexually active adolescent females: Evidence against exclusive sexual transmission. *Am. J. Obstet. Gynecol.* 1988;158:935-9.
113. Thomason JL, Gelbart SM, Wilcoski LM, Peterson AK, Jilly BJ, Hamilton PR. Proline ami-nopeptidase activity as a rapid diagnostic test to confirm bacterial vaginosis. *Obstet. Gynecol.* 1988;71:607-11.
114. Holst E et al. Bacterial vaginosis: Microbiological and clinical findings. *Eur. J. Clin. Microbiol.* 1987;6:536.

115. Barbone F, Austin H, Louv WC, Alexander WJ. A follow-up study of methods of contraception, sexual activity, and rates of trichomoniasis, candidiasis and bacterial vaginosis. *Am. J. Obstet. Gynecol.* 1990;163:510-4.

116. Wolner-Hanssen P. Risk factors for bacterial vaginosis. Abstract Presented at the Infectious Diseases Society for Obstetrics and Gynecology Annual Meeting. Seattle, WA. August 8–11, 1990.

117. Hammerschlag MR, Cummings M, Doraiswamy B, Cox P, McCormack WM. Nonspecific vaginitis following sexual abuse in children. *Pediatr.* 1985;75:1028-31.

118. Holst E. Reservoir of four organisms associated with bacterial vaginosis suggests lack of sexual transmission. *J. Clin. Microbiol.* 1990;28:2035-9.

119. Piot P et al. Biotypes of *Gardnerella vaginalis*. *J. Clin. Microbiol.* 1984;22:677-679.

120. Berger BJ et al. Bacterial vaginosis in lesbians: A sexually transmitted disease. *Clin. Infect. Dis.* 1995;21:1402-5.

121. Vejtorp M, Bollerup AC, Vejtorp L, Fanøe E, Nathan E, Reiter A, Andersen ME, Strømsholt B, Schrøder SS. Bacterial vaginosis: a double-blind randomized trial of the effect of treatment of the sexual partner. *Br. J. Obstet. Gynaecol.* 1988;95:920-6.

122. Moi H, Erkkola R, Jerve F, Nelleman G, Bymose B, Alaksen K, Tornqvist E. Should male consorts of women with bacterial vaginosis be treated? *Genitourin. Med.* 1989;65:263-8.

123. Vutyavanich T, Pongsuthirak P, Vannareumol P, Ruangsri R-A, Luangsook P. A randomized double-blind trial of tinidazole treatment of the sexual partners of females with bacterial vaginosis. *Obstet. Gynecol.* 1993;82:550-4.

124. Cook RL, Redondo-Lopez V, Schmitt C, Meriwether C, Sobel JD. Clinical, microbiological, and biochemical factors in recurrent bacterial vaginosis. *J. Clin. Microbiol.* 1992;30:870-7.

125. Hay PE, Morgan DJ, Ison CA, Bhide SA, Romney M, McKenzie P, Pearson J, Lamont RF, Taylor-Robinson D. A longitudinal study of bacterial vaginosis during pregnancy. *Br. J. Obstet. Gynecol.* 1994;101:1048-53.

126. Larsson P-G. Treatment of bacterial vaginosis. *Int. J. STD AIDS.* 1992;3:239-47.

127. Sobel JD, Schmitt C, Meriwether C. Long-term follow-up of patients with bacterial vaginosis treated with oral metronidazole and topical clindamycin. *J. Infect . Dis.* 1993;167:783-4.

128. Mårdh P-A. An overview of infectious agents in salpingitis, their biology, and recent advances in methods of detection. *Am. J. Obstet. Gynecol.* 1980;138:933.

129. Eschenbach DA, et al. Polymicrobial etiology of acute pelvic inflammatory disease. *N. Engl. J. Med.* 1975;293:166.

130. Soper DE, Brockwell NJ, Dalton HP, Johnson D. Observations concerning the microbial etiology of acute salpingitis. *Am. J. Obstet. Gynecol.* 1994;170:1008-17.

131. Sweet RL. Role of bacterial vaginosis in pelvic inflammatory disease. *Clin. Infect. Dis.* 1995;20(Suppl 2):S271-5.

132. Faro D, Martens M, Maccato M, Hammill H, Pearlman M. Vaginal flora and pelvic inflammatory disease. *Am. J. Obstet. Gynecol.* 1993;169:470-4.

133. Wolner-Hanssen P, Mårdh P-A, Møller B, Weström L. Endometrial infection in women with chlamydial salpingitis. *Sex. Trans. Dis.* 1982;9:84-8.

134. Wolner-Hassen P, Mårdh P-A, Svensson L, Westrom L. Laparoscopy in women with chlamydial infection and pelvic pain: A comparison of patients with and without salpingitis. *Obstet. Gynecol.* 1983;61:299-303.

135. Weström L, Mårdh P-A. Acute pelvic inflammatory disease. In Holmes KK, Mårdh P-A, Sparling PF, Wiesner PJ, Cates W Jr, Lemon SM, Stamm WE. Eds. *Sexually Transmitted Diseases.* Second Edition. San Francisco, CA. McGraw-Hill, 1990;593-613.

136. Mårdh P-A, Møller BR, Ingerselv HJ, Nesssler E, Weström L, Wolner-Hanssen P. Endometritis caused by *Chlamydia trachomatis*. *Br. J. Ven. Dis.* 1981;57:191-5.

137. Greenwood, SM, Moran JJ. Chronic endometritis: morphologic and clinical observations. *Obstet. Gynecol.* 1981;58:176-84.

138. Greenwood SM and Rotterdam H. Chronic endometritis. A clinical pathologic study. *Pathol. Ann.* 1978;13:209-31.

139. Wolner-Hanssen P, Kiviat NB, Holmes KK. Atypical pelvic inflammatory disease: subacute, chronic, or subclinical upper genital tract infection in women. In Holmes KK, Mårdh P-A, Sparling PF, Wiesner PJ, Cates W Jr, Lemon SM, Stamm WE. Eds. *Sexually Transmitted Diseases.* Second Edition. San Francisco, CA. McGraw-Hill, 1990;615-20.

140. Novak ER, Woodruff JD. Gynecology and obstetric pathology. With Clinical and Endocrine Relations. 8th edition Philadelphia, W.B. Saunders, 1979;239-59.

141. Kristiansen FV, Øster S, Frost L, Boustouller Y, Korsager B, Møller BR. Isolation of *Gardnerella vaginalis* in pure culture form the uterine cavity of patients with irregular bleeding. *Br. J. Obstet. Gynaecol.* 1987;94:979-84.

142. Larsson P-GB, Bergman BB. Is there a causal connection between motile curved rods, *Mobiluncus* species, and bleeding complications? *Am. J. Obstet. Gynecol.* 1986;154:107-8.

143. Korn AP, Bolan G, Padian N, Ohm-Smith M, Schachter J, Landers DV. Plasma cell endometritis in women with symptomatic bacterial vaginosis. *Obstet. Gynecol.* 1995;85:387-90.

144. Faro S. Prevention of infections after obstetric and gynecologic surgery. *J. Reprod. Med.* 1988;33(Suppl.):154-8.

145. Shapiro M, Munoz A, Tager IB, et al. Risk factors for infection at the operative site after abdominal or vaginal hysterectomy. *N. Engl. J. Med.* 1982;307:1661-6.

146. Larsson P-G, Platz-Christensen J-J, Försum U, Påhlson C. Clue cells in predicting infections after abdominal hysterectomy. *Obstet. Gynecol.* 1991;77:450-2.

147. Mårdh P-A, Stormby N, Weström L. Mycoplasma and vaginal cytology. *Acta Cytol.* 1971;15:310-5.

148. Mead PB. Cervical-vaginal flora of women with invasive cervical cancer. *Obstet. Gynecol.* 1978;52:601.

149. Thadepalli H, Savage EW, Roa B. Anaerobic bacteria associated with cervical neoplasia. *Gynecol. Oncol.* 1982;14:307.

150. Pavic N. Is there a local production of nitrosamines by vaginal microflora in anaerobic vaginosis/trichomoniasis. *Med. Hypoth.* 1984;15:433-6.

151. Van Tassel RL, MacDonald DK, Wilkins TD. Production of a fecal mutagen by *Bacteroides* spp. *Infect. Immun.* 1982;37:975.

152. Guijon F, Paraskevas M, Rand F, Heywood E, Brunham R, McNicol P. Vaginal microbial flora as a cofactor in the pathogenesis of uterine cervical intraepithelial neoplasia. *Int. J. Gynecol. Obstet.* 1992;37:185-91.

153. Platz-Christensen J-J, Sundström E, Larsson P-G. Bacterial vaginosis and cervical intraepithelial neoplasia. *Acta Obstet. Gynecol. Scand.* 1994;73:586-8.

154. Peters N, van Leeuwen AM, Pieters WJLM, Hollema H, Quint WGV, Burger MPM. Bacterial vaginosis is not important in the etiology of cervical neoplasia: A survey on women with dyskaryotic smears. *Sex. Trans. Dis.* 1995;22:296-302.

155. Voeller B. Heterosexual transmission of HIV. *JAMA* 1992;267:1917-8.

156. Saracco A, Musicco M, Nicolosi A, et al. Man-to-woman sexual transmission of HIV: Longitudinal study of 343 steady partners of infected men. *J. AIDS* 1993;6:497-502.

157. Cohen CR, Duerr A, Pruithithada N, Rugpao S, Hillier SL, Garcia P, Nelson K. Bacterial vaginosis and HIV seroprevalence among female commercial sex workers in Chiang Mai, Thailand. *AIDS* 1995;9:1093-7.

158. McDonald HM, O'Loughlin JA, Jolley P, Vigneswaran R, McDonald PJ. Vaginal infection and preterm labour. *Br. J. Obstet. Gynaecol.* 1991;98:427-35.

159. McDonald HM, O'Loughlin JA, Jolley PT, Vigneswaran R, McDonald PJ. Changes in vaginal flora during pregnancy and association with preterm birth. *J. Infect. Dis.* 1994;170(3):724-8.

160. Holst E, Goffeng AR, Andersch B. Bacterial vaginosis and vaginal microorganisms in idiopathic premature labor and association with pregnancy outcome. *J. Clin. Microbiol.* 1994;32:176-86.

161. Joesoef MR, Hillier SL, Wiknjosastro G, Sumampouw M, Linnan M, Utomo B. Intravaginal clindamycin treatment for bacterial vaginosis: Effects on preterm delivery and low birth weight. *Am. J. Obstet. Gynecol.* 1995;173:1527-31.

162. Hillier S, Krohn MA, Watts DH, Wolner-Hanssen P, Eschenbach D. Microbiologic efficacy of intravaginal clindamycin cream for the treatment of bacterial vaginosis. *Obstet. Gynecol.* 1990;76:407-13.

163. Krohn MA, Hillier SL, Nugent RP, Cotch MF, Carey JC, Gibbs RS, Eschenbach DA, for the Vaginal Infections and Prematurity Study Group. The genital flora of women with intraamniotic infection. *J. Infect. Dis.* 1995;171:1475-80.

164. Watts DH, Eschenbach DA, Kenny GE. Early postpartum endometritis: The role of bacteria, genital mycoplasmas, and *Chlamydia trachomatis. Obstet. Gynecol.* 1989;73:52-9.

165. Gibbs RS. Infection after cesarean section. *Clin. Obstet. Gynecol.* 1985;28:697-710.

166. Platz-Christensen JJ, Larsson P-G, Sundstrom E, Bondeson L. Detection of bacterial vaginosis in Papanicolaou smears. *Am. J. Obstet. Gynecol.* 1989;160:132-3.

167. Spiegel CA, Amsel R, Holmes KK. Diagnosis of bacterial vaginosis by direct gram stain of vaginal fluid. *J. Clin. Microbiol.* 1983;18:170-7.

168. Nugent RP, Krohn MA, Hillier SL. Reliability of diagnosing bacterial vaginosis is improved by a standardized method of gram stain interpretation. *J. Clin. Microbiol.* 1991;29:297-301.

169. Thomason JL, Gelbart SM, Wilcoski LM, Peterson AK, Jilly BJ, Hamilton PR. Proline aminopeptidase activity as a rapid diagnostic test to confirm bacterial vaginosis. *Obstet. Gynecol.* 1988;71:607-11.

170. Sheiness D, Dix K, Watanabe S, Hillier SL. High levels of *Gardnerella vaginalis* detected with an oligonucleotide probe combined with elevated pH as a diagnostic indicator of bacterial vaginosis. *J. Clin. Microbiol.* 1992;30:642-8.

171. Thomason JL, Schreckenberger PA, Spellacy WN et al. Clinical and microbiological characterization of patients with non-specific vaginosis having motile, curved anaerobic rods. *J. Infect. Dis.* 1984;149:801-809.

172. Thomason JL, Gelbart SM, Anderson RJ, Walt AK, Osypowski PJ, Broekhuizen FF. Statistical evaluation of diagnostic criteria for bacterial vaignosis. *Am. J. Obstet. Gynecol.* 1990;162:155-60.

173. Schnadig VJ, Davie KD, Shafer SK, Yandell RB, Islam MA, Hannigan EV. The cytologist and bacterioses of the vaginal-ectocervical area. Clues, commas and confusion. *Acta Cytol.* 1988;33(3):287-97.

174. Dunkelberg WE Jr. Diagnosis of *Hemophilus vaginalis* vaginitis by gram-stained smears. *Am. J. Obstet. Gynecol.* 1965;91:998-1000.

175. Joesoef MR, Hillier SL, Josodiwondo S, Linnan M. Reproducibility of a scoring system for gram stain diagnosis of bacterial vaginosis. *J. Clin. Microbiol.* 1991;29:1730-1.

176. Mazzulli T, Simor AE, Low DE. Reproducibility of interpretation of gram-stained vaginal smears for the diagnosis of bacterial vaignosis. *J. Clin. Microbiol.* 1990;28:1506-8.

177. Briselden AM, Hillier SL. Evaluation of Affirm VP microbial identification test for *Gardnerella vaginalis* and *Trichomonas vaginalis. J. Clin. Microbiol.* 1994;32:148-52.

178. Pheifer TA, Forsyth PS, Durfee MA, Pollock HM, Holmes KK. Nonspecific vaginitis. Role of *Haemophilus vaginalis* and treatment with metronidazole. *N. Engl. J. Med.* 1978;298:1429-34.

179. Centers for Disease Control. 1993 Sexually Transmitted Diseases Treatment Guidelines. *MMWR* 1993;42 (No. RR-14).

180. Blackwell, AL, Phillips I, Fox AR, Barlow D. Anaerobic vaginosis (non-specific vaginitis): Clinical microbiological and therapeutic findings. *Lancet* 1983:1379-82.

181. Eschenbach DA, Critchlow CW, Watkins H, Smith K, Spiegel CA, Chen KCS, Holmes KK. A dose-duration study of metronidazole for the treatment of nonspecific vaginosis. *Scand. J.Infect. Dis. Suppl.* 1983;40:73-80.

182. Swedberg J, Steiner JF, Deiss F, Steiner S, Driggers DA. Comparison of single-dose vs one-week course of metronidazole for symptomatic bacterial vaignosis. *JAMA* 1983;254:1046-9.

183. Ison CA, Taylor, RFH, Link C, Buckett P, Harris JRW, Easmon CSF. Local treatment for bacterial vaginosis. *BMJ* 1987;295:886.

184. Jerve F, Berdal TB, Bohman P, Smithe C, Evjen OK, Gjønnæss H, Gaasemyr M, Hausken L, Hesla K, Hoftvedt E, Høvik P, Kahn J, Karlsen RM, Lie S, Løvland HB, Nordmark P, Saltveit T, Sande Ø, Steier J, Winge T, Ystehede B, Qvigstad E. Metronidazole in the treatment of non-specific vaginitis (NSV). *Br. J. Vener. Dis.* 1984;60:171-4.

185. Jones BM, Geary I, Alawattegama AB, Kinghorn GR, Duerden BI. *In vitro* and *in vivo* activity of metronidazole against *Gardnerella vaginalis, Bacteroides* spp. and *Mobiluncus* spp. in bacterial vaginosis. *J. Antimicrob. Chemother.* 1985;16:189-97.

186. Balsdon MJ. treatment of *Gardnerella vaginalis* syndrome with a single 2 grams dosage of metronidazole. *Scand. J. Infect. Dis.* 1983;(Suppl. 40):101-2.

187. Mohanty KC, Deighton R. Comparison of two different metronidazole regimens in the treatment of *Gardnerella vaginalis* infection with or without trichomoniasis. *J. Antimicrob. Chemother.* 1985;16:799-803.

188. Blackwell A, Fox A, Phillips I, Barlow D. Metronidazole in treatment of non-specific vaginitis. Clinical and microbiological findings in ten patients given 2 grams of metronidazole. *Scand. J. Infect. Dis.* 1983;40:103-6.

189. Greaves WL, Chungafung J, Morris B, Haile A, Townsend JL. Clindamycin versus metronidazole in the treatment of bacterial vaginosis. *Obstet. Gynecol.* 1988;72:799-802.

190. Livengood CH III, Thomason JL, Hill GB. Bacterial vaginosis: Treatment with topical intravaginal clindamycin phosphate. *Obstet. Gynecol.* 1990;76:118-23.

191. Schmitt C, Sobel JD, Meriwither C. Bacterial vaginosis: treatment with clindamycin cream versus oral metronidazole. *Obstet. Gynecol.* 1992;79:1020-3.

192. Fischbach F, Petersen EE, Weissenbacher ER, Martius J, Hosmann J, Mayer H. Efficacy of clindamycin vaginal cream versus oral metronidazole in the treatment of bacterial vaginosis. *Obstet. Gynecol.* 1993;82:405-10.

193. Anders FJ, Parker R, Hosein I, Benrubi GI. Clindamycin vaginal cream versus oral metronidazole in the treatment of bacterial vaignosis: A prospective double-blind clinical trial. *S. Med. J.* 1995;85(11):1077-80.

194. Bistoletti P, Fredricsson B, Hagstrom B, Nord C-E. Comparison of oral and vaginal metronidazole therapy for nonspecific bacterial vaginosis. *Gynecol. Obstet. Invest.* 1986;21:144-9.

195. Bro F. Metronidazole pessaries compared with placebo in the treatment of bacterial vaginosis. *Scand. J. Prim. Health Care* 1990;8:219-23.

196. Brenner WE, Dingfelder JR. Metronidazole-containing vaginal sponges for the treatment of bacterial vaginosis. *Adv. Contracept.* 1986;2:363-9.

197. Edelman DA, North BB. Treatment of bacterial vaginosis with intravaginal sponges containing metronidazole. *J. Reprod. Med.* 1989;34:341-4.

198. Hillier SL, Lipinski C, Briselden AM, Eschenbach DA. Efficacy of intravaginal 0.75% metronidazole gel for the treatment of bacterial vaginosis. *Obstet. Gynecol.* 1993;81:963-7.

199. Livengood CH III, McGregor JA, Soper DE, Newton E, Thomason JL. Bacterial vaginosis: Efficacy and safety on intravaginal metronidazole treatment. *Am. J. Obstet. Gynecol.* 1994;170:759-64.

200. Hanson JM, McGregor JA, Hillier SL, Eschenbach DA, Kreutner AK, Galask R, Martens M. Metronidazole vaginal gel versus oral metronidazole for the treatment of bacterial vaginosis: Results of a multi-center trial, in press.

201. Ferris DG, Litaker MS, Woodward L, Mathis D, Hendrich J. Treatment of bacterial vaginosis: A comparison of oral metronidazole, metronidazole vaginal gel, and clindamycin vaginal cream. *J. Fam. Pract.* 1995;41(5):443-49.

202. Covino JM, Black JR, Cummings M, Zwickl B, McCormack WM. Comparative evaluation of ofloxacin and metronidazole in the treatment of bacterial vaginosis. *Sex. Trans. Dis.* 1993;20:262-4.

203. Durfee MA, Forsyth PS, Hale JA, Holmes KK. Ineffectiveness of erythromycin for treatment of *Haemophilus vaginalis*-associated vaginitis: Possible relationship to acidity of vaginal secretions. *Antimicrob. Agent Chemother.* 1979;16(5):635-7.

204. McDonald HM, O'Loughlin JA, Vigneswaran R, Jolley PT, McDonald PJ. Bacterial vaginosis in pregnancy and efficacy of short-course oral metronidazole treatment : A randomized controlled trial. *Obstet. Gynecol.* 1994;84:343-8.

205. Piper JM, Mitchel EF, Ray WA. Prenatal use of metronidazole and birth defects: No Association. *Obstet. Gynecol.* 1993;82:348-52.

206. Burtin P, Taddio A, Ariburnu O, Einarson TR, Koren G. Safety of metronidazole in pregnancy: A meta analysis. *Am. J. Obstet. Gynecol.* 1995;172:525-9.

207. Block FB, Llewelyn TH. The treatment of leukorrhea with lactic acid bacilli. *JAMA* 1917;6(24):2025-6.

208. Bibel DJ. Elie Metchnikoff's bacillus of long life. *Am. Soc. Microbiol. News.* 1988;54(12):661-5.

209. Thomas S. Döderlein's bacillus: Lactobacillus acidophilus. *J. Infect. Dis.* 1928;43:218-27.

210. Mohler RW, Brown CP. Döderlein's bacillus in the treatment of vaginitis. *Am. J. Obstet. Gynecol.* 1933;25:718-23.

211. Butler BC, Beakley JW. Bacterial flora in vaginitis. *Am. J. Obstet. Gynecol.* 1960;79:432-40.

212. Hallen A, Jarstrand C, Påhlson C. Treatment of bacterial vaginosis with lactobacilli. *Sex. Trans. Dis.* 1992;19:146-8.

213. Wood JR, Sweet RL, Catena A, Hadley WK, Robbie M. *In vitro* adherence of *Lactobacillus* species to vaginal eipthelial cells. *Am. J. Obstet. Gynecol.* 1985;153:740-3.

214. Hughes VL, Hillier SL. Microbiologic characteristics of *Lactobacillus* products used for colonization of the vagina. *Obstet. Gynecol.* 1990;75:244-8.

215. Thomason JL, Gelbart SM. *Bacterial Vaginosis. Current Concepts.* The Upjohn Company, Kalamazoo, MI. 1990.

chapter two

Sexually transmitted infections associated with chlamydia trachomatis

Michael A. Noble

2.1   Introduction..42
2.2   Infection in women..42
2.3   Infection in men 42
2.4   Epidemiology..42
    2.4.1   United States...43
    2.4.2   Canada 43
    2.4.3   Australia 43
    2.4.4   Japan..43
    2.4.5   Israel 44
    2.4.6   Sweden...44
2.5   Laboratory diagnosis 44
    2.5.1   Patient screening strategies 44
        2.5.1.1   Leukocyte esterase 45
        2.5.1.2   Sample collection...45
        2.5.1.3   Urine testing...45
2.6   Test sensitivity, specificity...46
    2.6.1   Gold standard vs. extended gold standard 46
    2.6.2   Techniques..46
        2.6.2.1   Culture 46
        2.6.2.2   Antigen detection...47
            2.6.2.2.1   Direct fluorescent antibody 47
            2.6.2.2.2   Enzyme immunoassay 47
            2.6.2.2.3   Clearview..48
        2.6.2.3   Nuceleic acid detection 48
            2.6.2.3.1   Probe...48
            2.6.2.3.2   Gene amplicfication 48
            2.6.2.3.3   Plasmid gene 48
        2.6.2.4   Serology 48
            2.6.2.4.1   Typing of isolates for epidemic investigation 49
2.7   Therapy and prevention 49
    2.7.1   Antibiotics 49
    2.7.2   Vaccines...50
References 50

2.1　Introduction

Genital infections with *Chlamydia trachomatis* are the most common bacteria-associated sexually transmitted infections reported.[1] Although the precise number of infections is not established, it was estimated in 1993 that there were more than 4 million infections annually. Many infections in both men and women are asymptomatic, however, *C. trachomatis* infection can be associated with significant unwellness in women, men, and infants.

2.2　Infection in women

The most common site of infection in women is the endocervix. Most infections in women are asymptomatic and are detected only by screening procedures at the time of pelvic examination. Although mild inflammation or ectropion may be present, it may not be sufficient to generate clinical signs.[2] The most common symptoms, when present, are vaginal discharge and dysuria. A diagnosis of mucopurulent cervicitis is supported when green or yellow mucopus is observed on a swab that has been inserted within the cervical os, or if at least 30 polymorphonuclear leukocytes (PMNs) are present per high power field on Gram stain of cervical secretions.[3]

Women with sterile pyuria may have urethral infection with *C. trachomatis*. This may occur in the absence of endocervical infection.[4]

It is estimated that 8% of women with endocervical *C. trachomatis* infection will progress to the spectrum of pelvic inflammatory disease including acute salpingitis,[5] pelvic peritonitis, periappendicitis, and perihepatitis. In a review by Paavonen, 25–67% of cases of pelvic inflammatory disease will have *C. trachomatis* isolated from any site.[6] It is estimated that eradication of genital chlamydial infections would eliminate 80% of tubal factor infertility and 50% of tubal pregnancies.[6] By animal model studies, progression to upper tract pathology is more associated with repeated infection.[7] The passage of *C. trachomatis* to the upper tract does not appear to be assisted by spermatozoa.[8]

Prior infection with *C. trachomatis* infection as measured by serology[9] is associated with female infertility. Asymptomatic endocervical infection detected by polymerase chain reaction (PCR) may be responsible for adverse outcomes with *in vitro* fertilization including implantation failure or spontaneous abortion.[10]

2.3　Infection in men

Chlamydial infection of the male urethra does not result in large numbers of complications, however, this group may represent a large reservoir for infection in women. Males may also be asymptomatic without urethral discharge. This is often associated with low numbers of inclusions and may be difficult to detect by enzyme immunoassay (EIA) techniques.[11] *C. trachomatis* urethritis may coexist with *Neisseria gonorrhoeae*, although in many low prevalence centers, the incidence of gonococcal infection has dropped so that coinfection is significantly less common. Rarely, chlamydial urethritis can progress to prostatitis[12,13] and epididymitis,[14] and is associated with male infertility. *C. trachomatis* infection is associated with 50% of cases of Reiter's syndrome that is not associated with gastrointestinal pathogens.[15-17]

2.4　Epidemiology

A large number of studies done around the world have examined the prevalence or incidence of genital *C. trachomatis* infections. Incidence studies are performed most frequently in sexually transmitted diseases (STD) clinics which represent high risk, high prevalence centers, or in student health or family planning clinics which are associated with lower risk and lower prevalence.

Because of the lack of a convenient and acceptable technique for examining the male urethra, there are few prevalence studies in males until recently.

2.4.1 United States

While estimates of prevalence of *C. trachomatis* in the U.S. range between 8 and 40%, no comprehensive national surveillance for chlamydia has been established.[18] Between 1987 and 1991 the number of states with legislation mandating chlamydia reporting increased from 18–36. Over the same time period, based on the combined states reports, the rate of reported cases rose from 91.4 cases per 100,000 population to 197.5 cases per 100,000 population. Of states reporting in 1991, Virginia had the highest (315.5) and New Jersey had the lowest (22.2) rate of reported infection per 100,000 population. Between 1987 and 1991, while the reported rate in men rose from 41.9 to 47.7 per 100,000 population, the reported rate in women rose from 138.0 to 281.2 per 100,000 population.

Counter to increases in reported rates, the San Diego County Department of Health Services reported the prevalence of *C. trachomatis* infection in women receiving family planning services in public health centers decreased between July 1989 and June 1993 from 10 to 1.9%. The prevalence of decline was minimal among black women, while steady among white and Hispanic women. Prevalence of infection was inversely related to age. Decreases were noted from 10.7% in 1986 to 6.9% in 1990 in urban family practice clinics throughout Milwaukee, WI.[19]

2.4.2 Canada

At the University of British Columbia Student Health Service between 1984 and 1988, women being seen for a reason that necessitated a gynecological examination were tested for the presence of *C. trachomatis*. Although the number of women seen annually remained constant, as did the percentage of those asymptomatic, the annual incidence rate fell from 7 to 4.4%.[20] Over the following 3 years until 1994, the rate continued to drop to 1.8%, where it has remained stable through 1994. At the Divisional Sexually Transmitted Disease Clinic in Vancouver, a decline in the number of patients with a diagnosis of *C. trachomatis* decreased from 3.9% of clinic visits (407 per 10,510 visits) to 2.6% of clinic visits (231 per 9,009 visits) between 1989 and 1993, despite a relatively constant patient population and constant clinical protocol.[21] In the province of Manitoba the incidence of genital *C. trachomatis* infection was observed to decline between 1988 and 1990 parallelling the declining trend in the prevalence of genital infections with *N. gonorrhoeae*.[22]

2.4.3 Australia

In a study by Garland et al., in 1980–82 chlamydial infections were reported in 3.2–14.6% of patients. By 1990 this had decreased to 2.7–5.5%.[23] A subsequent analysis[24] indicated a prevalence of 6.4% in patients attending the central STD clinic between 1990–1991.

2.4.4 Japan

For 13,000 women presenting for abortion in Hokkaido Japan, a prevalence rate of 5.6% was found in married women and 15.2% in unmarried women. No significant change in rate was detected in unmarried women between 1986 and 1994.[25]

2.4.5   Israel

Samra et al.[26] examined 64 women attending a methadone clinic in Tel Aviv for *C. trachomatis* by culture of genital swab. Twenty-five percent of the women were found to harbor *C. trachomatis*. Similarly, elevated numbers of patients positive for *C. trachomatis* were reported by Ghinsberg[27] from women attending outpatient clinics either with symptomatic complaints of vaginal discharge or requests for contraceptive advice. *C. trachomatis* is a common genital pathogen in Israel in all populations.

2.4.6   Sweden

Between 1985 and 1993, over 120,000 people were investigated for presence of *C. trachomatis*. Over this time period the rate of detection fell from 107.2 per 1000 women to 32.3 per 1000 women. A similar decline was detected in men.[28] Similar to other studies, positivity rates were highest among attendees to STD clinics and lowest in private practices. These trends were duplicated when results of serum sample testing were retrospectively analyzed between 1970 and 1993.[29]

2.5   Laboratory diagnosis

2.5.1   Patient screening strategies

In order to develop comprehensive information on the prevalence of *C. trachomatis* infection, it is necessary to develop strategies to screen populations at risk. The difficulties encountered when setting up such a strategy can be complicated by problems including the lack of an inexpensive widely available diagnostic test that is both sensitive and specific, limited resources, and lack of public health laws. The costs of untreated *C. trachomatis* infection must be viewed from two perspectives: those associated with diagnosis including clinic visit, diagnostic tests, medication, and its sequelae, and the costs associated with treatment of sequelae from untreated infection. Different approaches, either universal screening or selective screening with respect to patient selection strategies, have been examined in order to maximize capture of infected individuals. Multivariate analysis of cervical samples from 11,793 women in 22 family practice clinics in Colorado indicated that infection was significantly associated with endocervical bleeding, cervical mucopurulent discharge, a new sexual partner in the last 3 months, more than 3 sexual partners within the last year, pregnancy, use of oral contraceptives, and age.[30] Ramstedt et al. found age (18–23 years), duration of current relationship less than 1 year, non-use of condoms, and no previous history of sexually transmitted infection significantly related, however, screening based on these criteria would not effectively identify women at high risk.[9] Similarly Weinstock et al.[31] noted age less than 25 years, cervical friability, single marital status, new sexual partner within the last 3 months, and lack of condom use significantly associated with *C. trachomatis*, however, again no single factor or combination of factors could be used to capture all women with infection. They concluded that selective screening cannot be relied upon for detection of *C. trachomatis* in high risk populations. Based on the experience and analysis of universal screening with 11,141 women seen in family planning clinics, age less than 20 years, presence of cervicitis, a new sex partner in the last 60 days, two sex partners within the last 30 days, or a sex partner with symptoms could be selective screening criteria.[32] In family planning clinics, where asymptomatic presentation is common, if low cost, low sensitivity testing with direct fluorescent antibody (DFA) were used, selective screening would be cost effective if the clinic prevalence rate were 1.8% or less.[33] Within the same clinic if a higher cost, more sensitive assay (ligase chain assay) were used, selective screening would be cost effective if the prevalence rate was below 3.5%. For STD clinics, where asymptomatic presentation is much less common, the corresponding break-even prevalences were 4.1 and 7.7%.

Clinical screening criteria is an appealing technique to reduce the number of individuals being tested for *C. trachomatis* infection by laboratory techniques. In one study of over 6000 women attending a family planning clinic, significant relationships between *C. trachomatis* infection and age between 18 and 23 years, short-term relationships (less than 1 year), absence of previous genitourinary infection, and non-use of condoms, were identified; however, screening criteria fail to identify all women at risk. It is recommended to screen all sexually active young people.[9] Another study of 1000 women, in a similar setting, indicated that screening women with a new sex partner in the last year along with cervical friability, suspicious discharge, urinary frequency, and intermenstrual bleeding would reduce testing to 75.4% and detect 93.3% of cases.[34]

Examination of screening for *C. trachomatis* in women 18–34 years of age and at high risk for pelvic inflammatory disease demonstrates the utility and success of screening. A strategy of identifying, testing, and treating women at increased risk for cervical chlamydial infection was associated with a reduced incidence of pelvic inflammatory disease.[35]

2.5.1.1   Leukocyte esterase

The leukocyte esterase (LE) test detects enzymes released from PMNs. LE tests have widespread usage as urine dip sticks for the diagnosis of cystitis. Several studies have evaluated urine dip tests for predicting the presence of *C. trachomatis* or *N. gonorrhoeae* urethritis.[36–41] Sensitivity of the test has a broad range (51–94%). Factors such as timing of study (first void), time interval between sample collection and testing, and personnel performing the test (clinician vs. laboratory) may be influencing factors that affect test performance.

2.5.1.2   Sample collection

From the beginning, the specimen of choice for examination for genital *C. trachomatis* has been a swab collected either from the female cervix or from the male urethra. For specimens collected from women, it is necessary to first remove ectocervical mucus with a primary swab which can be discarded, and then with a fresh swab collect the sample by insertion into the cervical os for at least 10 s. When swabs are collected from the urethra, a fine flexible shafted swab is inserted 2-4 cm into the urethra and gently rotated 2 or 3 times. Transport to the laboratory is time and temperature sensitive. Ideally the swab should be transported in chlamydial transport medium on a cold pack at 2–8°C and arrive at the laboratory within 4 h. Swabs left at 4°C for more than 24 h have severe loss of growth. This is not evident with swabs stored at –70°C.[42] Cotton swabs with wooden shafts may result in poor growth recovery because of the introduction of inhibitory factors.[43] For non-culture techniques, swabs used for sample are collected in a similar fashion. Swab toxicity is not a factor and swabs can be transported at ambient temperature. Generally specimens can remain at ambient temperature for 2 days, or 4°C for a week prior to testing. Because cytobrushes are more efficient at removal of mucocolumnar junction cells, cytobrushes are associated with improved detection of *C. trachomatis* by culture or antigen technique.[44]

2.5.1.3   Urine testing

Swabbing the male urethra is an uncomfortable procedure and to date has been a major limiting factor blocking investigation of males with possible asymptomatic infection with *C. trachomatis*. Early considerations of urine as an alternate sample were thwarted because urine does not work as a candidate sample for culture. Early reports[45] suggested that urine may have utility as a candidate sample for chlamydia antigen detection in males. Subsequent to the early studies, urine has been demonstrated to be a valuable alternate sample for investigating both symptomatic and asymptomatic men when tested by a spectrum of assays. When tested by microparticle EIA urine testing on first void urine was 81.3%

sensitive and 95.7% specific as compared to urethral swab culture.[46] As compared to an expanded gold standard, the sensitivity was 80.8%, and the specificity was 100%. When tested by PCR, the sensitivity of urine testing after discrepant analysis was 87.1% and the specificity was 97.4%.[47] When tested by a range of EIAs, urine from symptomatic males ranged from 85–91% sensitive and 95–99% specific. For asymptomatic males, the sensitivity was 77%.[48] Another study examining the utility for EIAs found the sensitivity by one system to be 82.8% and by another 62.1%.[49] When tested by DFA the sensitivity of staining sediment from male first pass urine was 83%.[50] The composite of these results supports the concept that first catch urine is an acceptable, and perhaps, preferable sample for testing males for genital infection with *C. trachomatis* regardless of the test assay used.

By a similar process of wanting to find a noninvasive alternative to genital swabs, urine samples have been examined to replace the more cumbersome and uncomfortable endocervical and endourethral swabs used to collect samples from women. Early attempts to isolate *C. trachomatis* by cell culture from women were unsuccessful.[51] Similarly, some attempts to recover antigen from concentrated first void urine from women[52,53] were also unsuccessful, although others found examination of urine sediment by DFA to be equal to examination of endocervical swabs.[54] In a four-center study, comparing LCR examination of first void urine in women against culture from an endocervical swab,[55] as measured against an expanded gold standard, sensitivity and specificity of first void urine was 93.8 and 99.9%, respectively.

2.6   Test sensitivity, specificity

2.6.1   Gold standard vs. extended gold standard

Comparison studies for the determination of test sensitivity, specificity, and predictive value assume that the assay against which the experimental system is compared is accurate. Traditionally, for chlamydia-related studies, tissue culture has been considered the standard technique. Studies have frequently raised questions about the acceptability of culture as a gold standard. In some studies the sensitivity of chlamydia tissue culture has ranged from 33 to 86%.[56] Development of an extended gold standard as the basis of comparison has been raised. Common criteria for an extended gold standard include: (1) positive standard culture on primary isolation; (2) one positive non-culture test, confirmed by culture after multiple passages; (3) one positive non-culture test confirmed by at least one of the other non-culture techniques; and (4) positive PCR test confirmed by a different PCR method using different primers.[57,58]

2.6.2   Techniques

2.6.2.1   Culture

Chlamydia are obligate intracellular bacteria not sustainable on artificial cell-free media. Living host cells are required to support their growth. Two systems are available for propagation: embryonated hen's egg yolk sac and cell culture monolayer. The yolk sac system may be useful for production of high yields of fastidious *Chlamydia* isolates.[59] A number of cell lines have been successfully used to isolate *C. trachomatis* including McCoy cells, monkey kidney cells, HeLA cells, and L. cells.[60-62] The most common line used with clinical specimens is cyclohexamide-treated McCoy cells. A cell's monolayers may be established either in shell vials or in flat-bottomed, 96-well microtiter plates.[63] Isolation rates may be improved by the use of polyethylene glycol.[64] Culture is an unacceptable technique for recovery of *C. trachomatis* from urine.[65]

Table 1   Reported Sensitivity and Sensitivity of various Assays for the Detection of *C. trachomatis*

Assay	Sensitivity	Specificity	Ref.
Syva MicroTrak	96.3, 64.7, 63, 93.4, 100	99.4, 100, 98.1, 100	57, 68, 75, 77, 78
Abbott Chlamydiazyme	77.5, 87, 56	100, 100	68, 79, 80
Pharmacia Chlamydia EIA	77.0	100	79
Cell Culture	80.0, 95, 97.3, 66.7	100, 100, 100, 100	57, 77, 79, 81
VIDAS CHL	95	95	80
Clearview Chlamydia (Unipath)	67.3, 97.3	99.7, 100	81, 82
Magic Lite Chlamydia (CIBA)	48.1, 72.4	99.9, 97.1	82, 83
Baxter AntigEnz Chlamydia	88, 77.6	99, 99	75, 82

2.6.2.2   Antigen detection

2.6.2.2.1   Direct fluorescent antibody.   Direct staining of genital swab material was one of the first laboratory methods widely available for clinical laboratories to detect *C. trachomatis*.[66-72] Sample is applied to a standard microscope slide, methanol fixed, and incubated with fluorescent-linked antibody directed against genus-specific cell wall proteins. Following incubation and wash steps the slide can be viewed with a fluorescent microscope for the presence of apple green round elementary bodies. Slides with more than five elementary bodies are read as positive. Factors that can result in a false-negative result include inadequacy of sample or too thick an application of sample on the slide, making staining and reading difficult.

As a primary assay for detection of *C. trachomatis* DFA requires experienced technologists to detect well-formed apple green elementary bodies. Detection of positive samples takes a mean of 27 s of microscopic examination, while determination of negative samples takes a mean of 6 min.[73] Experience indicates that DFA may be an acceptable technique for small laboratories equipped with fluorescent microscopy provided that there is a maximum of 20 samples per run. Beyond that number, the procedure becomes too labor intensive and is frequently associated with eye discomfort on the part of the microscopist.

DFA is an acceptable technique for confirmation of positives by other assays.[74,75] The use of cytocentrifuges for application of materials on the slide results in superior detection.[71] As compared to chlamydia culture on McCoy cells, sensitivity for DFA staining ranged from 70–100%.[66-69] DFA may apply to detecting *C. trachomatis* in centrifuged urine sediment and may be a more sensitive assay for the detection of *C. trachomatis* than examination of cervical sample in the same individual by EIA.[68]

2.6.2.2.2   Enzyme immunoassay.   In many clinical laboratories, EIA for detection of *C. trachomatis* has become the procedure of choice. The assay is accurate, acceptably sensitive, specific and it lends itself to techniques that confirm the identification of *C. trachomatis*. The hardware involved has become progressively more automated, allowing for more samples to be processed with relatively few hands-on technologist hours. Confirmation of positive results either by application of blocking antibody[76] or by performance of a second assay[74,75] has reduced false-positive results to an absolute minimum. There is a broad range of equipment and reagents. Samples compatible with EIA technique include male and female genital samples and urine samples.

Literature contains many comparisons of the sensitivity, specificity, and predictive values of the commercial assays available. A partial summary of reported assay sensitivity and specificity is provided in Table 1.

2.6.2.2.3 Clearview. A more portable antigen capture technique, using a membrane-based diffusion card (Clearview, Wampole Laboratories, Cranbury NJ) has been developed. The card technique has distinct advantages, especially for smaller laboratories, in that it requires little specialized equipment and has an easily interpreted endpoint. When compared to culture as a gold standard, the Clearview card had a sensitivity of 78% and a specificity of 99.6%.[85] When compared to an extended gold standard (culture positive or positive by two non-culture techniques) the sensitivity was 72.9% and specificity was 98.9%.[81]

2.6.2.3 Nucleic acid detection

2.6.2.3.1 Probe. Nonisotopic DNA probe (Gen-Probe PACE; Gen-Probe Inc., San Diego CA) has been commercially available since 1990. Single-stranded DNA labeled with acridinium ester, complementary to the rRNA of *C. trachomatis*, is incubated with specimen in a 60°C water bath for one hour. Separation and elution reagents are added and the endproduct is measured for relative light units using a luminometer.[78,86,87] Sensitivity was 80–95.2% for detection of *C. trachomatis* in women compared to the gold standard,[86,87] but it was lower in males. The sensitivity of the assay for male urethra was improved by altering the collection swab and transport kit. Specificity of the nonisotopic probe can be raised to 100% by using competitive nucleic acid hybridization to differentiate true- and false-positive signals.[87]

2.6.2.3.2 Gene amplification. MOMP gene — Major outer membrane (MOMP) antigens are a target for detection of *C. trachomatis* by EIA methodology. In 1990 the detection of *C. trachomatis* by amplification by using primers in a conserved area of the MOMP gene was described.[88,89] Following amplification by PCR, detection of biotinylated RNA-DNA hybrids was performed by EIA. Detection of amplified DNA by EIA is 10- to 100-fold more sensitive than gel detection and is equal to ^{32}P hybridization of a Southern blot.[88] Detection of *C. trachomatis* using nested primers in the MOMP gene sequence can be more sensitive than shell vial culture. In one study of 787 patients of mixed populations culture was able to detect 37 positive samples (4.7%) as opposed to 46 (5.8%) by nested PCR.[90]

2.6.2.3.3 Plasmid gene. **Amplification of target RNA** — Detection of *C. trachomatis* by amplification of DNA has markedly improved sensitivity, however, like EIA, it suffers from being unable to determine viability. Based on amplification of target RNA by 3SR (self-sustaining sequence replication), a culture supplementing method for the detection of viable samples has been developed.[91] 3SR amplification has several key advantages as an efficient and powerful target amplification system. The technique is isothermal and can achieve 10^8-fold replication in 30 min.[92]

PCR and ligase chain reaction — Amplicor (Roche Molecular Systems) is a PCR amplification method for direct detection of *C. trachomatis* DNA in clinical specimens. Amplicor has been evaluated against culture and antigen detection assays for detection of *C. trachomatis*.[93-99] Amplification based on ligase chain reaction has similarly reached the level of commercial application (Lcx; Abbott Diagnostics).[4,38,53,99-102]

2.6.2.4 Serology

Antibody response can be observed by complement fixation (CF), microimmunofluorescence (MIF), indirect immunoperoxidase assay, and by ELISA. MIF testing uses antigen from *C. trachomatis*, *C. psittaci*, and *C. pneumoniae* individually dotted on a slide. Patient serum is incubated on the slide and is then re-incubated with either anti-human IgG, IgA, or IgM conjugated with fluorescein.[103-105]

C. trachomatis serology is not commonly examined in clinical medicine, because it will not provide timely or accurate information for the diagnosis of acute infections. That being

Table 2   Recommendations for Treatment of Confirmed or Suspected
Infection with *C. trachomatis*

Adolescents and adults

Recommended

       Doxycycline 100 mg orally 2 times per day for 7 days

       Azithromycin 1 g orally in a single dose

Alternatives

       Ofloxacin 300 mg orally 2 times per day for 7 days

or   Erythromycin base 500 mg orally 4 times per day for 7 days

or   Erythromycin ethyl succinate 800 mg orally for 7 days

or   Sulfisoxazole 500 mg orally 4 times per day for 10 days

Pregnant women

Recommended

       Erythromycin base 500 mg orally 4 times per day for 7 days

Alternatives

       Erythromycin base 250 mg orally 4 times per day for 14 days

or   Erythromycin ethyl succinate 800 mg orally for 7 days

or   Erythromycin ethyl succinate 400 mg orally for 14 days

or   Amoxicillin 500 mg orally 3 times per day for 7 days

From Centers for Disease Control and Prevention: 1993 Sexually transmitted
diseases treatment guidelines, *MMWR*, 42, 47, 1993.

said, serology is extremely useful in studies of pelvic inflammatory disease,[103] infertility,[106,107] where the active infection no longer exists, and where examining for antigens or nucleic acid is not possible.[108]

Infertility in women has been reported to be significantly associated with IgG and IgA titers against *C. trachomatis* as compared to controls.[106] No relationship is found between serology, male infertility, and the presence of *C. trachomatis* DNA or rRNA in semen.[107] Witkin et al.[108] found that presence of IgA antibodies in endocervical sample directed against *C. trachomatis* structural membrane components and recombinant *C. trachomatis* heat shock protein collected at the time of oocyte aspiration was significantly associated with embryo transfers that did not result in an ongoing pregnancy. Similar findings are not associated with the measurement of IgA antibody in serum.[109-111]

    2.6.2.4.1 Typing of isolates for epidemic investigation.   Typing of *C. trachomatis* isolates, while not a requirement for clinical laboratories, may be critical for epidemiological investigation and outbreak control. Serotyping based on monoclonal antibodies directed against antigens on the MOMP of strains initially recognized 15 serovars of *C. trachomatis*[112] which has been expanded by three additional serovars.[113,114] Additional techniques for differentiating between strains includes analysis of restriction enzyme analysis,[115] pulsed-field gel electrophoresis,[116] ribotyping,[117] and direct genotyping by PCR or nested PCR.[118-122]

2.7   Therapy and prevention

2.7.1   Antibiotics

Antibiotic therapy for *C. trachomatis* is used to prevent person-to-person transmission and to reduce risk of neonatal infection. Both symptomatic and asymptomatic infections require therapy. Current regimens for treatment of adolescents and adults is presented in Table 2.

2.7.2 Vaccines

Sexually transmitted diseases and eye infections caused by *C. trachomatis* are major health problems worldwide. A vaccine to prevent or control these diseases is badly needed. Although no vaccine candidate has reached the level of preparedness for human studies, considerable efforts have been made. Different preparations of *C. trachomatis* have been given by enteric administration prior to ocular challenge with live chlamydia were compared to the immunity that develops after recovery from ocular infection. Oral immunization with either live homologous serovar B or with formalin-killed heterologous serovar L2 did not influence the response to subsequent ocular challenge.[124] A relationship between degree of IgA stimulation and protection was noted. Further investigation has demonstrated that MOMP is a primary target antigen for the development of chlamydial vaccine.[125-132] This protein is composed of variable domains flanked by constant regions and some of the variable domains contain antigenic determinants that elicit a neutralizing antibody response. Parenteral immunization with a synthetic oligopeptide of MOMP is ineffective in preventing chlamydial genital tract infection. Local administration may be required.[125]

A peptide of 12 amino acids from a conserved region of MOMP is a primary T-cell epitope in both mice and humans.[126] Intradermal injection of peptide conferred some protection in susceptible C3H mice against the development of salpingitis. A poliovirus hybrid construct which included a sequence from variable domain I of the MOMP was highly immunogenic in rabbits. Antisera from immunized animals neutralized chlamydial infectivity both *in vitro* and passively *in vivo*. Because poliovirus infection induces a strong mucosal immune response in primates and humans, these results indicate that poliovirus-chlamydia hybrids could become powerful tools for the study of mucosal immunity to chlamydial infection and for the development of recombinant chlamydial vaccines.[127]

References

1. Centers for Disease Control and Prevention, Recommendations for the prevention and management of *Chlamydia trachomatis* infections. *MMWR*, 42(RR-12), 1, 1993.
2. Noble M.A., Barteluk R.L., Farquhar D.J., and Percival Smith R., *Chlamydia trachomatis* antigen in the cervix and its clinical correlates: prevalence in a student population. *Can. Fam. Physician,* 34, 1687, 1988.
3. Katz B.P., Caine V.A., and Jones R.B., Diagnosis of mucopurulent cervicitis among women at rist for *Chlamydia trachomatis* infection. *Sex. Trans. Dis.,* 16, 103, 1989.
4. Chernesky M.A., Jang D., Lee H., Burczak J.D., Hu H., Sellors J., Tomazic-Allen S.J., and Mahony J.B., Diagnosis of *Chlamydia trachomatis* infections in men and women by testing first-void urine by ligase chain reaction. *J. Clin. Microbiol.,* 32, 2682, 1994.
5. Cates W. Jr., and Wasserheit J.N., Genital *Chlamydia trachomatis* infections, Epidemiology and reproductive sequellae. *Am. J. Obstet. Gynecol.,* 164, 1771, 1991.
6. Paavonen J., Genital *Chlamydia trachomatis* infection in the female. *J. Infect.,* 25 Supp.1, 39, 1992.
7. Rank R.G., Sanders M.M., and Patton D.L., Increased incidence of oviduct pathology in the guinea pig after repeat vaginal inoculation with the chlamydial agent of guinea pig inclusion conjunctivitis. *Sex. Transm. Dis.,* 22, 48, 1995.
8. Patton D.L., Wolner-Hanssen P., Zeng W., Lampe M., Wong K., Stamm W.E., and Holmes K.K., The role of spermatozoa in the pathogenesis of *Chlamydia trachomatis* salpingitis in a primate model. *Sex. Trans. Dis.,* 20, 214, 1993.
9. Ramstedt K., Forssman L., Giesecke J., and Granath F., Risk factors for *Chlamydia trachomatis* infection in 6810 young women attending family planning clinics. *Int. J. STD AIDS,* 3, 117, 1992.
10. Bass C.A., Junkind D.L., Silverman N.S., and Bondi J.M., Clinical evaluation of a new polymerase chain reaction assay for detection of *Chlamydia trachomatis* in endocervical specimens. *J. Clin. Microbiol.,* 31, 2648, 1993.

11. Moncada J., Schachter J., Bolan G., Nathan J., Shafer M.A., Clark A., Schwebke J., Stamm W., Mroczkowski T., Seliborska Z., and Martin D.A., Evaluation of Syva's enzyme immunoassay for the detection of *Chlamydia trachomatis* in urogenital specimens, *Diagn. Microbiol. Infect. Dis.*, 15, 663, 1992.

12. Shortliffe L.M., Sellers R.G., and Schachter J., The characterization of nonbacterial prostatitis: search for an etiology. *J. Urol.*, 148, 1461, 1992.

13. Tekgul S., Aktepe O., Sahin A., Ergen A., and Remzi D., Genital infections in men associated with *Chlamydia trachomatis*. *Int. Urol. Nephrol.*, 24, 167, 1992.

14. Fisher M.A., *Chlamydia trachomatis* genital infections. *W. V. Med. J.*, 89, 331, 1993.

15. Kirchner J.T., Reiter's syndrome. A possibility in patients with reactive arthritis. *Postgrad. Med.*, 97, 111, 1995

16. Rahman M.U., Cantwell R., Johnson C.C., Hodinka R.L., Schumacher H.R., and Hudson A.P., Inapparent genital infection with *Chlamydia trachomatis* and its potential role in the genesis of Reiters syndrome. *DNA Cell Biol.*, 11, 215, 1992.

17. Beutler A.M., Schumacher H.R. Jr., Whittum-Hudson J.A., Salameh W.A., and Hudson A.P., Case report: *in situ* hybridization for detection of inapparent infection with *Chlamydia trachomatis* in synovial tissue of a patient with Reiter's syndrome. *Am. J. Med. Sci.*, 310, 206, 1995.

18. Webster L.A., Greenspan J.R., Nakashima A.K., and Johnson R.E., An evaluation of surveillance for *Chlamydia trachomatis* infection in the United States, 1987-1991. *MMWR*, 42, 21, 1993.

19. Addis D.G., Vaughn M. L., Ludka D., Pfister J., and Davis J.P., Decreased prevence of *Chlamydia trachomatis* infection associated with a selective screening program in family practice clinics in Wisconsin. *Sex. Trans. Dis.*, 20, 28, 1993.

20. Noble M.A., Barteluk R.L., and Percival Smith R.K.L., Yearly incidence of *Chlamydia trachomatis* infection of the cervix in a university student health service population over four years — British Columbia. *Can. Dis. Weekly Rep.*, 15, 181, 1989.

21. BC Ministry of Health and Ministry Responsible for Seniors. 1994. Sexually Transmitted Disease Control: Division of British Columbia Centre for Disease Control.

22. Orr P., Sherman E., Blanchard J., Fast M., Hammond G., and Brunham R., Epidemiology of infection due to *Chlamydia trachomatis* in Manitoba, Canada. *Clin. Infect. Dis.*, 19, 876, 1994.

23. Garland S.M., Gertig D.M., and McInnes J.A., Genital *Chlamydia trachomatis* infection in Australia. *Med. J. Aust.*, 159, 90, 1993.

24. Hart G., The epidemiology of genital chlamydial infection in South Australia. *Int. J. STD AIDS*, 4, 204, 1993.

25. Koroku M., Kumamoto Y., Hirose T., Nishimura M., Sato T., Hayashi K., Tsukamoto T., Minami K., and Yoshio H., Epidemiologic study of *Chlamydia trachomatis* infection in pregnant women. *Sex. Trans. Dis.*, 21, 329, 1994.

26. Samra Z., Dan M., Segev S., Fintsi Y., Bar-Shany S., Weinberg M., and Gutman R., Prevalence of sexually transmitted pathogens among women attending a methadone clinic in Israel. *Genitourin. Med.*, 67, 133, 1991.

27. Ghinsberg R.C., and Nitzan Y., *Chlamydia trachomatis* direct isolation, antibody prevalence and clinical symptoms in women attending outpatient clinics. *New Microbiol.*, 17, 231, 1994.

28. Herrmann B., and Egger M., Genital *Chlamydia trachomatis* infections in Uppsala County, Sweden, 1985-1993: declining rates for how much longer? *Sex. Trans. Dis.*, 22, 253, 1995.

29. Persson K., Mansson A., Jonsson E., and Nordenfelt E., Decline of herpes simplex virus type 2 and *Chlamydia trachomatis* infections from 1970 to 1993 indicated by a similar change in antibody pattern. *Scand. J. Infect. Dis.*, 27, 195, 1995.

30. Humphreys J.T., Henneberry J.F., Rickard R.S., and Beebe J.L., Cost-benefit analysis of selective screening for *Chlamydia trachomatis* infection attending Colorado family planning clinics. *Sex. Trans. Dis.*, 19, 47, 1992.

31. Weinstock H.S., Bolan G.A., Kohn R., Balladares C., Back A., and Oliva G., *Chlamydia trachomatis* infection in women: a need for universal screening in high prevalence populations? *Am. J. Epidemiol.*, 135, 41, 1992.

32. Sellor J.W., Pickard L., Gafni A., Goldsmith C.H., Jang D., Mahony J.B., and Chernesky M.A., Effectiveness and defficiency of selective vs. universal screening for chlamydial infection in sexually active young women. *Arch. Intern. Med.*, 152, 1837, 1992.

33. Ramstedt K., Forssman L., Giesecke J., and Granath F., Risk factors for *Chlamydia trachomatis* infection in 6810 young women attending flamily planning clinics. *Int. J. STD AIDS*, 3, 117, 1992.

34. Sellors J.W., Pickard L., Gafni A., Goldsmith C.H., Jang D., Mahony J.B., and Chernesky M.A., Effectiveness and efficiency of selective vs. universal screening for chlamydia infection in sexually active young women. *Arch. Intern. Med.*, 152, 1837, 1992.

35. Scholes D., Stergachis A., Heidrich F.E., Andrilla H., Holmes K.K., and Stamm W.E., Prevention of pelvic inflammatory disease by screening for cervical chlamydial infection. *N. Engl. J. Med.*, 334, 1362, 1996.

36. Sellors J.W., Mahony J.B., Pickard L., Jang D., Groves D., Luinstra K.E., and Chernesky M.A., Screening urine with a leukocyte esterase strip and subsequent chlamydial testing of asymptomatic men attending primary care practitioners. *Sex. Trans. Dis.*, 20, 152, 1993.

37. Tyndall M.W., Nasio J., Mathia G., Ndinya-Achola J.O., Plummer F.A., Sellors J.W., Luinstra K.E., Jang D., Mahony J.B., and Chernesky M.A., Leukocyte esterase urine strips for the screening of men with urethritis — use in developing countries. *Genitourin. Med.*, 70, 3, 1994.

38. Anestad G., Berdal B.P., Scheel O., Mundal R., Odinsen O., Skaug K., Khalil O.S., Plier P., and Lee H., Screening urine samples by leukocyte esterase test and ligase chain reaction for chlamydial infections among asymptomatic men. *J. Clin. Microbiol.*, 33, 2483, 1995.

39. Patrick D.M., Rekart M., and Knowles L., Unsatisfactory performance of the leukocyte esterase test of first voided urine for rapid detection of urethritis. *Genitourin. Med.*, 70, 187, 1994.

40. Mayaud P., Changalucha J., Grosskurth H., Ka-Cina G., Rugemalila J., Nduba J., Newell, J., Hayes R., and Mabey D., The value of urine specimens in screening for male urethritis and its microbial aetiologies in Tanzania. *Genitourin. Med.*, 68, 361, 1992.

41. O'Brien S.F., Bell T.A., and Farrow J.A., Use of a leukocyte esterase dipstick to detect *Chlamydia trachomatis* and *Neisseria gonorrhoeae* urethritis in asymptomatic adolescent male detainees. *Am. J. Public Health*, 78, 1583, 1992.

42. Mahony J.B., and Chernesky M.A., Effect of swab type and storage temperature on the isolation of *Chlamydia trachomatis* from clinical specimens. *J. Clin. Microbiol.*, 22, 865, 1985.

43. Baron E.J., Cassell G.H., Duffy L.B., Eschenbach D.A., Greenwood J.R., Harvey S.M., Maddinger N.E., Perterson E.M., and Waites K.B. Laboratory diagnosis of female genital infections in Cumitech 17A. Edited by E.J. Baron. American Society for Microbiology, 1993.

44. Ciotti R.A., Sondheimer S.J., and Nachamkin I., Detecting *Chlamydia trachomatis* by direct immunofluoresce using a Cytobrush sampling technique. *Genitounrin. Med.*, 64, 245, 1988.

45. Cherrnesky M.A., Castriciano S., Sellors J., Stewart I., Cunningham I., Landis S., Seidelman W., Grant L., Devlin C., and Mahony J., Detection of *Chlamydia trachomatis* antigens in urine as an alternative to swabs and cultures. *J. Infect. Dis.*, 161, 124, 1990.

46. Chernesky M.A., Jang D., Sellors J., Coleman P., Bodner J., Hrusovsky I., Chong S., and Mahony J.B., Detection of *Chlamydia trachomatis* antigens in male urethral swabs and urines with a microparticle enzyme immunoassay. *Sex. Trans. Dis.*, 22, 55, 1995.

47. Wiesenfeld H.C., Uhrin M., Dixon B.W., and Sweet R.L., Diagnosis of male *Chlamydia trachomatis* urethritis by polymerase chain reaction. *Sex. Trans. Dis.*, 21, 268, 1994.

48. Moncada J., Schachter J., Shafer M.A., Williams E., Gourlay L., Lavin B., and Bolan G., Detection of *Chlamydia trachomatis* in first catch urine from symptomatic and asymptomatic males. *Sex. Trans. Dis.*, 21, 8, 1994.

49. Jensen I.P., A comparison of urine sample to rethral swab for detection of *Chlamydia trachomatis* in asymptomatic young men using two enzyme immuoassays. *Sex. Trans. Dis.*, 19, 165, 1992.

50. Hay P.E., Thomas B.J., McKenzie P., and Taylor Robinson D., Detection of *Chlamydia trachomatis* in men. Sensitive tests for sensitive urethras. *Sex. Trans. Dis.*, 20, 1, 1993.

51. Morris R.E., Legault J., and Baker C., Prevalence of isloated urethral asymptomatic *Chlamydia trachomatis* infection in the absence of cervical infection in incarcerated adolescent girls. *Sex. Trans. Dis.*, 20, 198, 1993.

52. Sellors J.W., Mahony J.B., Jang D., Pickard L., Goldsmith C.H., Gafni A., and Chernesky M.A., Comparison of cervical, urethral, and urine specimens for the detection of *Chlamydia trachomatis* in women. *J. Infect. Dis.*, 164, 205, 1991.

53. Svensson L.O., Mares I., and Olsson S.E., Detection of *Chlamydia trachomatis* in urinary samples from women, *Genitourin. Med.*, 67, 117, 1991.

54. Taylor-Robinson D., Thomas B.J., and Osborn M.F., Evaluation of enzyme immunoassay (Chlamydiazyme) 0 for detecting *Chlamydia trachomatis* in genital tract specimens. *J. Clin. Pathol.*, 40, 194, 1987.

55. Lee H.H., Chernesky M.A., Schachter J., Burczak J.D., Andrews W.W., Muldoon S., Leckie G., and Stamm W.E., Diagnosis of *Chlamydia trachomatis* genitourinary infection in women by ligase chain reaction assay in urine. *Lancet*, 345, 213, 1995.

56. Kellog J.A., Clinical and laboratory considerations of culture vs. antigen assays for detection of *Chlamydia trachomatis* from genital specimens. *Arch. Pathol. Lab. Med.*, 113, 453, 1989.

57. Thejls H., Gnarpe J., Gnarpe H., Larrson P.-G., Platz-Christensen J.-J., Ostergaard L., and Victor A., Expanded gold standard in the diagnosis of *Chlamydia trachomatis* in a low prevalence population: diagnostic efficasy of tissue culture, direct immunofluorescence, enzyme immunoassay, PCR and serology. *Genitourin. Med.*, 70, 300, 1994.

58. Jang D., Sellors J.W., Mahony J.B., Pickard L., and Chernesky M.A., Effects of broadening the gold standard on the performance of a chemiluminometric immunoassay to detect *Chlamydia trachomatis* antigens in centrifuged first void urine and urethral swab samples from men. *Sex. Trans. Dis.*, 19, 315, 1992.

59. Schachter J. and Wyrick, P.B., Culture and isolation of *Chlamydia trachomatis*. *Methods Enzymol.*, 236, 377, 1994.

60. Johnston S.L.G. and Siegal C., Comparison of buffalo green monkey kidney cells and McCoy cells for the isolation of *Chlamydia trachomatis* in shell vial centrifugation culture. *Diagn. Microbiol. Infect. Dis.*, 15, 355, 1992.

61. Naamazaki K., Suzuki K., and Chiba S., Replication of *Chlamydia trachomatis* and *C. pneumoniae* in the human monocytic cell line U-937. *J. Med. Microbiol.*, 42, 1191, 1995.

62. Munday G.R.G., Johnson A.P., Thomas B.J., and Taylor-Robinson D., A comparison of immunofluorescence and Giemsa for staining *Chlamydia trachomatis* inclusions in cyclohexamide-treated McCoy cells. *J. Clin. Pathol.*, 33, 177, 1980.

63. Schachter J., Chlamydiae, in A. Balows, W.J. Hausler, Jr., K.L. Herrmann, H.D. Isenberg, and H.J. Shadomy (ed) *Manual of Clinical Microbiology*, 5th edition, American Society for Microbiology, Washington D.C., p.1045–1053, 1991.

64. Gibson J.P.R., Egerer M., and Wiedbrauk D.L., Improved isolation of *Chlamydia trachomatis* from a low-prevalence population by using polyethylene glycol. *J. Clin. Microbiol.*, 31, 292, 1993.

65. Smith T.F., and Weed L.A., Comparison of urethral swabs, urine and urinary sediment for the isolation of Chlamydia. *J. Clin. Microbiol.*, 2, 134, 1975.

66. Lipkin E.S., Moncada J.V., Schafer M.A., Welson T.E., and Schachter J., Comparison of monoclonal antibody staining and culture in diagnosing cervical chlamydiae infection. *J. Clin. Microbiol.*, 23, 114, 1986.

67. Stamm W.E., Harrison H.R., Alexander E. R., Cles L.D., Spence M.R., and Quinn T.C., Diagnosis of *Chlamydia trachomatis* infection by direct immunofluorescence staining of genital secretions. *Ann. Intern. Med.*, 101, 638, 1986.

68. Thomas B.J., MacLeod E.J., Hay P.E., Horner P.J., and Taylor-Robinson D., Limited value of two widely used enzyme immuoassays for the detection of *Chlamydia trachomatis* in women. *Eur. J. Clin. Microbiol.*, 13, 651, 1994.

69. Noble M.A., Kwong A., Barteluk R.L., and Percival Smith R., Laboratory diagnosis of *Chlamydia trachomatis* using two immundiagnostic methods. *Am. J. Clin. Pathol.*, 90, 205, 1988.

70. Rahm V.A., Gnarpe H., and Odlind V., Evaluation of a direct fluorescence assay as a screening method in asymptomatic young women. *Sex. Trans. Dis.*, 19, 84, 1992.

71. Thompson C., Jones R., Smith B., Brogan O., Smith I.W., and Carrigan D., Evaluation of a microdot immunofluorescent antigen detection test for *Chlamydia trachomatis*. *Genitourin. Med.*, 70, 262, 1994.

72. Quinn T.C., Warfield P., Kappus E., Barbacci M., and Spence M., Screening for *Chlamydia trachomatis* infection in an inner-city population: a comparison of diagnostic methods. *J. Infect. Dis.*, 152, 419, 1985.

73. Barteluk R., and Noble M.A., Clinical laboratory assessment of detection of *Chlamydia trachomatis* using direct immunofluorescent technique (Syva MicroTrak). Scientific Meeting on Sexually Transmitted Diseases, Ottawa, Ontario. October, 1985 (abstract).

74. Beebe J.L., Rau M.P., and Albrecht K.D., Confirmatory testing of *Chlamydia trachomatis* Syva enzyme immuoassay gray zone specimens by Syva direct fluorescent antibody test. *Sex. Trans. Dis.*, 20, 140, 1993.

75. Chan E.L., Brandt K., and Horsman G.B., A 1-year evaluation of Syva MicorTrack *Chlamydia* enzyme immuoassay with selective confirmation by direct fluorescent antibody assay in a high-volume laboratory. *J. Clin. Microbiol.*, 32, 2208, 1994.

76. Olsen M.A., and Sambol A.R., Confirmation of positive results for chlamydial antigen by the Chlamydiazyme assay, value of repeated testing a blocking antibody assay. *J. Clin. Microbiol.*, 31, 1892, 1993.

77. Clark A., Stamm W.E., Gaydos C., Welsh L., Quinn T.C., Schachter J., and Moncada J., Multicenter evaluation of the AntigEnz Chlamydia enzyme immuoassay for diagnosis of *Chlamydia trachomatis* genital infection. *J. Clin. Microbiol.*, 30, 2762, 1992.

78. Stary A., Teodorowicz L., Horting-Muller I., Nerad S., and Storch M., Evaluation of the Gen-Probe PACE 2 and the Microtrack enzyme immuoassay for diagnosis of *Chlamydia trachomatis* in urogenital samples. *Sex. Trans. Dis.*, 21, 26, 1994.

79. Warren R., Dwyer B., Plackett M., Petit K., Rizvi N., and Baker A., Comarative evaluation of detection assays for *Chlamydia trachomatis*. *J. Clin. Microbiol.*, 31, 1663, 1993.

80. Steingrimsson O., Olafsson J. H., Sigvaaldaddottir E., and Palsdottir R., Clinical evaluation of an automated enzyme-linked fluorescent assay for the detection of chlamydial antigen in specimens from high-risk patients. *Diagn. Microbiol. Infect. Dis.*, 18, 101, 1994.

81. Blanding J., Hirsch L., Stranton N., Wright T., Aarnaes S., de la Maza L. M., and Peterson E. M., Comparison of the Clearview Chlamydia, the PACE 2 assay, and culture for the detection of *Chlamydia trachomatis* from cervical specimens in a low-prevalence population. *J. Clin. Microbiol.*, 31, 1622, 1993.

82. Klutytmans, J.A. J.W., Goessens W.H.F., Mouton J.W., van Rijsoort-Vos J.H., Niesters H.G.M., Quint W.G.V., Habbema L.H., Stolz E., and Wagenvoort J.H.T., Evaluation of Clearview and Magic Lite tests, polymerase chain reaction, and cell culture for detection of *Chlamydia trachomatis* in urogenital specimens. *J. Clin. Microbiol.*, 31, 3204, 1993.

83. Scieux C, Bianchi A., Vassias I., Meouchy R., Felten A., Morel P., and Perol Y., Evaluation of a new chemluminometric immunoassay, Magic Light Chlamydia, for detecting *Chlamydia trachomatis* antigen from urogenital specimens. *Sex. Trans. Dis.*, 19, 161, 1992.

84. Mumtaz G., Clark S., Ridgway G.L., Miller C.J., Johal B., and Allason Jones E., Comparison of an enzyme immuoassay (Antigenz Chlamydia) with cell culture for the detection of genital chlamydial infection in high and low risk populations. *Genitourin. Med.*, 69, 119, 1993.

85. Skulnick M., Small G.W., Simor A.E., Low D.E., Khosid H., Fraser S., and Chua R., Comparison of the Clearview Chlamydia test, Chlamydiazyme, and cell culture for detection of *Chlamydia trachomatis* in women with a low prevalence of infection. *J. Clin. Microbiol.*, 29, 2086, 1991.

86. Woods G., Young A., Scott Jr. J.C., Blair T.M.H., and Johnson A.M., Evaluation of a nonisotopic probe for detection of *Chlamydia trachomatis* in endocervical specimens. *J. Clin. Microbiol.*, 28, 370, 1990.

87. Kluytmans J.A.J., Goessens W.H.F., van Rijsoort-Vos J.H., Niesters H.G.M., and Stolz E., Improved performance of PACE 2 with modiffied collection system in combination with probe competition assay for detection of *Chlamydia trachomatis* in urtethral specimens from males. *J. Clin. Microbiol.*, 32, 568, 1994.

88. Bobo, L., Coutlee F., Yolken R., Quinn T., and Viscidi R., Diagnosis of *Chlamydia trachomatis* cervical infection by detection of amplified DNA with an enzyme immunoassay. *J. Clin. Microbiol.*, 28, 1968, 1990.

89. Bobo, L., PCR detection of *Chlamydia trachomatis* in Diagnostic Molecular Microbiology, Principles and Applications. Edited by D.H. Persing, T.F. Smith, F.C. Tenover, and T.J. White. American Society for Microbiology. Washington D.C. pp. 235, 1993.

90. Frost E.H., Deslandes S., and Bourgaux-Ramoisy D., Sensitive detection and typing of *Chlamydia trachomatis* using nested polymerase chain reaction. *Genitourin. Med.*, 69, 290, 1993.

91. Hadock P.V., and Kochik S.A., 3SR detection of *Chlamydia trachomatis* in *Diagnostic Molecular Microbiology, Principles and Applications.* Edited by D.H. Persing, T.F. Smith, F.C. Tenover, and T.J. White. American Society for Microbiology. Washington D.C., 241–246.

92. Gingeras, T.R., and Kwoh D.Y., *In vitro* nucleic acid target amplification techniques, issues and benefits. *Praxis. Biotechnol.*, 4, 403, 1992.

93. Mahony J.B., Luinstra K.E., Sellors J.W., Pickard L., Chong S., Jang D., and Chernesky M.A., PCRs in determining performance of Chlamydia Amplicor PCR with endocervical specimens from women with a low prevalence of infection. *J. Clin. Microbiol.*, 32, 2490, 1994.

94. de Barbeyrac B., Peellet I, Dutilh B., Bébéar B., Géniaux M., and Bébéar C.H., Evaluation of the *Amplicor Chlamydia trachomatis* test versus culture in genital samples in various prevalence populations. *Genitourin. Med.*, 70, 162–166, 1994.

95. Bianchi A., Scieux C., Brunat N., Vexiau D., Kermanach M., Pezin P., Janier M., Morel P., and Lagrange P.H., An evaluation of the polymerase chain reaction amplicor *Chlamydia trachomatis* in male urine and female urogenital specimens. *Sex. Trans. Dis.*, 21, 196, 1994.

96. Kessler H.H., Pierer K., Stuenzner D., Auer-Grumbach P., Haller E.M., and Marth E., Rapid detection of *Chlamydia trachomatis* in conjunctival, pharyngeal, and urethral specimens with a new polymerase chain reaction assay. *Sex. Trans. Dis.*, 21, 191, 1994.

97. Wiesenfeld H.C., Uhrin M., Dixon B.W., and Sweet R.L., Diagnosis of male *Chlamydia trachomatis* urethritis by polymerase chain reaction., *Sex. Transm. Dis.*, 21, 268, 1994.

98. Wu C.H., Lee M.F., Yin S.C., Yang D.M., and Cheng S.F., Comparison of polymerase chain reaction, monoclonal antibody based enzyme immuoassay, and cell culture for detection of *Chlamydia trachomatis* in genital specimens. *Sex. Trans. Dis.*, 19, 193, 1992.

99. Bauwens J.E., Clark A.M., and Stamm W.E., Diagnosis of *Chlamydia trachomatis* endocervical infections by a commercial polymerase chain reaction assay. *J. Clin. Microbiol.*, 31, 3023, 1993.

100. van Doornum G.J.J., Buimer M., Prins M., Henquet C.J.M., Coutinho R.A., Plier R.K., Tomazic-Allen S., Hu H., and Lee H., Detection of *Chlamydia trachomatis* infection in urine samples from men and women by ligase chain reaction. *J. Clin. Microbiol.*, 33, 2042, 1995.

101. Schachter J., Stamm W. E., Quinn T.C., Andrews W.W., Burczak J.D., and Lee H.H., Ligase chain reaction to detect *Chlamydia trachomatis* infection of the cervix. *J. Clin. Microbiol.*, 32, 2540, 1994.

102. Chernesky M.A., Lee H., Schachter J., Burczak J.D., Stamm W.E., McCormack W.M., and Quinn T.C., Diagnosis of *Chlamydia trachomatis* urethral infection in symptomatic and asymptomatic men by testing first-void urine in a ligase chain reaction assay. *J. Infect. Dis.*, 170, 1308, 1994.

103. Mattila A., Miettinen A., Heinonen P.K., Teisala K., Punnonen R., and Paavonen J., Detection of serum antibodies to *Chlamydia trachomatis* in patients with chlamydial and nonchamydial pelvic inflammatory disease by the IPAzyme Chlamydia and enzyme immuoassay. *J. Clin. Microbiol.*, 31, 998, 1993.

104. Ossewaarde J.M., de Vries A., van den Hoek J.A.R., and Loon A.M., Enzyme immuoassay with enhanced specificity for detection of antibodies to *Chlamydia trachomatis*. *J. Clin. Microbiol.*, 32, 1419, 1994.

105. Moss T.R., Darougar S., Woodland R.M., Nathan M., Dines R.J., and Cathrine V., Antibodies to Chlamydia species in patients attending a genitourinary clinic and the impact of antibodies to *C. pneumoniae* and *C. psittaci* on the sensitivity and the specificity of *C. trachomatis* serology tests. *Sex. Trans. Dis.*, 20, 61, 1993.

106. Sarov I., Kleinman D., Holcberg G., Potashnick G., Insler V., Cevenini R., and Sarov B., Specific IgG and IgA antibodies to *Chlamydia trachomatis* in infertile women. *Int. J. Fertil.*, 31, 193, 1986.

107. Dieterle S., Mahony J. B., Luinstra K.E., and Stibbe W., Chlamydial immunoglobulin IgG and IgA antibodies in serum and semen are not associated with the presence of *Chlamydia trachomatis* DNA or rRNA in semen from male partners of infertile couples. *Hum. Reprod.*, 10, 315, 1995.

108. Witkin S.S., Kligman I., Grifo J.A., and Rosenwaks Z., *Chlamydia trachomatis* detected by polymerase chain reaction in cervices of culture-negative women correlates with adverse *in vitro* fertilization outcome. *J. Infect. Dis.*, 171, 1657, 1995.

109. Soffer Y., IgA antichlamydia antibodies as a diagnostic tool for monitoring of active chlamydial infection. *Eur. J. Epidemiol.*, 8, 882, 1992.

110. Tasdemir I., Tasdemir M., Kodama H., Sekine K., and Tanaka T., Effect of chlamydial antibodies on the outcome of *in vitro* fertilization (IVF) treatment. *J. Assist. Reprod. Genet.*, 11, 104, 1994.

111a. Claman P., Amimi M.N., Peeling R.W., Toye B., and Jessamine P., Does serologic evidence of remote *Chlamydia trachomatis* infection and its heat shock protein (CHSP 60) affect *in vitro* fertilization-embryo transfer outcome? *Fertil. Steril.,* 65, 146, 1996.

111b. Lim J.S., Jones W.E., Yan L., Wirthwein K.A., Flaherty E.E., Haivanis R.M., and Rice P.A., Underdiagnosis of *Chlamydia trachomatis* infection. Diagnostic limitations in patients with low-level infection. *Sex. Trans. Dis.,* 19, 259, 1992.

112. Moulder J.W., Hatch T.T., Kuo C.C., Schacter J., and J. Storz, Order II. Chlamydiales. Storz and Page 1971, 334, p. 729–739. In N.R. Krieg, and J.G. Holt (ed), *Bergey's Manual of Systemic Bacteriology, Vol 1.* Williams & Wilkins, Baltimore, 1984.

113. Ossewaarde J.M., Rieffe M., de Vries A., Derksen-Nawrocki R.P., Hooft H.J., van Doornum G.J.J., and van Loon A.M., Comparison of two panels of monoclonal antibiodies for determination of *Chlamydia trachomatis* serovars. *J. Clin. Microbiol.,* 32, 2968, 1994.

114. Rodriquez P., de Barbeyrac B., Persson K., Dutilh B., and Bébéar C., Evaluation of molecular typing for epidemiological study of *Chlamydia trachomatis* genital infections. *J. Clin. Microbiol.,* 31, 2238, 1993.

115. Peterson E.M., and de la Maza L.M., Restriction endonuclease analysis of DNA for *Chlamydia trachomatis* biovars. *J. Clin. Microbiol.,* 26, 625, 1988.

116. Rodriquez P., Allardet-Servent A., de Barbeyrac B., Ramuz M., and Bébéar C., Genetic variability among *Chlamydia trachomatis* reference and clinical strains analyzed by pulsed-field gel electrophoresis. *J. Clin. Microbiol.,* 32, 292, 1994.

117. Scieux C, Grimont F., Regnault B., and Grimont P.A.D., DNA fingerprinting of *Chlamydia trachomatis* by use of ribosomal RNA, oligonucleotide and randomly cloned DNA probes. *Res. Microbiol.,* 143, 755, 1992.

118. Dean D., Schachter J., Dawson C.R., and Stephens R.S., Comparison of the major membrane protein variant sequence regions of B/Ba isolates: a molecular epidemiologic approach to *Chlamydia trachomatis* infections. *J. Infect. Dis.,* 166, 383, 1992.

119. Gaydos C.A., Bobo L., Welsh L., Hook E.W. 3rd, Viscidi R., and Quinn T.C., Gene typing of *Chlamydia trachomatis* by polymerase chain reaction and restriction endonuclease digestion. *Sex. Trans. Dis.,* 19, 303, 1992.

120. Lan J., Ossewaarde J M., Walboomers J.M.M., Meijer C.J.L.M., and van den Brule A.J.C., Improved PCR sensitivity for direct genotyping of *Chlamydia trachomatis* serovars by using a nested PCR. *J. Clin. Microbiol.,* 32, 528, 1994.

121. Sayada C., Denamur E., Xerri B., Orfila J., Catalan F., and Elion J., Rapid genotyping of the *Chlamydia trachomatis* major outer membrane protein by the polymerase chain reaction. *FEMS Microbiol. Lett.,* 83, 73, 1991.

122. Lan J., Ossewaarde J.M., Walbroomers J.M.M., Meijer C.J.L.M., and van den Brule A.J.C., Improved PCR sensitivity for direct genotyping of *Chlamydia trachomatis* serovars by using a nested PCR. *J. Clin. Microbiol.,* 32, 528, 1994.

123. Centers for Disease Control and Prevention: 1993 sexually transmitted diseases treatment guidelines. *MMWR,* 42, 47, 1993.

124. Taylor H.R., Young E., MacDonald A.B., Schachter J., and Prendergast R.A., Oral immunization against chlamydial eye infection. *Invest. Ophthalmol. Vis. Sci.,* 28, 249, 1987.

125. Su H., Parnell M., and Caldwell H.D., Protective efficacy of a parenterally administered MOMP-derived synthetic oligopeptide vaccine in a murine model of *Chlamydia trachomatis* genital tract infection: serum neutralizing IgG antibodies do not protect against chlamydial genital tract infection. *Vaccine,* 13, 1023, 1995.

126. Knight S.C., Iqball S., Woods C., Stagg A., Ward M.E., and Tuffrey M., A peptide of *Chlamydia trachomatis* shown to be a primary T-cell epitope *in vitro* induces cell-mediated immunity *in vivo. Immunology,* 85, 8, 1995.

127. Murdin A.D., Su H., Klein M.H., and Caldwell H.D., Poliovirus hybrids expressing neutralization epitopes from variable domains I and IV of the major outer membrane protein of *Chlamydia trachomatis* elicit broadly cross-reactive *C. trachomatis*-neutralizing antibodies. *Infect. Immun.,* 63, 1116, 1995.

128. Su H., and Caldwell H.D., Immunogenicity of a synthetic oligopeptide corresponding to antigenically common T-helper and B-cell neutralizing epitopes of the major outer membrane protein of *Chlamydia trachomatis. Vaccine,* 11, 1159, 1993.

129. Murdin A.D., Su H., Manning D.S., Klein M.H., Parnell M.J., and Caldwell H.D., A poliovirus hybrid expressing a neutralization epitope from the major outer membrane protein of *Chlamydia trachomatis* is highly immunogenic. *Infect. Immun.*, 61, 4406, 1993.

130. Campos M., Pal S., O'Brien T.P., Taylor H.R., Prendergast R.A., and Whittum-Hudson J.A., A chlamydial major outer membrane protein extract as a trachoma vaccine candidate. *Invest. Ophthalmol. Vis. Sci.*, 36, 1477, 1995.

131. Villeneuve A., Brossay L., Paradis G., and Hebert J. Characterization of the humoral response induced by a synthetic peptide of the major outer membrane protein of *Chlamydia trachomatis* serovar B. *Infect. Immun.*, 62, 3547, 1994.

132. Brossay L., Villeneuve A., Paradis G., Cote L., Mourad W., and Hebert J., Mimicry of a neutralizing epitope of the major outer membrane protein of *Chlamydia trachomatis* by anti-idiotypic antibodies. *Infect. Immun.*, 62, 341, 1994.

chapter three

Chancroid

Brian P. Currie

3.1 Introduction..59
    3.1.1 Overview 59
    3.1.2 Microbiology of *Haemophilus ducreyi*......................................60
3.2 Epidemiology of chancroid 62
    3.2.1 Geographic and temporal variation in disease prevalence 62
    3.2.2 Risk factors...63
    3.2.3 Relationship to HIV-1 disease...63
    3.2.4 Recent developments...64
3.3 Pathogenesis...65
    3.3.1 Clinical course and pathology 65
    3.3.2 Complications...67
    3.3.3 Disease variants..68
    3.3.4 Diagnosis 68
3.4. Treatment..70
    3.4.1 Approach to treatment 70
    3.4.2 Response to therapy 71
    3.4.3 Public health issues..72
References...72

3.1 Introduction

3.1.1 Overview

Chancroid is a sexually transmitted disease (STD) caused by infection with *Haemophilus ducreyi*. It is characterized by painful genital ulcerations and inguinal lymphadenopathy and the disease must be differentiated from the other sexually transmitted genital ulcerative diseases including syphilis, genital herpes, lymphogranuloma venereum, and donovanosis. Unfortunately, the clinical diagnosis of chancroid is not reliable and until recently, definitive diagnosis required the culture of *H. ducreyi* from clinical material. This in turn was further complicated by the fact that *H. ducreyi* is difficult to culture. The organism is fastidious with nutritional requirements that probably vary between strains and many clinical laboratories do not have extensive experience in isolating the organism. As a consequence, a wide range of culture recovery rates of *H. ducreyi* from clinically typical chancroid ulcers or lymph node aspirates have been reported (47 to 90%). Both the poor predictive performance of clinical and culture diagnosis of chancroid have complicated

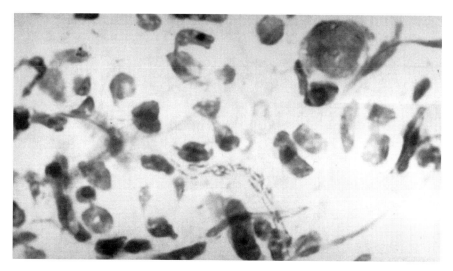

Figure 1   Gram-stain preparation of chancroid ulcer exudate exhibiting "railroad tracking." (Photo courtesy of Edward Bottone, Ph.D.)

past efforts to characterize the natural history and epidemiology of the disease. The recent development of potentially accurate non-culture diagnostic tests for chancroid may resolve many of these issues.

3.1.2   *Microbiology of* Haemophilus ducreyi

H. ducreyi is a small somewhat pleomorphic Gram-negative coccobacillus without an extracellular capsule. The average bacillus is 1.2 to 1.5 µm in length and approximately 0.5 µm in width, with rounded ends. When specimens derived from clinical material are Gram-stained, the organism exhibits a streptobacillary form and classically forms long parallel chains of bacteria along mucous threads referred to as "railroad tracks" (see Figure 1). When Gram-stained after culture, a more complicated arrangement of bacteria referred to as "school of fish" or "fingerprints" may result (see Figure 2). Some have suggested that a presumptive identification of *H. ducreyi* could be made on these morphological characteristics alone, although the sensitivity and specificity of this approach have not been demonstrated to be acceptable for routine use.[1-3]

Small, nonmucoid, yellow-gray, semi-opaque, adherent colonies are characteristic after growth on various solid-agar-based formulations used for the primary isolation of *H. ducreyi*. Colonies may be pushed intact across the agar surface, are not associated with pitting, and may be associated with zones of alpha-hemolysis on some blood agars.[2] Interestingly, *H. ducreyi* also exhibits agglutination in suspension. Although there is strong evidence that the cell surface is responsible for the observed colony cohesiveness and inability to grow in liquid culture without autoagglutination, there is a clear lack of information regarding cell surface structure and composition of this organism. Extremely limited electron microscopy data suggest that *H. ducreyi* demonstrates typical Gram-negative cell wall features; however, additional studies have identified a novel lipooligosaccharide cell wall component.[2,4,5] There are strong suggestions that *H. ducreyi* exhibits a variety of surface carbohydrates and outer membrane proteins.[2,5] In addition, apparently all strains exhibit pili which appear as very fine surface appendages.[6] The role of any of these features in pathogenesis remains poorly defined.

The organization and control of metabolic pathways in *H. ducreyi* remain uncharacterized except for those related to differential characteristics used for identification.[5] Long identified as a microaerophilic fastidious organism, it is now well appreciated that primary

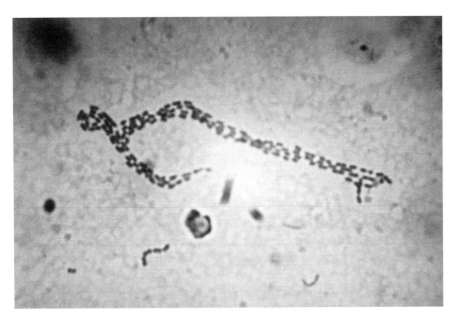

Figure 2 Gram-stain preparation of chancroid from culture exhibiting "school of fish" pattern. (Photo courtesy of Kenneth Borchardt, Ph.D.)

isolation growth is pH, moisture, CO_2 temperature, and media dependent. In addition, nutritional differences may exist between strains.[5] Optimal conditions include a pH of 6.5 to 7.0, a water saturated atmosphere, CO_2 enrichment, and temperature of 28 to 35°C.[2,7] A base medium containing acid-hydrolyzed protein, such as Mueller-Hinton agar or enzymatically hydrolyzed protein, such as GC medium base, supplemented with hemin, albumin, selenium, and L-glutamine appears to support growth, as well as other nutritionally complex media, such as chocolatized blood agar with IsoVitale X.[2] Previous studies have reported a wide range of recovery of *H. ducreyi* in culture form clinical material (47–94%), but all of these studies have been hampered by the lack of a "gold standard" for the presence of *H. ducreyi* infection.[7] Recovery of the organism appears to be maximized by tandem culture on more than one type of medium (i.e., enriched GC base and Mueller-Hinton agar) with reported recovery rates of 75 to 90% in some research studies.[7] Use of multiple media in the clinical setting is not practical and even if used, recovery rates of *H. ducreyi* in clinical laboratories without substantial experience in isolating the organism are likely to be much lower than those reported. Recent evidence suggests that thioglycolate-hemin-based media containing various combinations of selenium dioxide, glutamine, and albumin can be used as transport media with *H. ducreyi* recovery rates of 71 to 75% when specimens were maintained at 4°C for 4 days.[5]

Very little has been ascertained regarding the genetics of *H. ducreyi*. In contrast to the lack of chromosomal genetic information available, a wide variety of plasmids have been well characterized in *H. ducreyi* that appear to be similar to those seen in Pasteurellacae and Enterobacteriaceae.[2,5,7] Transfer of conjugative plasmids and mobilization of nonconjugative plasmids have both been demonstrated in *H. ducreyi*. Geographic and temporal differences in antimicrobial susceptibilities for strains have been appreciated and many can be related to the presence or absence of resistance plasmids that encode resistance to sulfonamides, aminoglycosides, tetracyclines, chloramphenicol, and β-lactams.[2,5,7] It is not unusual for a single *H. ducreyi* isolate to contain multiple resistance plasmids, including more than one conferring resistance to β-lactam antibiotics. In the U.S., 30% of strains isolated between 1982 and 1990 were shown to lack resistance plasmids.[8,9] Some strains lacking plasmids have also been demonstrated to exhibit decreased susceptibility to trimethoprim/sulfamethoxazole, ciprofloxacin, and ofloxacin, suggesting chromosomally mediated resistance to these agents. Other data indicating increased penicillin MICs among β-lactamase-negative strains of *H. ducreyi* also suggest the development of chromosomally mediated penicillin resistance.[8] Recent studies suggest the production of an extracellular cytotoxin by some *H. ducreyi* isolates that is heat and pronase sensitive.[5] Further characterization of this cytotoxin is required in order to understand any potential role it may have in the pathogenesis of tissue necrosis and ulcer formation in chancroid and to understand its genetics.

3.2 Epidemiology of chancroid

3.2.1 Geographic and temporal variation in disease prevalence

The lack of widespread availability of suitable culture media, the technical difficulties in primary isolation of *H. ducreyi,* and the poor predictive value of clinical diagnosis of chancroid have all probably contributed to an underestimation of the disease. In underdeveloped countries, these factors are coupled with marginal surveillance systems for disease reporting and subsequently it has been difficult to accurately characterize the incidence of disease. Even in developed countries, such as the U.S., the same three factors have had significant impact on limiting assessment of disease incidence. Only 10% of 5409 cases of chancroid reported in the U.S. from 1981 to 1990 were confirmed by culture.[10] In 1990, only 14% of 115 STD clinics surveyed in the U.S. had culture media for primary *H. ducreyi* isolation and only 8% had the capability to perform a diagnostic evaluation of genital ulcer disease (darkfield microscopy and syphilis serology capability; as well as ability to culture *H. ducreyi* and herpes simplex virus; HSV).[10] It has also been reported by the Centers for Disease Control and Prevention that several U.S. chancroid outbreaks since the mid-1980s went unreported because of lack of culture confirmation.[10] In conclusion, chancroid surveillance in the U.S. is also likely to significantly underestimate the incidence of disease. Nonetheless, there are sufficient data to allow broad characterization of the epidemiology of the disease.

Although chancroid has a worldwide distribution, there is significant geographic variation in the prevalence of the disease. Chancroid is much more common in the tropics and in developing countries. Numerous studies have documented the predominance of chancroid as a cause of genital ulcer disease in sub-Saharan Africa (including Kenya, Rwanda, Zimbabwe, and South Africa), the Indian subcontinent, Southeast Asia (including Thailand, Malaysia, and Singapore), Central Asia, South America, Central America, and the Caribbean.[7,11-15]

In contrast, chancroid is much less common in developed areas of the world. Until recently, the incidence of chancroid in developed countries was primarily related to epidemic chancroid in the military and to sporadic imported cases from individuals returning from tropical countries. Chancroid emerged as an important clinical disease in the U.S. military forces in the 1940s and by 1947 the U.S. incidence of chancroid peaked at 6.4 cases/100,000.[16] The annual incidence decreased markedly between 1950 and 1984 to incidence rates of 0.2 to 0.6 cases/100,000 with clusters of chancroid microepidemics at seaports generated by imported cases.[17] This trend was abruptly reversed from 1985 to 1987 when the incidence of reported cases rose 10-fold from 0.2 to 2.1/100,000.[17,18] During this time period, localized outbreaks in a handful of states consistently accounted for the majority of reported cases. New York, California, Texas, Florida, and Georgia accounted for 92% of cases from 1981 to 1986 and New York, Texas, Florida, Georgia, and Louisiana accounted for 92% of cases in 1990.[18] The focal nature of these outbreaks was further underscored by the fact that in 1990, 62% of all U.S. cases of chancroid were reported from four U.S. cities — Dallas, Houston, New Orleans, and New York City.[18] These focal outbreaks of chancroid involved traditional STD core populations, but were also highly associated with crack use and the exchange of drugs or money for sex and appeared to mirror the urban epidemic of crack cocaine use. Interestingly, reported cases of chancroid began to decrease after 1987 and the decline accelerated from 1990 to 1994, when the U.S. incidence rate fell to 0.3/100,000.[13,18] The reasons for this decline remain unclear.

3.2.2 Risk factors

Chancroid has historically been linked with prostitution on a worldwide basis and female prostitutes probably serve as a sustained source of disease. Unlike other STDs, which are transmitted primarily by asymptomatic or minimally symptomatic individuals, chancroid is believed to be primarily transmitted by contact with genital ulcers which are often painful.[7,14] The economic imperatives of prostitution may promote continued activity in the presence of painful ulcers. In addition, intravaginal ulcers in prostitutes may be asymptomatic and difficult to detect, especially in settings of limited access to health care, and contacts of prostitutes are difficult to trace and treat. The association between chancroid and prostitution appears to have been recently modified in North America and perhaps in the Caribbean and Latin America, by drug addiction, especially to crack cocaine.[7,19,20] Again, the economics of addiction, which often involve the exchange of sex for drugs or money, could drive continued sex activity in the face of painful ulcerative disease. Drug addiction is associated with reduced access to health care which could also increase the significance of asymptomatic vaginal ulcers and interfere with effective control activities. In summary, chancroid appears to have established a closer association with prostitution and drug use throughout the world than any other traditional STD.

In the U.S., most cases of chancroid have occurred in heterosexual African-Americans or Hispanics.[17,19,20] There is a preponderance of cases among men, with male-to-female ratios of disease in most U.S. outbreaks ranging between 3:1 to 25:1.[17,19,20] This observation could be explained by asymptomatic and overlooked lesions among female prostitutes, or more likely by the fact that infected symptomatic female prostitutes have large numbers of male contacts. The risk of disease appears to be higher for uncircumcised men.[7,20] It has been suggested that the less cornified epithelium of the glans and foreskin may be more susceptible to *H. ducreyi* invasion and that the preputial sac may serve as a reservoir for prolonged exposure of uncircumcised men to infected genital secretions of their partners.[7]

3.2.3 Relationship to HIV-1 disease

Genital ulcer disease has been closely and consistently linked with the acquisition of HIV-1 disease.[21-28] Retrospective epidemiologic studies in Africa have shown that HIV-infected men more commonly have a history of genital ulcer disease compared to uninfected men. A study of 340 men seeking treatment for an STD in a Nairobi clinic indicated that HIV-1 seroconverters reported a greater frequency of prostitute exposure, were seven times more likely to have a presenting diagnosis of genital ulcer disease, and were ten times more likely to be uncircumcised relative to non-seroconverters.[23] Similarly, a case-control study of HIV-1 seroconverting female prostitutes indicated no differences in regard to sexual practices or non-sexual HIV risk factors relative to non-seroconverters, but indicated that genital ulcer disease was the most significant risk factor for seroconversion.[25] Over 60% of seroconverting women experienced at least one episode of genital ulcer disease prior to seroconversion and women who converted had a significantly greater frequency of ulcer episodes per month relative to non-seroconverters.[23] When 422 HIV-seronegative men attending a Nairobi STD clinic were followed prospectively, it was determined that an initial presentation to the clinic with a genital ulcer and being uncircumcised were the strongest predictors of subsequent HIV-1 seroconversion.[24] Finally, in a New York City STD clinic, the risk of HIV-1 acquisition among 462 patients who presented with genital ulcer disease was 2.4 times greater than in those without ulceration and the relative risk rose to 3.5 among patients with ulcerative disease whose only other risk factor for HIV-1 infection was heterosexual activity.[26]

Chancroid has been implicated as a cause of HIV-1 acquisition more than other etiologies of genital ulcerative disease. However, most of the epidemiologic studies linking HIV-1 and chancroid were conducted where chancroid is a prevalent cause of ulcerative disease. In New York City, a clinical diagnosis of chancroid was significantly associated with HIV-1 acquisition, but most cases of chancroid were not confirmed by culture, nor was HSV cultured.[26] On the other hand, the recent detection of HIV-1 virus by culture or DNA amplification in the culture-confirmed chancroid ulcers of HIV-1 positive men and women would seem to support the acquisition and transmission of HIV-1 disease via chancroid ulcers.[27,28]

The mechanism of enhanced transmission of HIV-1 disease by chancroid is unknown. Ulceration may simply increase exposure to or secretion of HIV-1 infected fluids, the inflammatory ulcerative lesion may activate cellular mechanisms which permit enhanced viral multiplication and enhanced viral secretion, or alternatively the activation of cellular mechanisms may provide cells that are susceptible viral targets for infection.[21] A second hypothesis is that the recruitment of immune cells, particularly neutrophils, into the genital area upregulates viral production.[29] This recruitment of neutrophils by an STD could provide a common pathway for increased HIV viral replication and transmission by all STDs and could account for the epidemiologic evidence that also associates non-ulcer forming STDs (*Trichomonas*, *Chlamydia trachomatis*, and Candida) with increased risk of HIV-1 infection.[29]

3.2.4   Recent developments

The difficulty in establishing a clinical or culture diagnosis of chancroid has driven the development of a variety of non-culture diagnostic tests for the disease. These include the development of polyclonal and monoclonal antibodies for use in assays for direct immunofluorescence detection of *H. ducreyi* from clinical smears, DNA probes to detect *H. ducreyi* from lesion exudates, and polymerase chain reaction (PCR)-based DNA amplification technologies to be used to detect the presence of *H. ducreyi* from swabs of chancroid ulcers.[30-35] Perhaps the most promising of these diagnostic tests is the development of a commercial multiplex PCR assay that can simultaneously amplify and subsequently detect DNA from *H. ducreyi*, *Treponema pallidum*, and HSV from a single swab specimen.[35] Preliminary data indicate that the test is sensitive and specific, and its application at a Mississippi STD clinic identified previously unsuspected high levels of coinfection with chancroid and syphilis among patients with genital ulcer disease.[35] The multiplex PCR assay has the potential to assist in accurately assessing the incidence of chancroid disease, to unravel the controversy surrounding an asymptomatic carrier state of chancroid, and to provide an understanding of the significance of coinfections among patients with symptomatic chancroid.

An understanding of the epidemiology of chancroid has also been limited by the lack of sensitive methods to differentiate strains of *H. ducreyi*. The recent development of DNA strain typing techniques for *H. ducreyi* based on ribotyping and their application to focal outbreaks of chancroid indicate that this type of analysis may prove to be a powerful tool in epidemiological investigations in the future.[20] Molecular epidemiologic studies can provide information useful in characterizing the epidemiology of the disease in a community, including tracing the origin of an epidemic and targeting control efforts.

3.3 *Pathogenesis*

3.3.1 *Clinical course and pathology*

The existence of *H. ducreyi* as a non-pathogenic colonizer of the human genital tract is debatable.[7,14,36] It is now widely believed that the development of clinical chancroid results from sexual exposure to individuals with overt chancroid ulceration or from exposure to individuals with asymptomatic ulceration in less sensate locations, such as the cervix or the proximal vaginal mucosa.[7,14,36]

The pathogenesis of *H. ducreyi* infection remains obscure, primarily due to the lack of an *in vitro* or *in vivo* model accurately reflecting human disease. Numerous cell culture models have been developed utilizing a variety of epithelial cell lines.[37-40] Studies utilizing adult foreskin cells have demonstrated that the cells can support limited *H. ducreyi* growth, that *H. ducreyi* cell attachment occurs, and that production of *H. ducreyi* bacterial strain-specific cytopathic effects can occur.[37,38] Evidence suggests intracellular penetration between cultured foreskin cells, with variable documentation of cell invasion.[38-40] Past attempts at *in vivo* disease models have involved intradermal injection of *H. ducreyi* in rabbits and mice, which resulted in lesions that did not resemble human chancroid.[41,42] A recently described model using genital inoculation of pigtailed macaques appears promising; however, only male animals appear to develop clinical disease after inoculation.[43]

Although experimental human challenge studies exist that are decades old, conclusions were compromised by limitations in the understanding of the microbiology of *H. ducreyi*. Interestingly, after an almost 40-year hiatus, human challenge studies have resurfaced. Recent studies have produced mildly painful lesions of the exterior of the human upper arm 3 days after an inoculum of 10^5 or greater colony forming units of *H. ducreyi* were administered in areas of abraded skin and viable organisms could be recovered from the lesions.[44] Further characterization of this model could provide a means to better understand the pathogenesis of chancroid.

While *H. ducreyi* bacteria have been demonstrated to adhere to human epithelial cells, the surface component mediating adherence is not known. Whether the organism can subsequently invade epithelial cells is controversial and it remains to be established whether a novel lipooligosaccharide or cytotoxin subsequently results in cell death, tissue necrosis, and ulcer formation.[5]

The incubation period is notable for the absence of prodromal symptoms and is usually 4 to 10 days in duration (range 2 to 35 days), after which a painless papule on an erythematous base develops at the presumed inoculation site.[3,7] Over the course of 24 to 48 h the lesion becomes pustular, eroded, and ulcerated, but disease progression never involves vesicle formation. Chancroid ulcers are variable in size, ranging from 1mm to several centimeters in diameter and are most commonly 1 to 2 cm in diameter. The ulcer is painful, can be variable in shape, has sharp margins which are frequently undermined, is not indurated, and the friable granulomatous base of the ulcer is covered by a gray or yellow necrotic purulent exudate (see Figures 3–5).

The chancroid ulcer has been described histologically and classically consists of three zones: (1) a narrow superficial zone of necrotic tissue, red cells, fibrin, degenerate neutrophils, and numerous *H. ducreyi* bacteria, (2) a middle zone characterized by edematous inflammatory tissue with microvascularization and strands of endothelial cells, and (3) a deep zone with dense plasma cell infiltrates and lymphocytes.[45]

Men typically present with fewer ulcers than women and a third of men will have disease characterized by a single ulcer (see Figures 3 and 4).[7,14-16] The lesions are most commonly located on the prepuce, coronal sulcus, and glans and less frequently on the penile shaft, the scrotum, and perineum.[16] In uncircumcised men, greater than 50% of

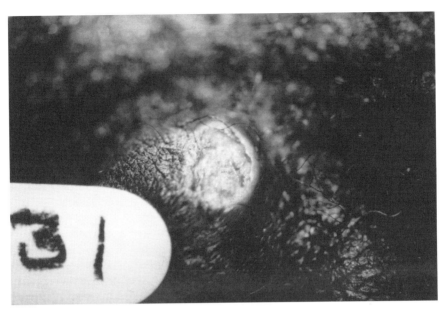

Figure 3   Classic penile chancroid ulcer. (Photo courtesy of Jeffrey Gilbert, M.D.)

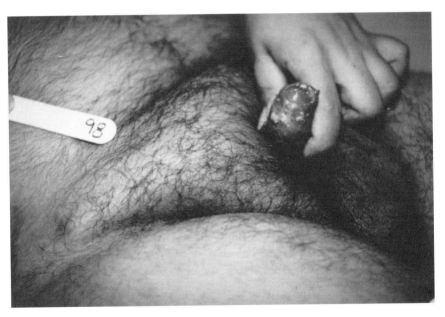

Figure 4   Male patient with chancroid and condyloma acuminata coinfection. Coronal chancroid ulcer is not visible as phimosis prevents foreskin retraction. Note huge right inguinal bubo and condyloma acuminata studding the internal foreskin surface. (Photo courtesy of Jeffrey Gilbert, M.D.)

ulcers occur on the prepuce and are equally divided between the internal and external surface.[36] Edema of the prepuce is common. Local autoinoculation to opposing skin or mucosal surfaces can occur with resulting "kissing lesions," most often seen between the glans and prepuce.[16,36]

Women typically present with multiple lesions; in one study of prostitutes at a Kenyan clinic, female patients presented with an average of 4.5 ulcers (see Figure 5).[7,14-16,46] In women chancroid ulcers are most commonly located at the entrance to the vagina and

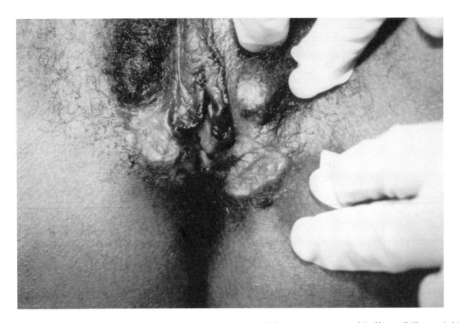

Figure 5 Typical chancroid ulcers in a female patient. (Photo courtesy of Jeffrey Gilbert, M.D.)

include lesions on the fourchette, labia, vestibule, and clitoris.[16] Longitudinal ulcers at the posterior fourchette, periurethral ulcers, perianal involvement, and involvement of the medial aspect of the thighs are common.[16] Perianal involvement does not necessarily result from anal intercourse.[15,46] Vaginal wall ulcers rarely occur, usually by extension from the introitus and are often painless.[7,16] Painless cervical lesions also can occur, and although considered uncommon, limited data suggest they may be present in 9% of female patients with chancroid.[7,16,47]

Acute painful inguinal lymphadenitis will occur in approximately 40% of infected patients one to two weeks after the primary lesion has appeared.[16] It is unilateral in two thirds of cases and bilateral in the remainder.[14,16] If untreated the adenopathy progresses to develop central necrosis, liquefaction, and suppuration with periadenitis involving the overlying skin. The resulting abscess or bubo may spontaneously rupture if not treated and drained and can lead to the formation of chronic draining sinuses (see Figure 4). Bubo pus is thick, creamy, and viscous and both Gram stain and culture of the material are frequently negative for *H. ducreyi*.[7,16] The factors responsible for initiating inguinal lymphadenopathy, suppuration, and bubo formation remain obscure.

Before the era of antimicrobial therapy, chancroid was a protracted illness with slow resolution.[15,16] Significant tissue destruction might occur, but disease did not spread beyond the genital tract.[15,16] Patients eventually healed their infection after several months, but often with subsequent scarring.[15] Occasionally, genital ulcers and inguinal abscesses were reported to persist for years.[16]

Chancroid has not been documented to cause systemic infection, even in immuno-comprised hosts.[15,16] Extragenital chancroid (oral, fingers, breasts) is rare and is believed to result from local inoculation of the disease.[2,3] Neonatal disease has not been described among infants born to mothers with active chancroid at the time of delivery.[16]

3.3.2 Complications

Occasionally, superinfection of chancroidal ulcers with anaerobic bacteria, particularly *Fusobacterium* sp. or *Bacteroides* sp., can lead to gangrenous phagedenic ulceration and extensive destruction of genital tissue.[16]

Acute prepuce edema resulting from ulcerative disease of the foreskin in uncircumcised men can result in a temporary phimosis.

Late complications of chancroid can include the formation of chronic draining inguinal sinuses after bubo rupture, rectovaginal fistulas in women, urethral fistulas of the glans in men, and cicatrix formation of the foreskin resulting in permanent phimosis requiring circumcision.[16,48]

3.3.3   Disease variants

Only about 50% of chancroid ulcers have typical features and among atypical presentations there are a number of well-described disease variants.[36] They include giant chancroid, follicular chancroid, papular chancroid, dwarf chancroid, transient chancroid, and a form of chancroid that can mimic granuloma inguinale.[36,48,49] Giant chancroid starts as a single small ulcer, but it is characterized by rapid and superficial peripheral extension of disease following rupture of an inguinal abscess. The disease spreads from the ruptured bubo to the suprapubic region and thigh by extension or autoinoculation, and although it may involve a large area, the disease is not deeply destructive. Follicular chancroid is restricted to hair-bearing areas, such as the external vulva, and involves direct infection of the pilar apparatus. It can closely resemble a simple pyogenic folliculitis. Papular chancroid starts as a papule and becomes ulcerated, however, the lesion later becomes raised, particularly around the margins. These lesions can resemble condylomata lata of secondary syphilis. Dwarf chancroid is characterized by multiple small painful ulcers and can closely resemble herpetic infection. In transient chancroid, the initial chancroid ulceration resolves rapidly in 4 to 6 days and is then followed by acute regional lymphadenitis with suppuration in 10 to 20 days. Because of its presentation, the disease may be difficult to differentiate from lymphogranuloma venereum. Finally, chancroid can present with red "beefy" ulcers on the prepuce that can mimic granuloma inguinale infection (see Figure 6).[49] Urethritis may be an uncommon manifestation of chancroid in men with documented genital ulcers. Among 456 men with culture-confirmed chancroid ulcers, 1.9% were documented to have a culture-confirmed *H. ducreyi* symptomatic urethritis.[50]

Anecdotal reports have suggested that HIV-infected patients may exhibit a different clinical course of chancroid than immunocompetent patients. Unusual manifestations of disease including multiple ulcerations and extragenital lesions, systemic symptoms, delayed healing, and treatment failure have all been noted, but further population-based investigations are necessary to evaluate the potential impact of HIV coinfection on the course of chancroid.[51-53]

3.3.4   Diagnosis

The combination of a painful genital ulcer with tender inguinal adenopathy is suggestive of chancroid and when accompanied by suppurative inguinal adenopathy is almost pathognomonic.[54] In general, four or less painful genital ulcers should suggest chancroid, particularly if they are classic in appearance. Genital herpes, although also causing painful ulcers, is suggested when multiple ulcers (greater than four) are involved and disease progression involves vesicle formation. Chancroid lesions are painful and are not indurated; painless indurated lesions are suggestive of syphilis. Although the classic presentation of the chancroid ulcer is common, it is important to appreciate the wide variation in chancroid presentation that may occur and the relatively high frequency of coinfection reported for genital ulcer disease. Approximately 50% of culture-confirmed cases of chancroid have atypical presentations and coinfection with syphilis and chancroid have been reported in as high as 10% of patients with genital ulcer disease.[36,54] The sensitivity and specificity of a clinical diagnosis of chancroid will vary depending on the relative

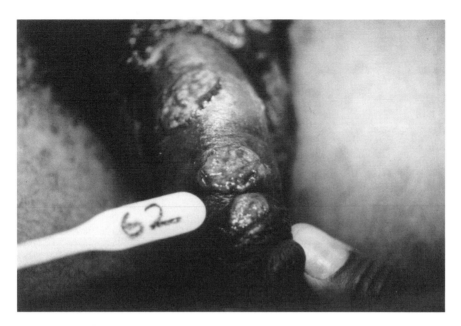

Figure 6   Chancroid ulcers that mimic granuloma inguinale. Penile ulcers were red and "beefy." (Photo courtesy of Jeffrey Gilbert, M.D.)

frequency of chancroid as a cause of genital ulcer disease within any given geographic area. Even in areas such as South Africa, where chancroid causes 70% of genital ulcer disease, the accuracy of a clinical diagnosis of chancroid is only 80%.[7] In areas where chancroid is less common (etiology of 9% of genital ulcer disease), the accuracy of a clinical diagnosis can drop to 47%.[7] In geographic areas where the frequency of chancroid as a cause of genital ulcer disease is low, for instance in the U.S. where herpes is the most common cause of genital ulcer disease, both the sensitivity and specificity of a clinical diagnosis of chancroid can be highly suspect. In conclusion, the clinical diagnosis of chancroid is usually very unreliable.

Gram stain of ulcer exudate has been used as a diagnostic aid to identify *H. ducreyi* based on its distinct morphologies. Used with some success to attempt to confirm a clinical diagnosis, it now is generally accepted to have a sensitivity of only 50% or less.[16] Specificity is also a problem in that ulcer exudates are polymicrobial in nature, and Gram stain of exudate can be difficult to interpret. Gram stain of bubo pus is very insensitive and its specificity has never been established.[7]

Currently, a definitive diagnosis of chancroid requires *H. ducreyi* culture confirmation. As previously discussed, culture sensitivity of "classic" chancroid lesions probably varies between 47 and 75% and frequently is not available.

Effective evaluation of genital ulcer disease currently requires access to: (1) either culture or antigen detection assay for HSV, (2) darkfield microscopy or direct immunofluorescence test for syphilis detection and syphilis serological testing, and (3) Gram stain and culture for chancroid.[54] Utilization of these laboratory diagnostic aids, as are epidemiologically required, should result in increased sensitivity and specifity of chancroid diagnosis, as well as better detection of coinfections. Even in this setting at least one quarter of patients with genital ulcer disease will have no laboratory-confirmed diagnosis after evaluation, and a clinician will treat for the diagnosis considered most likely.[54] Many experts recommend treatment for both chancroid and syphilis if the diagnosis is unclear or if the patient resides in an area known to be endemic for chancroid, especially when diagnostic capabilities for the two diseases are not ideal.[54]

Table 1 Recommended Treatment for Chancroid

Recommended Regimens
Azithromycin 1 g orally in a single dose
or
Ceftriaxone 250 mg intramuscularly in a single dose
or
Erythromycin base 500 mg orally 4 times a day for 7 days
Alternative Regimen
Ciprofloxacin 500 mg orally 2 times a day for 3 days

From *The Medical Letter on Drugs and Therapeutics*, 37, 117, 1995.

In summary, definitive diagnosis of chancroid currently requires culture confirmation. A probable diagnosis can be made if a patient has one or more genital ulcers, and (1) darkfield examination of the ulcer is negative or a syphilis serology test is negative when performed at least 7 days after the onset of ulcers and (2) either the clinical presentation of disease is not typical of herpes or herpes test results of ulcers are negative.[54]

Clearly, if non-culture diagnostic tests for chancroid can be developed that are sensitive, specific, cost effective, and easy to use, the accuracy of the diagnosis of chancroid could be substantially improved. Release of a commercial multiplex PCR assay for simultaneous detection of chancroid, syphilis, and herpes could potentially revolutionize the evaluation of genital ulcer disease.

3.4   Treatment

3.4.1   Approach to treatment

The treatment of chancroid includes effective antibiotic therapy, appropriate management of buboes, and improved wound hygiene. Antibiotic therapy of the disease has been complicated by the continual development of antibiotic resistance among *H. ducreyi* isolates which necessitates periodic review of recommended treatment guidelines. In addition, therapy is further complicated by recent data which suggest that HIV-infected patients may not respond to therapy as well as patients who are not infected.

Recently recommended and alternative regimens for the treatment of chancroid among non-HIV infected patients are summarized in Table 1.[54-56] Resistance to azithromycin or ceftriaxone has not been reported for *H. ducreyi* and a recent study indicated that both drugs were equally effective in treating chancroid (100% response rate for both).[57] In addition, both drugs offer the advantage of single dose therapy. The safety of azithromycin for use in pregnant and lactating women has not been established. In spite of the fact that erythromycin has been widely recommended and used for chancroid therapy for twenty years, only two *H. ducreyi* isolates resistant to erythromycin have been described;[7] both were reported more than a decade ago and no further erythromycin resistance has been reported since then.[7,53] *In vivo* studies continue to document the drug as highly effective chancroid therapy when used for 7 days.[7,53] A 3-day course of ciprofloxacin was first introduced by the Centers for Disease Control as an alternative chancroid therapy in 1988, when initial data indicated cure rates of 95 to 100%.[7,53] Recent large scale *in vivo* studies evaluating ciprofloxacin therapy of chancroid are not available and this regimen has received only limited attention in the U.S. *H. ducreyi* isolates remain sensitive to fluoroquinolones (including ciprofloxacin, ofloxacin, fleroxacin, enoxacin, and rosaxcin) and ciprofloxacin resistance has only been documented in Thailand.[7] Ciprofloxacin therapy is contraindicated for pregnant and lactating women, children, and adolescents less than 17 years of age. Previously recommended alternative regimens of amoxicillin/clavulanate and trimethoprim/sulfonamide should no longer be used due to the development of resistance among *H. ducreyi* isolates, particularly in the U.S.[7,55]

Recent data suggest that HIV-infected patients may have higher failure rates for antimicrobial treatment of chancroid, especially when single dose ceftriaxone or 3-day courses of fluoruquinolones are utilized (cure rates of 55 to 65%).[51,53] Seven-day courses of erythromycin or azithromycin result in cure rates of 79% in HIV-infected patients and 94% in non-HIV-infected patients.[58] Longer courses of ceftriaxone or fluoroquinolones have not been evaluated for the treatment of HIV-infected patients. As a consequence, many experts recommend regimens of either azithromycin or seven-day courses of erythromycin with close follow up when treating HIV-infected patients.[54-56]

When presumptive therapy is given for non-herpetic genital ulcer disease in areas where both chancroid and syphilis are known to be endemic, it is recommended that patients receive simultaneous ceftriaxone and benzathine penicillin treatment. Syphilis and chancroid coinfection rates may be as high as 10%, and treatment with only penicillin will result in failure to cure chancroid, and may also result in failure to cure syphilis due to β-lactamase production by *H. ducreyi* bacteria coinfecting genital lesions.[56,59]

Bubo management consists of drainage of buboes greater than 5 cm in diameter, as previous studies have documented that buboes of that size are likely to spontaneously rupture or require drainage to improve symptoms or allow a more rapid cure.[16] Buboes that rupture can lead to sinus formation and scarring. In general, buboes less than 5 cm in diameter will resolve with only antibiotic therapy. Drainage of fluctuant nodes can be accomplished by closed-needle aspiration or surgical incision and drainage with packing. If closed-needle aspiration is attempted, the needle should be introduced through adjacent uninvolved skin into the bubo to prevent fistula formation or rupture. Traditionally, closed-needle aspiration has been thought to be superior to surgical incision and drainage in that it prevented superinfection and chronic sinus formation. However, incision and drainage is probably safe when used with currently recommended antibiotic therapy.[7] Recent limited evidence suggests that either modality is an effective means of bubo drainage, although needle aspiration may require retreatment more often.[60]

Wound hygiene, such as gentle cleansing with soap and water or the local application of saline soaks, can relieve symptoms, remove necrotic debris, and promote ulcer healing.[16,36]

Management of any patient with chancroid should include instruction regarding safe sex practices, HIV-1 testing and counseling, and syphilis serology testing at the initial visit. If initial results are negative, both tests should be repeated in three months.

3.4.2 Response to therapy

Patients should be re-examined 3 to 7 days after initiation of therapy. Successful treatment results in symptomatic improvement of ulcers in 3 days and objective improvement of ulcers after 7 days.[54] Lack of improvement should prompt consideration of misdiagnosis, coinfection with another STD, HIV infection of the patient, non-compliance with therapy, or infection with antibiotic resistant *H. ducreyi*. The time required for complete healing of an ulcer is related to the size of the ulcer. Large ulcers may require greater than two weeks to heal. Clinical resolution of buboes can lag far behind that of ulcers, even during successful therapy.

Patients coinfected with HIV-1 should be closely monitored for response and may experience treatment failure more often than other patients. Successful treatment may require more prolonged courses of therapy than those recommended for general use and patients may exhibit delayed healing of ulcers.

3.4.3   Public health issues

Prevention of chancroid has assumed a new importance given the potential for enhanced acquisition and transmission of HIV-1 disease via chancroid ulcers. The relatively short incubation period of chancroid suggests that contact tracing should be an effective way of controlling disease transmission. Any person known to have had sexual contact with a patient diagnosed with chancroid within the 10 days before the onset of the patient's symptoms should be examined and treated. The examination and treatment should be performed even if contact patients are asymptomatic.

References

1. Borchardt, K. A. and Hoke, A. W., Simplified laboratory technique for diagnosis of chancroid, *Arch. Derm.*, 102, 188, 1970.
2. Albritton, W. L., Biology of *Haemophilus ducreyi*, *Microbiol. Rev.*, 53, 377, 1989.
3. Hand, W. L., Haemophilus species (including chancroid), in *Principles and Practice of Infectious Diseases*, 4th edition, Mandell, G. L., Bennett, J. E. and Dolin, R., Eds., Churchill Livingstone, New York, 1995, Chapter 202.
4. Kilian, M. and Theilade, J., Cell wall ultrastructure of strains of *Haemophilus ducreyi* and *Haemophilus piscium*, *Int. J. Syst. Bacteriol.*, 25, 351, 1975.
5. Trees, D. L. and Morse, S. A., Chancroid and *Haemophilus ducreyi*: an update, *Clin. Microbiol. Rev.*, 8, 357, 1995.
6. Spinola, S. M., Castellazzo, A., Shero, M. and Apicella, M. A., Characterization of pili expressed by *Haemophilus ducreyi*, *Microb. Path.*, 9, 417, 1990.
7. Marrazzo, J. M. and Handsfield, H. H., Chancroid: new developments in an old disease, in *Current Clinical Topics in Infectious Diseases*, Vol. 15, Remington, J. S. and Swartz, M. N., Eds., Blackwell Science, Boston, 1995, Chapter 6.
8. Motley, M. S., Sarafian, K., Knapp, J. S., Zaidi, A. A. and Schmid, G., Correlation between *in vitro* antimicrobial susceptibilities and β-lactamase plasmid contents of isolates of *Haemophilus ducreyi* from the United States, *Antimicrob. Agents Chemother.*, 36, 1639, 1992.
9. Sarafian, S. K. and Knapp, J. S., Molecular epidemiology, based on plasmid profiles of *Haemophilus ducreyi* infections in the United States: results of surveillance, 1981–1990, *Sex. Trans. Dis.*, 19, 35, 1992.
10. Schulte, J. O., Martich, F. A. and Schmid, G. P., Chancroid in the United States, 1981–1990: evidence for underreporting of cases, *MMWR*, 41-SS3, 47, 1992.
11. Betts, C. and Zacarias, F., Regional assessment of STD trends in Latin America and the Caribbean, *Sex. Trans. Dis.*, 21 (Suppl.), S108, 1994.
12. Tan, T., Rajan, V. S., Koe, S. L., Tan, N. J., Tan, B. H. and Goh, A. J., Chancroid: a study of 500 cases, *Asian J. Infect. Dis.*, 1, 27, 1977.
13. Ronald, A., Chancroid, in *Atlas of Infectious Diseases, Vol. V — Sexually Transmitted Diseases*, Mandell, G. L. and Rein, M. F., Eds., Churchill Livingstone, New York, 1996, Chapter 16.
14. Ronald, A. R. and Plummer, F. A., Chancroid and *Haemophilus ducreyi*, *Ann. Int. Med.*, 102, 705, 1985.
15. Schmid, G. P., Chancroid, in *Bacterial Infections of Humans: Epidemiology and Control*, Evans, A. S. and Brachman, P. S., Eds., Plenum Medical Book Company, New York, 2nd edition, 1991, Chapter 8.
16. Ronald, A. R. and Albritton, W., Chancroid and *Haemophilus ducreyi*, in *Sexually Transmitted Diseases*, 2nd edition, Holmes, K. K., Mardh, P., Sparling, P. F. and Weisner, P. J., Eds., McGraw-Hill, New York, 1990, Chapter 24.
17. Schmid, G. P., Lawrence, L. S., Blount, J. H. and Alexander, E. R., Chancroid in the U.S. — reestablishment of an old disease, *JAMA*, 258, 3265, 1987.
18. Division of STD Prevention, Sexually transmitted disease surveillance, 1994, U.S. Department of Health and Human Services, Public Health Service, Atlanta: Centers for Disease Control and Prevention, September, 1995.

19. DiCarlo, R. P., Armentor, B. S. and Martin, D. H., Chancroid epidemiology in New Orleans men, *J. Inf. Dis.*, 172, 446, 1995.

20. Flood, J. M., Sarafian, S. K., Bolan, G. A., Lammel, C., Engelman, J., Greenblatt, R. M., Brooks, G. F., Back, A. and Morse, S. A., Multistrain outbreak of chancroid in San Francisco, 1989–1991, *J. Inf. Dis.*, 167, 1106, 1993.

21. Jessamine, P. G., Plummer, F. A., Ndinya-Achola, J. O., Wainberg, M. A., Wamola, I., D'Costa, L. J., Cameron, D. W., Simonsen, J. N., Plourde, P. and Ronald, A. R., Human immunodeficiency virus, genital ulcers and the male foreskin: synergism in HIV-1 transmission, *Scand. J. Inf. Dis.*, Suppl. 69, 181, 1990.

22. Wasserheit, J. N., Epidemiological synergy: interrelationships between human immunodeficiency virus and other sexually transmitted diseases, *Sex. Trans. Dis.*, 19, 61, 1992.

23. Simonsen, J. N., Cameron, D. W., Gakinya, M. N., Ndinya Achola, J. O., D'Costa, L. J., Karasira, P., Cheang, M., Ronald, A. R., Piot, P. and Plummer, F. A., Human immunodeficiency virus infection among men with sexually transmitted diseases — experience from a center in Africa, *N. Eng. J. Med.*, 319, 274, 1988.

24. Cameron, D. W., Simonsen, J. N., D'Costa, L. J., Ndinya-Achola, J. O., Piot, P. and Plummer, F. A., Female to male transmission of human immunodeficiency virus type 1: risk factors for seroconversion in men, *Lancet*, 2, 403, 1989.

25. Plummer, F. A., Cameron, D. W., Simonsen, J. N., Bosire, M., Kreiss, J., Waiyaki, P. and Ronald, A. R., Cofactors in male to female transmission of HIV, *JID*, 163, 233, 1991.

26. Telzak, E. E., Chiasson, M. A., Bevier, P. J., Stoneburner, R. L., Castro, K. G. and Jaffe, H. W., HIV-1 seroconversion in patients with and without genital ulcer disease: a prospective study, *Ann. Intern. Med.*, 119, 1181, 1993.

27. Plummer, F. A., Wainberg, M. A., Plourde, P., Jessamine, P., D'Costa, L. J., Wamola, I. A. and Ronald, A. R., Detection of human immunodeficiency virus type 1 (HIV-1) in genital ulcer exudate of HIV-1 infected men by culture and gene amplification, *JID*, 161, 810, 1990.

28. Kreiss, J. K., Coombs, R., Plummer, F., Holmes, K. K., Nikora, B., Cammeron, W., Ngugi, E., Ndinya-Achola, J. O. and Corey, L., Isolation of human immunodeficiency virus from genital ulcers in Nairobi prostitutes, *JID*, 160, 380, 1989.

29. Ho, J. L., The influence of coinfections on HIV transmission and disease progression, *AIDS Reader*, July-August, 114, 1996.

30. Desjardins, M., Thompson, C. E., Filion, L. G., Ndinya-Achola, J. O., Plummer, F. A., Ronald, A. R., Piot, P. and Cameron, D. W., Standardization of an enzyme immunoassay for human antibody to *Haemophilus ducreyi*, *J. Clin. Microbiol.*, 30, 2019, 1992.

31. Karim, Q. N., Finn, G. Y., Easmon, C. S., Dangor, Y., Dance, D. A. B., Ngeow, Y. F. and Ballard, R. C., Rapid detection of *Haemophilus ducreyi* in clinical and experimental infections using monoclonal antibody: a preliminary evaluation, *Genitourin. Med.*, 65, 361, 1989.

32. Parsons, L. M., Shayegani, M., Waring, A. L. and Bopp, L. H., DNA probes for the identification of *Haemophilus ducreyi*, *J. Clin. Microbiol.*, 27, 1441, 1989.

33. Rossau, R., Duhamel, M., Jannes, G., Decourt, J. L. and Heuverswyn, H. V., The development of specific rRNA-derived oligonucleotide probes for *Haemophilus ducreyi*, the causative agent of chancroid, *J. Gen. Microbiol.*, 137, 277, 1991.

34. Johnson, S. R., Martin, D. H., Cammarata, C. and Morse, S. A., Development of a polymerase chain reaction assay for the detection of *Haemophilus ducreyi*, *Sex. Trans. Dis.*, 21, 13, 1994.

35. Centers for Disease Control and Prevention, Chancroid detected by polymerase chain reaction — Jackson, Mississippi, 1994–1995, *MMWR*, 44, 567, 1995.

36. Ronald, A. R. and Alfa, M. J., Chancroid, lymphogranuloma venereum, and granuloma inguinale, in *Infectious Diseases*, Gorbach, S. L., Bartlett, J. G. and Blacklow, N. R., Eds., W. B. Saunders Co., Philadelphia, 1992, Chapter 120.

37. Alfa, M. J., Cytopathic effect of *Haemophilus ducreyi* for human foreskin cell culture, *J. Med. Microbiol.*, 37, 43, 1992.

38. Alfa, M. J., Degagne, P. and Hollyer, T., *Haemophilus ducreyi* adheres but does not invade cultured human foreskin cells, *Infect. Immun.*, 61, 1735, 1993.

39. Shah, L., Davies, H. A. and Wall, R. A., Association of *Haemophilus ducreyi* will cell-culture lines, *J. Med. Microbiol.*, 37, 268, 1992.

40. Totten, P. A., Lara, J. C., Norn, D. V. and Stamm, W. E., *Haemophilus ducreyi* attaches to and invades human epithelial cells *in vitro*, *Infect. Immun.*, 62, 5632, 1994.
41. Purcell, B. K., Richardson, J. A., Radolf, J. D. and Hansen, E. J., A temperature-dependent rabbit model for production of dermal lesions by *Haemophilus ducreyi*, *J. Infect. Dis.*, 164, 359, 1991.
42. Trees, D. L., Arko, R. J. and Morse, S. A., Mouse subcutaneous chamber model for *in vivo* growth of *Haemophilus ducreyi*, *Microb. Pathog.*, 11, 387, 1991.
43. Toten, P. A., Morton, W. R., Knitter, G. H., Clark, A. M., Kiviat, N. B. and Stamm, W. E., A primate model for chancroid, *J. Infect. Dis.*, 169, 1284, 1994.
44. Spinola, S. M., Wild, L. M., Apicella, M. A., Gaspari, A. A., and Campagnari, A. A., Experimental human infection with *Haemophilus ducreyi*, *JID*, 169, 1146, 1994.
45. Freinkel, A. L., Histological aspects of sexually transmitted genital lesions, *Histopathology*, 11, 819, 1987.
46. Plummer, F. A., D'Costa, L. J., Nsanze, H., Karasira, P., MacLean, I. W., Piot, P. and Ronald, A. R., Clinical and microbiologic studies of genital ulcers in Kenyan women, *Sex. Trans. Dis.*, 12, 193, 1985.
47. Hammond, G. W., Slutchuk, M., Scatliff, J., Sherman, E., Wilt, J. C. and Ronald, A. R., Epidemiologic, clinical, laboratory and therapeutic features of an urban outbreak of chancroid in North America, *Rev. Infect. Dis.*, 2, 867, 1980.
48. Gaisin, A. and Heaton, C. L., Chancroid: alias the soft chancre, *Int. J. Dermatol.*, 3, 188, 1975.
49. Kraus, S. J., Werman, B. S., Biddle, J. W., Sottnek, F. O. and Ewing, E. P., Pseudogranuloma inguinale caused by *Haemophilus ducreyi*, *Arch. Dermatol.*, 118, 494, 1982.
50. Kunimoto, D. Y., Plummer, F. A., Namaara, W., D'Costa, L. J., Ndinya-Achola, J. O. and Ronald, A. R., Urethral infection with *Haemophilus ducreyi* in men, *Sex. Trans. Dis.*, 15, 37, 1988.
51. Tyndall, M., Malisa, M., Plummer, F. A., Ombetti, J., Ndinya-Achola, J. D. and Ronald, A. R., Ceftriaxone no longer predictably cures chancroid in Kenya, *JID*, 167, 469, 1993.
52. Quale, J., Atypical presentation of chancroid in a patient infected with HIV, *Am. J. Med.*, 88(5N), 43N, 1990.
53. Schulte, J. M. and Schmid, G. P., Recommendations for treatment of chancroid, 1993, *Clin. Inf. Dis.*, Supplement 1, S39, 1995.
54. Centers for Disease Control and Prevention, 1993, Sexually transmitted diseases treatment guidelines, *MMWR*, 42, 1, 1993.
55. The Medical Letter, Inc., Drugs for sexually transmitted diseases, The *Medical Letter on Drugs and Therapeutics*, 37, 117, 1995.
56. Bureau of Sexually Transmitted Disease Control, Sexually transmitted diseases treatment guidelines — 1994, New York State Department of Health, Albany, New York, 1994.
57. Martin, D. H., Sargent, S. J., Wendel, G. D., McCormack, W. M., Spier, N. A. and Johnson, R. B., Comparison of azithromycin and ceftriaxone for the treatment of chancroid, *Clin. Inf. Dis.*, 21, 409, 1995.
58. Tyndall, M. W., Agoki, E., Plummer, F. A., Malisa, W., Ndinya-Achola, J. O. and Ronald, A. R., Single dose azithromycin for the treatment of chancroid: a randomized comparison with erythromycin, *Sex. Trans. Dis.*, 21, 231, 1994.
59. Gilbert, J., Sham, M. J., Miles, J. R. and Nowicki, C., Treatment of chancroid with ceftriaxone in New York City, *City Health Information*, 6, 1, 1987.
60. Ernst, A. A., Marvez-Valls and Martin, D. H., Incision and drainage versus aspiration of fluctuant buboes in the emergency department during an epidemic of chancroid, *Sex. Trans. Dis.*, 22, 217, 1995.

chapter four

Current concepts in the laboratory diagnosis of gonorrhea

Michael H. Levi

4.1   Introduction..76
4.2   Epidemiology of gonococcal infections in the United States 76
4.3   Pathogenesis of *N. gonorrhoeae* infections 79
    4.3.1   Role of pili...79
    4.3.2   Role of outer membrane-bound proteins and lipooligosaccharides
         (LOS)..80
    4.3.3   Auxotyping and serotyping 81
4.4   Clinical manifestations of infection with *N. gonorrhoeae* 82
    4.4.1   Infections in men..82
    4.4.2   Infections in women 83
    4.4.3   Complications of infection with *N. gonorrhoeae* 84
4.5   Laboratory diagnosis of *N. gonorrhoeae* infections...............................85
    4.5.1   Collection of specimens 85
    4.5.2   Media...87
    4.5.3   Gram stains 88
    4.5.4   Direct detection of *N. gonorrhoeae* antigen or DNA from specimens 89
    4.5.5   Identification and culture confirmation of *N. gonorrhoeae*................90
4.6   *N. gonorrhoeae* antimicrobial resistance and susceptibility testing....................91
    4.6.1   Current epidemiology of antibiotic resistance 92
    4.6.2   Beta lactam antibiotics...93
    4.6.3   Alternative antimicrobial agents active against *N. gonorrhoeae*....................95
References...98

"Young Larch would stare at his pus until Dr. Ernst would arrive
and greet his little living experiments all over the lab [as if they were
his old baseball teammates].

" ' Honestly, Larch,' " the famous bacteriologist said one morning,
" ' the way you look into that microscope, you appear to be plotting
revenge!' "

from *The Cider House Rules* by John Irving

0-8493-9476-7/97/$0.00+$.50
© 1997 by CRC Press LLC

4.1 Introduction

N. gonorrhoeae, the etiologic agent of gonorrhea, was first described in 1879 by Albert Neisser.[1] Working as an assistant in dermatology at the University of Breslau, Germany, Neisser made astute observations of diplococci in patients with symptoms of gonococcal urethritis, cervicitis, and conjunctivitis. Today we recognize the Family, Neisseriaceae, which contains the genera, *Neisseria, Moraxella, Acinetobacter, Eikenella, Simonsiella, Alysiella,* and *Kingella.*[2,3] All members are aerobic, nonmotile, non-sporeforming, Gram-negative cocci or rods. The genus *Neisseria* is composed of 10 species of human origin all of which (excluding *N. elongata*) are cocci 0.6–1.5 µm in diameter occurring singly or more often in pairs with adjacent sides flattened (coffee bean shaped). Although most of the *Neisseria* species can colonize in man, *N. gonorrhoeae* is always considered a pathogen and clinically significant.[3] All species rapidly oxidize dimethyl or tetramethylparaphenylene diamine (oxidase test). *N. gonorrhoeae* is the most fastidious member of the genus and has complex growth requirements for vitamins, amino acids, and iron which is supplied by enriched media.[3,4] Enriched and selective media, which enhance the growth of *N. gonorrhoeae* from specimens while reducing contamination by normal microbial flora, are now routinely used in clinical laboratories. The optimum temperature for growth of *N. gonorrhoeae* is 36–37°C with a high relative humidity (~50%) and 3–10% CO_2. *N. gonorrhoeae* colonies are usually 0.6–1.0 mm in diameter and when examined using oblique light, five colony morphologies (T_1–T_5) have been recognized. T_1 colonies are small, raised, slightly viscous, and dew drop-like with entire edges. T_2 colonies are friable, with defined or crenated edges. Both T_1 and T_2 represent strains with pili and are virulent for human volunteers. Non-virulent T_3–T_5 colonies are larger, slightly convex with a colorless or slight brown tinge. Further cultural and identification techniques will be discussed below.

4.2 Epidemiology of gonococcal infections in the United States

Gonorrhea is a sexually transmitted disease whose signs and symptoms can be vastly different in men and women. Men tend to have self-limited symptomatic disease and usually seek medical attention. Women may have only mild symptoms that may go unnoticed. It is estimated that at least 50% of women fall into the asymptomatic category.[5] When asymptomatic *N. gonorrhoeae* infections are coupled with inadequate detection methods (screening) and treatment, 10–40% of infected women may develop pelvic inflammatory disease (PID).[5] PID is believed to cause infertility in 20%, ectopic pregnancy in 9%, and chronic pelvic pain in 18% of these women.[5] These facts have focused gonorrhea prevention on three issues: safer sexual practices, contact investigation, and notification of sexual partners and routine screening of high risk women. Although eradication of gonorrhea in the U.S. is an unlikely goal, control programs have significantly reduced the number of reportable cases.[6-8]

The overall success of the U.S. gonorrhea control programs is demonstrated by the decline in the number of reported cases since the mid-1970s. Currently gonorrhea is at the lowest levels in 30 years and levels below the year 2000 objective (Figure 1). In 1994, 418,068 cases of gonorrhea and 448,984 cases of *Chlamydia trachomatis* infections were reported in the U.S. This was the first year in which *C. trachomatis* outnumbered those of gonorrhea. The highest rates of gonorrhea are reported in the South and Southeastern regions of the U.S. (Figure 2). The 1994 data excludes the state of Georgia which has high rates of gonorrhea; if gonorrhea rates were similar to those reported by this state in 1993 levels, the overall 1994 gonorrhea rates would not be significantly different.[5] It should be noted that the rate of decline in 1994 was less then in previous years, but the significance of this is not yet known.

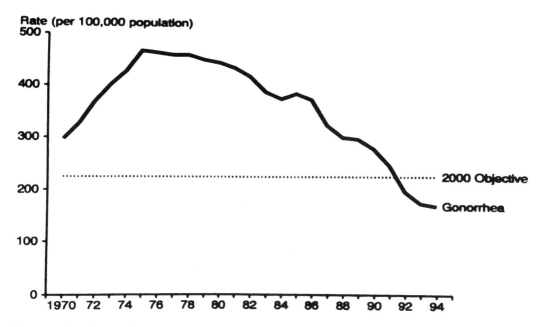

Figure 1   Incidence of reported cases of gonorrhea in the United States. (From Division of STD prevention. *Sexually Transmitted Disease Surveillance, 1994.* U.S. Department of Health and Human Services, Public Health Service. Atlanta: Centers for Disease Control and Prevention, September 1995.)

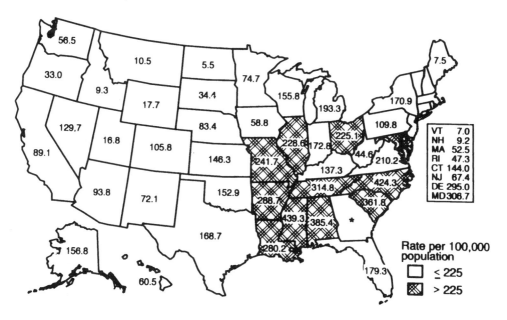

Figure 2   Rates of reported gonorrhea per state during 1994. (From Division of STD prevention. *Sexually Transmitted Disease Surveillance, 1994.* U.S. Department of Health and Human Services, Public Health Service. Atlanta: Centers for Disease Control and Prevention, September 1995.)

Scrutiny of the specific gonorrhea rates allows one to better understand the epidemiology of this infection. To a great extent gonorrhea has become a disease localized in the cites, where women, members of non-white minorities, and users of illicit drugs have

Table 1   Reported Cases and Incidence Rates of Gonorrhea According to
Race/Ethnicity in the United States, 1994[a]

Racial/ethnic group	Reported cases	Cases per 100,000 population
White, non-Hispanic	52,332	30.1
Black, non-Hispanic	309,404	1,219
Hispanic	17,331	84.5
Native American	2,150	104.7
Asian/Pacific Islander	1,682	22.4
Total	382,899	166.8/100,000

[a] Data excludes New York City and New York State, which do not report cases
according to race/ethnicity; including New York, 30,997 cases (170.0 cas-
es/100,000) were reported in 1994.

Adapted from Division of STD prevention. *Sexually Transmitted Disease Surveillance,
1994.* U.S. Department of Health and Human Services, Public Health Service. Atlanta: Centers for Disease Control and Prevention, September 1995.

increased the risk of infection.[5,6,8] The overall gonorrhea rates in large cities (>200,000 persons) declined in 1994, but 39 (62%) of these urban areas still had rates above the year 2000 goal. Although the total rates in men and women were below the year 2000 goal, womens' rates increased from 147.1/100,000 to 153.7/100,000. Screening of high risk women and appropriate treatment has been the key to lowering gonorrhea rates in this group. This is supported by the male-to-female rate ratio for gonorrhea, which has declined between 1980 and 1994 from 1.5 to 1.2 in 1994.

Adolescents (10 to 19 year olds) and young adults (20 to 24 year olds) are at highest risk for acquiring sexually transmitted diseases (STDs). These age groups tend to have multiple sex partners, engage in unprotected sexual intercourse, and have a greater risk of selecting another person at high risk. Rates of gonorrhea in young adolescents (<19 year olds) declined from the mid-1980s through 1993. In 1994, this group demonstrated a 7% increase in gonorrhea, which is the first increase since 1985 and is almost entirely attributed to increased cases in females.[5] These increases included all ethnic groups. Young males of similar age demonstrated declines in gonorrhea between 1993 and 1994.

In the U.S., race and ethnicity are associated with an increased risk for STDs.[5] This disparity is associated with factors that influence health status, e.g., poverty level, access to quality health care, health-care seeking behavior, illicit drug use, and living in high risk areas (Table 1).[5] In 1994 African-Americans accounted for 81% of the total reported cases of gonorrhea with adolescents and young adults at greatest risk. Overall, rates of gonorrhea in African-American adolescents did not demonstrate any significant declines until the early 1990s. In 1994 African-American 15- to 19-year-old women had an extremely high rate of gonorrhea (4911.9 cases/100,000 population) and demonstrated a 5.5% increase over 1993. African-American men in the same age group also have a high rate (4007.5 cases/100,000 population), but demonstrated a 2.2% decrease over 1993. These rates are about 28-fold higher than those for white adolescents of the same age. Similar high rates for 20- to 24-year-old blacks were also reported in 1994. Knowledge of this disparity in gonorrhea rates by race/ethnicity is crucial for communities to organize and focus on this problem.

In an era of shrinking federal health-care funds and the risk of HIV infection, control of all STDs must have programs aimed at high risk populations. The data discussed above clearly demonstrate that gonorrhea control programs need to be continued and should focus special efforts on inner city youth. These programs must couple prevention with education and reliable screening programs.

Table 2 Surface Components of *N. Gonorrhoeae* that may have a Role in Virulence

Designation	Location and characteristics	Contribution to virulence
Pilin	Pili PilE -major pilin protein PilC-involved in pilin maturation (?) Phase/antigenic variation	Initial binding to epithelial cells
P.I (Por)	Outer membrane porin P.IA-antigenic form found on most invasive strains P.IB-antigenic form found on strains that cause localized infection	May prevent phagolysosome fusion in PMN's and/or reduce oxidative burst
P.II (Opa)	Outer membrane protein Phase/antigenic variation	Intimate attachment, contributes to (but is not sufficient for) invasion of host cells; involved in microcolony formation
P.III	Outer membrane protein; analog of OmpA (porin)	Antibodies directed against P.III block bactericidal antibodies against P.I, LOS
LOS	Outer membrane lipooligosaccharide	Mediates bacterium-bacterium attachment (microcolony formation); elicits inflammatory response, triggers TNFa release that causes scarring of fallopian tubes
Tbp1, Tbp2	Receptor for human transferrin	Iron acquisition
Lbp	Receptor for human lactoferrin	Iron acquisition

From Salyers, A.A. and Whitt, D.D., *Bacterial Pathogenesis: A Molecular Approach,* ASM Press, Washington, D.C. 1994, Chap. 20. With permission.

4.3   *Pathogenesis of* N. gonorrhoeae *infections*

The pathogenesis of gonococcal infections can be broken down into three specific steps: first, the attachment of the bacterium to epithelial cells; second, the penetration either through or between epithelial cells, and finally destruction of epithelial cells.[9] The bacterium's outer cell membrane contains most of the specific surface appendages that are important in these steps. Considering their importance in pathogenesis, many of these structures have been the targets for vaccine development (Table 2). Unfortunately *N. gonorrhoeae* has complex genetic mechanisms to alter these proteins and lipopolysaccharides. In turn, this reduces the effect of the host's opsonizing antibodies and explains why natural infection does not lead to immunity. Organism control of surface structures is accomplished by two mechanisms. The first is antigen variation which allows the bacterium to change the gene sequence that is transcribed, resulting in different proteins. The second mechanism is phase variation which refers to the organism's ability to switch a gene on or off. Although antigenic or phase variations are present in a fraction of the total infecting population (10^{-2}–10^{-4}), these strains will not be recognized by host antibodies, allowing them to become the dominant strain. A discussion of the crucial steps in pathogenesis follows below.

4.3.1   *Role of pili*

Pili are filamentous protein surface structures of *N. gonorrhoeae* that are crucial for attachment to epithelial cells. *Neisseria* pili are made of repeating identical subunits (pilins) of about 17-21 kDa and belong to the type IV class shared by various other Gram-negative bacilli.[10,11] Structurally pili have three regions. First, there is a highly conserved area of 53 amino acid residues close to the outer membrane that plays a role in pilus assembly and host cell recognition. Second, there is a central pilin region that contains single amino acid changes (semivariable region). Finally, there is a highly variable carboxy terminal region that differs dramatically from strain to strain. A single *N. gonorrhoeae* is genetically capable of producing antigenically different pilin variants. Human volunteer studies have shown that pilin antigenic variation occurs throughout the infection cycle and that multiple pilin variants can be present during a single infection.[12]

Pilin expression is controlled at the *pilE* locus which contains the intact pilin gene and promoter sequences.[10,11] The chromosome also has several copies of variant *pil* loci (*pil S*) which are transcriptionally inactive because they lack the promotor region and 5′-coding sequences. Antigenic variation occurs from the recombination of a *pil S* and *pilE* gene. The level of *pilE* expression can also be controlled by the regulatory genes *pilA* and *pilB*.[11] These genes are members of a two-component system that regulates expression in response to environmental stress. The former is a transcriptional activator, while the latter acts as a sensor for nitrogen levels and phosphorylates *pilA* in response to nitrogen starvation. The result would be increased pilin production during periods of nitrogen starvation.

Phase variation from an organism with pili (P$^+$) to one without (P$^-$) is controlled by a number of different mechanisms.[10,11] Post-translational modification of the Pil E protein can result in P$^+$ when the protein assembles into membrane-bound pili. If this protein is nicked at another site and lacks the hydrophobic region needed for assembly, pili will not form on the surface. Instead Pil^s is formed which is soluble and is excreted into the extracellular medium. Homologous recombination between *pilE* and *pilS* can also result in the production of an aberrant protein that cannot be assembled into pili, thus producing a Pil$^-$ phenotype. Finally, Pil$^+$ to Pil$^-$ can also be influenced by PilC proteins. PilC1 and PilC2 proteins are produced by closely related genes and yield two high MW proteins. The genes *pilC1* and *pilC2* are subject to frameshift mutations within a poly (G) region at the 5′ end of both genes. It is not exactly known how these mutations result in phase variation, but three explanations have been made: (1) variant protein C results in reduction in pilin assembly, (2) antigenic variation resulting in Pil^s, and (3) reduction in adherence but not necessarily piliation.

4.3.2   Role of outer membrane-bound proteins and lipooligosaccharides (LOS)

A group of membrane-bound proteins and LOS participate in bacterial attachment and invasion of host cells. Por (Porin) protein (Protein I) provides a channel for the passage of low molecular aqueous solutes. [13] Purified Por has several interesting features. First, when added to cultured epithelial cells it inserts into the cell membrane and collapses the membrane potential. Secondly, it binds to the calcium-binding protein, calmodulin. By diminishing the oxidative burst and preventing phagolysosomal fusion, Por may affect polymorphonuclear leukocyte (PMN) killing of *N. gonorrhoeae*. There are two different Por alleles: *P.IA* and *P.IB*. Strains which carry the former are usually associated with systemic gonorrhea, while the latter are usually associated with localized disease. Por demonstrates stable interstrain antigenic variation and is the basis of strain serotyping (see below).[13] Por is membrane bound close to LOS and not well exposed on the bacterial surface. Nonetheless because P.IA and P.IB contain conserved regions, they are considered possible vaccine candidates.[11]

Opa/class five proteins (Opacity proteins) are important in adherence and invasion of pathogenic *Neisseria*, but are not sufficient for attachment.[10,11] Colonies expressing this protein are more opaque when isolated on culture media, while Opa negative are clear and relatively easy to isolate. *In vitro* work with *N. gonorrhoeae* Opa negative mutants and nonphagocytic cells demonstrates that these mutants cannot adhere as well to cells. When the gene for Opa is transferred to *E. coli*, the organisms show increased adherence to epithelial cells.[10] Human male volunteer studies have shown that infecting strains tend to be those that express Opa phenotype.[14] Ironically, cervical isolates from menstruating women or from normally sterile sites (fallopian tubes, blood, synovial fluid) tend to lack Opa expression.[13] Opa also plays a role in microcolony formation by binding of Opa to another cell's LOS. This process of microcolony formation may have a role in initial attachment of *N. gonorrhoeae* to epithelial cells.

Opa proteins are also susceptible to phase and antigenic variation. This structure is composed of a family of proteins produced from 11 *opa* genes. Each gene is intact and constitutively expressed and prone to antigenic variation by homologous recombination events.[11] Phase variation results from frameshift mutation (slipped strand mispairing) of highly repetitive pentameric repeat signal sequence (CTCTT). Frameshifts in one or all the genes coding for Opa produce aberrant (nonfunctional) proteins.[10]

P.III is a porin protein that is usually present on the surface of *N. gonorrhoeae* and elicits a specific antibody response. Antibody against P.III has the ability to block antibodies against P.I. and LOS. Antibody against P.III blocks the bactericidal action of these antibodies, by increasing the risk of reinfection.[15] IgA proteases are produced by *N. gonorrhoeae* but not nonpathogenic Neisseriae. This enzyme is thought to also protect the bacterium from secretory immunoglobulin, but the role of this enzyme is still unclear.[13]

LOS of *N. gonorrhoeae* is composed of lipid A and a core oligosaccharide which lacks the O-anitgenic side chains present in other Gram-negative bacteria. LOS is important in the pathogenesis of gonococcal disease by several mechanisms. LOS triggers an intense inflammatory response and is responsible for many symptoms associated with gonococcal infections. LOS is known to activate complement, induce "sloppy" phagocytosis, aid bacterial adherence to cells, and lyse host cells.[10,11] The mucoid character of gonococcal discharge is due to DNA and cellular material from lysis of PMNs and epithelial cells. LOS is also known to induce local production of TNFα which is believed to be responsible for most of the tissue damage of salpingitis.[11]

Activation of complement by a serum-sensitive strain is beneficial to the host. Complement activation produces C3b, which opsonizes the bacteria, C5a, which is chemotactic for PMNs and finally results in the membrane attack complex (MAC), which will lyse the serum-sensitive gonococci. Compared to the small number which phagocytize gonococci, it is not known why so many PMNs are recruited, nor if PMNs kill gonococci. Serum killing is probably the most important of the host protective factors. Serum-resistant gonococcal strains are responsible for systemic disease in immunologically competent hosts.[11] Serum resistance is directly related to antigenic variation of the LOS by sialylation of the terminal LOS galactose residues.[10] Gonococci use the enzyme 2,3,-sialytransferase, to attach CMP *N*-acetylneruaminic acid which is found in host secretions, serum, and red cells. Since sialic acid is a ubiquitous host antigen, modified LOS now mimics host cells and does not activate complement. Sialylation of LOS also blocks bactericidal antibodies from binding to P.I.[11]

Iron acquisition is important for the viability of *N. gonorrhoeae*. Because free iron is scarce in host tissue, *N. gonorrhoeae* can directly bind transferrin, lactoferrin, and heme, to specific receptor proteins (Table 2). The receptors for transferrin and lactoferrin are produced in greatest concentrations during periods of iron deprivation; little is known about the mechanism for binding heme. Additionally, very little is known about the mechanisms by which the organism removes iron from the iron-binding compounds.

4.3.3   *Auxotyping and serotyping*

The transmission and eradication of specific *N. gonorrhoeae* strains have been studied using phenotypic and genotypic markers. Three phenotypic markers which have been useful are auxotyping, serotyping, and antimicrobial susceptibility testing patterns. Auxotyping groups of organisms by matching stable strain-dependent nutritional requirements and has been a useful typing method.[16] There are 13 distinct autxtypes depending on growth responses to seven organic chemicals: thiamin pyrophosphate, thiamin, proline, arginine, methionine, isoleucine, and hypoxanthine. It has been clearly shown that strains which require arginine, hypoxanthine, and uracil (AUH strains) are associated with decreased penicillin minimum inhibitory concentrations (MICs) and disseminated infection.[17,18] Proline, citrulline, and uracil auxotrophs are associated with asymptomatic carriage in males. These strains would have a selective advantage and have now been reported from Canada, U.S., and Sweden.[19] Outer membrane protein I has been used to divide strains into three serogroups: W-I that contains protein IA and W-II/W-III that contains protein IB. IA can be further divided into 24 serovars, IA-1 to 24 and IB into 32 serovars, IB-1-32. IA serotype is clearly associated with disseminated gonococcal disease and cervical isolates, while rectal isolates are serotype IB. Although the association with IA and dissemination is not understood, IB porin is thought to provide protection for the transportation of toxic compounds and antibiotics.[17-19] Auxotyping and serotyping are usually done in the research or public health setting and are not part of the routine clinical laboratory.

Plasmid analysis is not highly discriminatory, but it can be useful in following the spread of plasmid-mediated antibiotic resistance.[20] Restriction endonuclease analyses of the bacterial chromosome have also been used to determine the relationship between *N. gonorrhoeae* isolates.[20-21] Studies have found that organisms within one serogroup and serotype can be further divided by restriction of the chromosome. DNA amplification fingerprinting has also been shown to be very sensitive in discriminating strains.[22]

4.4   Clinical manifestations of infection with N. gonorrhoeae

4.4.1   Infections in men

Signs and symptoms of *N. gonorrhoeae* infection occur following organism attachment to columnar epithelial cells lining the urethra, rectum, oropharynx, or conjunctiva (Table 3). In men, the most common presentation of gonococcal infection is in an abrupt onset of anterior urethritis (dysuria and discharge).[23-25] Complicating the diagnosis of a male with urethritis is the fact that many other organisms can cause similar symptoms. The other infections, commonly grouped together as nongonococcal urethritis (NGU), are caused by *C. trachomatis* (30–50%), *Ureaplasm urealyticum* (20–25%), and *Trichomonas vaginalis*, Herpes simplex, and *Candida* sp. (1–5%), and 20–30% of NGU cases are idiopathic.[24] Gonococcal urethritis differs from NGU by incubation period, character of the urethral discharge, and presence of dysuria.[15] In gonococcal urethritis 75% of men develop symptoms within 4 days and 80–90% of men will develop symptoms within two weeks of exposure. Most men have a spontaneous purulent discharge.[23,25] Incubation period for NGU is usually between 7–14 days with a range of 2–35 days; 50% of men with NGU will develop urethral symptoms within 4 days. Urethral discharge in NGU is cloudy or mucoid without gross purulence in 50% of males and 10–50% of men with NGU have a clear or only moderately visible discharge. Dysuria is present in 73–88% of males with gonorrhea, but only 53–75% of those with NGU. Therefore a male who presents with overt purulent urethral discharge and dysuria is more likely to have an infection with *N. gonorrhoeae*. On the other, hand a male with either dysuria or mucoid discharge is more likely to have NGU. Despite the clinical differences, accurate diagnosis cannot be made solely by clinical factors. Diagnosis requires microscopic examination of the discharge and usually, culture or antigen detection.[23]

Pharyngitis caused by *N. gonorrhoeae* is usually asymptomatic (90%) and occurs in 3–7% of heterosexuals and 10-25% of homosexual males.[26,27] Homosexual males are also at increased risk of *N. gonorrhoeae* proctitis (30–55%) which may have associated mucopurulent

Table 3   Clinical Manifestations of Gonorrhea

Population	Clinical manifestation	
	Uncomplicated	Complicated
Men	Urethritis	Prostatitis
	Pharyngitis	Epididymitis lymphangitis
	Proctitis	Seminal vesiculitis
	Conjunctivitis	DGI
Women	Cervicitis	PID
	Pharyngitis	Endometritis and parametritis
	Proctitis	Salpingitis and oophoritis
	Bartholinitis	Pelvic peritonitis
	Cystitis	Tubal or tubo-ovarian abscess
	Urethritis	Bartholins gland abscess
	Conjunctivitis	Perihepatitis and perisplenitis
		Periappendicitis
		DGI[a]
Neonates	Oropharyngeal infection	Ophthalmia neonatorum
		Neonatal sepsis
		Neonatal arthritis

[a] May include the following: arthritis-dermatitis syndrome, tenosynovitis, endocarditis, myocarditis, and meningitis.

From Evangelista, A.T. and Beilstein, H.R., Cumitech 4A, *Laboratory Diagnosis of Gonorrhea*, coordinating ed., Abramson, C., American Society for Microbiology, Washington, D.C., 1993. With permission.

rectal discharge, anorectal bleeding, tenesmus, and constipation.[26,27] Ocular infection in adult males is rare and usually due to autoinoculation. *N. gonorrhoeae* infections of the eye can be highly destructive and require aggressive treatment.[28]

Since the arrival of effective antimicrobial agents, complicated infections in men are rare.[13,27] About 10% of acute epididymitis is the result of *N. gonorrhoeae* urethritis, although it is a more frequent cause of epididymitis in males <35 years of age. Other complications such as penile lymphangitis, periurethral abscess, acute prostatitis, seminal vesiculitis, and urethral stricture are extremely rare in the industrialized nations.[27] Interestingly, it is likely that some of the gonococcal urethral stricture was actually caused by pre-antibiotic treatment with intraurethral caustic compounds.

4.4.2   Infections in women

Gonococcal infections in women are complicated because of the many anatomical sites which can be infected, frequent coinfections, and a wide range of clinical presentations from asymptomatic to symptomatic (Table 3). Symptomatic women with a lower genitourinary tract infection with *N. gonorrhoeae* may have vaginal discharge, intermenstrual uterine bleeding, and lower abdominal discomfort (often associated with PID). Since coinfection with *C. trachomatis*, *Candida albicans*, *T. vaginalis*, HSV, etc. are not uncommon, the specific symptoms associated with *N. gonorrhoeae* are not clear.[27,29] Additionally despite mucopurulent drainage from the endocervical canal, >25% of women with *N. gonorrhoeae* lower genitourinary tract infections will be asymptomatic. Recent information shows that certain auxotrophs of *N. gonorrhoeae* may result in 90% asymptomatic carriage of *N. gonorrhoeae*.[13] Therefore, in women the microscopic exam and identification of *N. gonorrhoeae* are critical to the diagnosis of gonorrhea.

N. gonorrhoeae is isolated most frequently from the cervix when purulent or mucopurulent discharge from the endocervical canal is present.[26] *N. gonorrhoeae* rarely infects the vaginal squamous epithelium in postpubescent women. The incubation period for gono-coccal cervicitis is around 10 days.[13] The physical exam may be normal, but many women will have cervical abnormalities with drainage and easily induced mucosal bleeding.[30] Patients with documented cervical infections may also have infections of the urethra and Skene's and Bartholin's glands. Urethral stripping may yield purulent material for Gram stain and culture.[29] Urethral infection is not usually found without *N. gonorrhoeae* cervicitis, except in women with prior hysterectomy.[27] Sexually active women with acute urethral syndrome (dysuria, frequency, and pyuria) should be examined for *N. gonorrhoeae* urethri-tis. Culture of a centrifuged urine specimen may contain small numbers of *N. gonorrhoeae* (10^2 CFUs/ml). Gonococcal proctitis is common and found in 35–50% of women with cervicitis with similar symptoms to those seen in males. Gonococcal pharyngitis is also present in 10-20% of heterosexual women with urogenital infection.

4.4.3   Complications of infection with N. gonorrhoeae

PID results from ascending cervical infections into the uterus and fallopian tubes.[13,27,29] Women usually experience persistent abdominal pain, although infections within the fallopian tubes (salpingitis) may be asymptomatic. Salpingitis can result in irreversible damage to the tubes, infertility, and ectopic pregnancy. Perihepatitis can also be present in women with salpingitis (Fitz-Hugh-Curtis syndrome). Patients usually complain of a sudden onset of pain in the right upper abdominal quadrant. If laparoscopy is performed patients demonstrate "violin string" adhesions between the liver and the anterior abdom-inal wall. A full discussion of these syndromes is beyond the scope of this discussion, but these severe sequelae of *N. gonorrhoeae* infections highlight the importance of sensitive diagnostic techniques, especially in the asymptomatic women.

Pregnant women with gonococcal infections have a higher incidence of intrapartum complications and can transmit the disease to their babies.[9] Clinical presentation of gon-orrhea in pregnant women is similar to those found in nonpregnant woman. Intrapartum gonococcal infection increases the risk for spontaneous abortion, acute chorioamnionitis, premature rupture of fetal membranes, delayed delivery after rupture of membranes, and premature delivery.[9,31] The prevalence of gonorrhea in pregnant women in industrialized nations is low (about 1%). In the developing countries it is estimated to be between 3–15% with >50% of infections with penicillinase-producing *N. gonorrhoeae* (PPNG).[32,33] Maternal infections in the U.S. may be underestimated, especially in the 15 to 19-year-old age group. A recent study in Dallas, TX found in adolescents going to an STD clinic pregnant women were just as likely to have gonorrhea as nonpregnant.[34] The implication is that neonates remain at substantial risk for gonococcal infections in groups where intrapartum infection is high. This fact plus the high percentage of asymptomatic infections, are strong argu-ments for enhanced screening programs for adolescent women at risk for gonorrhea.[9]

Pediatric gonococcal infections can be divided into those with maternal and perinatal sources and those infections acquired beyond infancy. Gonococcal infections of the new-born are uncommon in the U.S. and directly related to the effectiveness of screening programs for the pregnant mother.[9] Although exposure of the neonate to *N. gonorrhoeae* can result in many clinical presentations, gonococcal ophthalmia neonatorum is the most common syndrome. In the U.S. *C. trachomatis* is probably the most common cause of neonatal infectious conjunctivitis, and *N. gonorrhoeae* is the least common.[9] Clinically there is an overlap in symptoms and incubations periods, between gonococcal conjunctivitis and other forms of infectious conjunctivitis.[9] Therefore it is imperative that gonococcal infection is considered in all cases of neonatal conjunctivitis. Worldwide the incidence of neonatal gonococcal conjunctivitis may be as high as 23%.[33] Considering that worldwide there are 80 million births annually, prevention of gonococcal conjunctivitis would have a major impact on reduction of blindness.[32,33]

Infections beyond the first year of life are indications of early sexual activity or child abuse.[9] The nonestrogenized alkaline vaginal mucosa of prepubescent women can be infected with *N. gonorrhoeae* and should also be cultured in this group.[26] Child abuse is a critical issue in pediatric gonococcal infections. Accordingly, the laboratory must confirm all positive results with the use of two medically and legally accepted standards for the identification of *N. gonorrhoeae*.[35]

Disseminated gonococcal infection (DGI) occurs in 0.5–3% of persons with *N. gonorrhoeae* infections.[13] Dissemination can occur in persons with complement deficiencies and/or infection with virulent strains, e.g., AHU⁻ auxotypes, Por IA serovars, or serum-resistant strains. The effect of HIV infection on gonococcal disease is unclear, although acute gonococcal sepsis in HIV infected women have been reported.[36] DGI is the most common cause of infectious arthritis in young adults and must always be considered in the differential of septic arthritis. Women are at greater risk then men, especially during menstruation and in the second and third trimesters of pregnancy.[29] Gonococcal arthritis often has a biphasic arthritis-dermatitis syndrome.[13,25] Within a week of the onset of a DGI, patients will show migratory polyarthralgias involving the knees, elbows, and distal joints. In these patients joint effusions are rare and when an infusion is present it will have less than 20,000 WBC/mm³ and is usually sterile.[29] The skin may show sparse tender papules about 5–15 mm in diameter with pustular, hemorrhagic, or necrotic centers. Between 5 and 40 lesions are usually present and are found on the extremities.[13] Although often culture negative, skin lesions should have Gram stains and cultures. Mucosal cultures in 80% of patients with DGI will be positive and 50% of patients will have positive blood cultures.[29,37] In the second week skin lesions resolve, but arthritis progresses in one or two joints, usually the knee, ankle, elbow, or wrist.[13] The hallmark of this stage of the disease is a clinical presentation and purulent synovial fluid with 50,000–100,000 WBC/mm³ with 90% neutrophils. Blood cultures are usually negative, but synovial cultures are often positive.[25] Although rare some persons will develop either endocarditis or meningitis following DGI.[13,29]

4.5 *Laboratory diagnosis of* N. gonorrhoeae *infections*

Bacteriologic isolation of *N. gonorrhoeae* is still considered the gold standard laboratory technique to diagnose gonococcal disease. Interestingly, new data show that direct and amplified genetic probes may be more sensitive and specific than culture and may become a reasonable alternative.[38] Therefore when designing protocols for the diagnosis of gonorrhea, laboratorians must consider the clinical needs of an institution, the prevalence of the disease in the community, and the cost-benefit analysis of tests. Test performance is critical in choosing a diagnostic test for gonorrhea.[39] When a community has 1% prevalence of gonorrhea, a test with a sensitivity of 90% and a specificity of 99% will only have a positive predictive value (PPV) of 50%. This test in populations with low prevalence of gonorrhea, e.g., suburban women being screened at prenatal exam, would result in inappropriate use of antibiotics and psychological distress. A similar test in a high prevalence area might have a PPV of 91% and an NPV of 98.8%. False-positive tests would occur less frequently in this setting, e.g., urban STD clinic, and might be cost effective and useful in the reduction off gonococcal disease.

4.5.1 *Collection of specimens*

Successful culture of *N. gonorrhoeae* requires that the appropriate specimen be obtained from the correct anatomical site (Table 4). As discussed above, *N. gonorrhoeae* is a fastidious and fragile bacterium that will not tolerate drying or temperatures below 37°C. The most efficient way to maintain organism viability is to have the clinician inoculate bacteriologic

Table 4   Specimen Collection for Culturing *N. gonorrhoeae*

Patient category	Primary specimen site(s)	Additional specimen site(s)
Men heterosexual	Urethra	Oropharynx[a]
Men homosexual or bisexual	Urethra Anorectal region Oropharynx	
Women	Endocervix	Anorectal region[b] Urethra Oropharynx[a] Bartholin's gland Endometrium
Men and women with DGI	Blood (men and women) Urethra (men) Endocervix (women)	Oropharynx[a] Anorectal region[b] Joint aspirate[c] Skin lesion
Neonates	Conjunctiva	Orogastric aspirate Oropharynx Blood
Children (1–10 years)	Same as for adults	Same as for adults

[a] When there is a history of orogenital contact.

[b] When there is a history of anogenital contact.

[c] When an infected joint is suspected.

From Evangelista, A.T. and Beilstein, H.R., Cumitech 4A, *Laboratory Diagnosis of Gonorrhea*, coordinating ed., Abramson, C., American Society for Microbiology, Washington, D.C., 1993. With permission.

media when the specimen is obtained ("bedside inoculation"). This requires their cooperation and appreciation of the microbial nature of *N. gonorrhoeae*.

Before obtaining specimens it is important to make sure that the patient has not urinated in the last 2 h. Urine will reduce the organism load in the urethra and produce false-negative results. When obtaining a urethral specimen, male patients can be in a standing or supine position. Avoiding contamination from the external skin, a blatant purulent discharge can be obtained on swab. If a discharge is not readilty apparent the urethra can be gently stripped as described by McCormack.[23] This may produce a specimen adequate for Gram stain and culture. If no discharge is present the swab should be inserted into the urethra about 1–2 cm, left in place for 10–20 s, and gently rotated as it is removed (Figure 3A).[40] Sterile non-bacteriostatic saline can be used as lubricant. A small calcium alginate (Calgiswab) on a nylon or dacron swab with a plastic or aluminum shaft should be used. Routine transport swabs (Cary-Blair, Ames, etc.) should not be used for *N. gonorrhoeae* culture since it has been shown that the organisms die rapidly.[41]

Cervical specimens are obtained with aid of a speculum; warm water, not lubricant should be used to help place the speculum. Upon examination of the cervix excessive cervical mucus should be removed, followed by introducing a non-cotton swab into the cervical canal (Figure 3B).[40] The swab should be moved from side to side and left in place for 10–30 s and rolled on a culture plate. Urethral sampling may be helpful, especially in women who have had prior hysterectomy.[13] A purulent exudate may also be expressed from the female via gentle movement of a finger along the urethra. If no discharge is expressed, a swab may also be inserted into the urethra following the same instructions for a male urethral specimen.

Rectal swabs should be inserted about 3–4 cm, but fecal contamination should be avoided. Oropharyngeal swabs are taken from the posterior pharynx and tonsils.

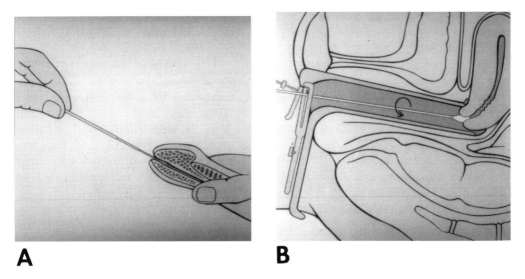

Figure 3 Obtaining specimens for culture of *N. gonorrhoeae*. (A) Obtaining specimen from the male urethra and (B) obtaining specimen from cervical os. (From Zenilman, J.M., Gonorrhea: clinical and public health issues, *Hosp. Prac.*, 28, 29, 1993. The McGraw-Hill Companies. Illustration by Nancy Lou Makris Riccio. With permission.)

Although less than 50% of patients with DGI will have positive blood cultures, the chance of recovery is best earlier in the course of the disease.[37] All *Neisseriae* are inhibited by the anticoagulant sodium polyanetholsulfonate which is in most commercial blood culture bottles. This inhibition can be overcome by the addition of 1% gelatin.[26] Joint aspirates should be rapidly transported to the laboratory for culture. Joint fluid should not be inoculated into blood culture bottles since it will decrease the sensitivity of the Gram stain and increases the chance of having a contaminant overgrow the *Neisseria*. Although prostatic fluid is usually negative for *N. gonorrhoeae*, culture should be done.

4.5.2 Media

It will be helpful to clinicians performing gonorrhea cultures if they have a simple culture system. Gonococcal media and their use are discussed in detail in many other publications and will be briefly discussed below.[26,42] The maximum culture sensitivity is achieved when a nonselective chocolate agar medium is used in addition to a selective media, e.g., Modified Thayer-Martin (MTM), Martin Lewis, GC-Lect, and NYC medium. Unfortunately, this is usually not practical or cost effective and most laboratories rely on a single selective gonococcal agar. Specimens from normally sterile sites, e.g., synovial, peritoneal, amniotic fluids, etc. do not require selective media and should be rapidly transported to the lab in an appropriate transport vial. All the selective media contain several antibiotics to inhibit normal genitourinary, pharyngeal, or rectal flora. MTM is probably the most widely used and commercially available medium, but lacks serum and has vancomycin concentrations (3 µg/mL) and 3–10% of *N. gonorrhoeae* strains will have their growth inhibited by this concentration of vancomycin.[43] Vancomycin inhibition of *N. gonorrhoeae* should be considered when smear-positive specimens fail to be confirmed by culture.[44] NYC medium is a clear formulation that incorporates horse blood and is more reliable for the recovery of unusual auxotrophs such as AUH⁻ strains.[45] Although NYC medium is commercially available, batch-to-batch variation can occur and it is about double the price of MTM media. GC-Lect medium is similar to MTM, but improves the recovery of fastidious strains.[46] This is accomplished by lowering the amount of vancomycin (2 µg/mL) and providing an enriched medium. In the STD clinic setting, any medium can be used cost effectively and efficiently by placing cultures in a humidified candle extinction jar that can be stored in a 35–37°C incubator. All gonorrhea media must be stored at 4°C and allowed to reach room temperature (25°C) before use. (Note: In a busy STD clinic it is not uncommon to see well-trained clinicans warming media in their pockets!)

In other settings, especially where gonorrhea cultures are taken intermittently, the JEMBEC (John E. Martin Biological Environmental Chamber) style plate is the most effiecint culture system.[47] This is a rectangular plate that can be filled with any gonococcal agar and provides a sufficient surface for specimen inoculation. A CO_2-generating tablet (sodium bicarbonate and citric acid) is placed within a designated area of the plate and the entire unit is placed into a small ziplock bag. The moisture from the plate, captured by the ziplock bag, activates the tablet thus producing a 5% CO_2 atmosphere. Gonococcal viability is well maintained using either the candle jar or the JEMBEC systems. If transport includes extreme temperatures, an insulated carrier should be used. If the cultures must be transported over long distances, cultures should be incubated 18–24 h before shipment and should arrive within 48 h. In the laboratory, JEMBEC can be removed from the ziplock bags and placed in the CO_2 incubator. Microbiologists can review JEMBEC cultures at a rapid pace (75–100 plates/h) and remove suspicious cultures for further identification. From the laboratory point of view, use of JEMBEC plates is an extremely cost-effective methodology.

4.5.3   *Gram stains*

Even in the best coordinated facilities some false-negative results occur due to fastidious organisms, vancomycin susceptibility, loss of viability in transport, and improper specimen collection. This makes the Gram stain of purulent material expressed from the urethra, cervix, rectum, or conjunctiva an important adjunct test in the diagnosis of gonorrhea. Gram stains from the other sites have not been evaluated.[27] When one considers a specimen with many PMNs and intracellular Gram-negative diplococci as positive for *N. gonorrhoeae* (Figure 4) and the absence of Gram-negative diplococci as negative, then a Gram stain can provide immediate diagnosis in many settings (Table 5).[27] The sensitivity and specificity of the Gram stain for positive smears obtained from males with symptomatic purulent urethritis are excellent, making culture an option. On the other hand, symptomatic males with small numbers of PMNs or extracellular Gram-negative diplococci require culture.[48] In asymptomatic males (contacts or tests of cure) the sensitivity and PPVs are lower and require culture. It is also a common misconception that Gram stain cannot be performed on cervical smears. As shown in Table 5, cervical Gram stain from symptomatic females has a relatively low sensitivity, but a high specificity for gonorrhea. Anorectal Gram stains are similar in test performance to cervical smears. This demonstrates that positive smears in patients at risk for gonococcal infection can also provide immediate diagnostic information. Additionally, smears that show extracellular organisms only are less likely to be culture confirmed as *N. gonorrhoeae*.[44] In all situations interpretation of smears must also take into consideration the likelihood of gonorrhea in a given population.

Because gonorrhea is an emotionally charged diagnosis, I think it is prudent to confirm all smears with a second diagnostic test. The smear provides an immediate result from which a clinician can make treatment decisions for patients they may not see a second time. Culture is cost effective when performed as described above, has the highest specificity, and provides an indicator on the quality of work being done in a medical facility. Cultures also enable a laboratory to identify the organism and to perform antimicrobial susceptibility testing. Meningococci have been shown to produce similar syndromes, especially in homosexual males, but could not be differentiated from gonococci on the basis of a smear.

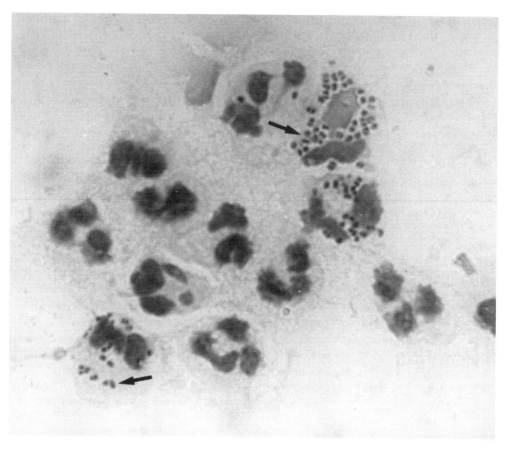

Figure 4   Gram stain from a symptomatic male with a purulent urethral exudate, STD Clinic, Pittsburgh, PA. Arrow = intracellular diplococci.

Table 5   Sensitivity and Specificity of Gram-Stained Smears for the Detection of Genital and Anorectal Gonorrhea

Site and clinical setting	Sensitivity	Specificity
Urethra:		
Men with symptomatic urethritis	90–95	95–100
Men with asymptomatic urethral infection	50–70	95–100
Endocervix:		
Uncomplicated gonorrhea	50–70	95–100
Pelvic inflammatory disease	60–70	95–100
Anorectum:		
Blind swabs	40–60	95–100
Anoscopically obtained specimens	70–80	95–100

From Hook, E.W. and Handsfield, H.H., Gonococcal infections in the adult, in *Sexually Transmitted Diseases*, K.K. Holmes, P.-A. Mardh, P.F. Sparling, P.J Wiesner, W Cates, S.M. Lemon, and WE. Stamm, Eds., McGraw-Hill, New York 1990, Chap. 14. With permission.

4.5.4   Direct detection of N. gonorrhoeae *antigen or DNA from specimens*

N. gonorrhoeae antigen or DNA detection methods have been developed as alternatives to routine Gram stains and cultures.[13,26,42] Three main assays are commercially available: (1) Gonozyme (Abbott Laboratories, North Chicago, IL) an enzyme immunoassay (EIA)

detection of *N. gonorrhoeae* outer membrane proteins, (2) Gonostat (Biotech Diagnostics, Baton Rouge, LA) which detects *N. gonorrhoeae* DNA in urethral, endocervical, and anorectal specimens by genetic transformation, and (3) Pace 2 (Gen-Probe, San Diego, CA), a direct DNA probe for *N. gonorrhoeae* rRNA. These diagnostic tests can be done rapidly, can be automated, and are not prone to problems of transport. The Gonozyme assay was one of the first antigen assays and one for which there is a sizable amount of data.[42] The Gonozyme performance was equivalent to the Gram stain for urethral specimens from symptomatic men. For asymptomatic males the sensitivity was about 70% and specificity was >95%. This indicates that a culture must also be included in the asymptomatic group and shows that this test would have a poor PPV in low incidence areas. In women, Gonozyme is more sensitive than Gram stains, 76% vs. 48%, respectively, but less sensitive and specific than culture.[26,42] Gonozyme does not have the sensitivity of a true screening test, nor the specificity of a confirmatory test, and its use should be limited where the cost can be justified due to insurmountable specimen transport problems. Gonostat uses a dry specimen swab from which DNA is extracted and used to transform a temperature-sensitive mutant strain that will not normally grow at 37°C. If *N. gonorrhoeae* DNA is present in the specimen the mutant will grow in 24–48 h indicating a positive result. Specimens must be sent to a central laboratory for analysis and they have not been as readily available for study, but appear to have good sensitivity and specificity.[26]

Pace 2 is a chemiluminescent DNA probe directed against *N. gonorrhoeae* ribosomal RNA. A specimen taken for the Pace 2 probe can be tested with both the *N. gonorrhoeae* and the *C. trachomatis* probes. A new Pace 2C combines probes against *N. gonorrhoeae* and *C. trachomatis* into one test. If the sensitivity and specificity for this product prove to be as good as the individual tests, this assay may become an extremely attractive screening test for two common STD problems. In symptomatic males the concordance between Pace 2 and Gram stain was 99.5%, but with an increased cost for Pace 2 of $5.00 per specimen.[48] Pace 2 did detect some extra cases in men who had few or no PMNs and may be justified in those cases. In one study of symptomatic and asymptomatic women the sensitivitiy and specificity of the Pace 2 was not different from culture and was better when screening a low prevalence group.[50]

The combo probe 2C performed very well with endocervical specimens with sensitivity and specificity of 96 and 98.8%, respectively.[51] This probe is designed to serve as a screen for both *N. gonorrhoeae* and *C. trachomatis* from which positive specimens can be confirmed using a specific probe or culture. All the discrepancies with negative culture and positive 2C probe (FP) were resolved using the DNA probe for the specific agent. The 2C only missed one *N. gonorrhoeae* and *C. trachomatis* (FN). A recently described ligase chain reaction outperformed culture in high and low prevalence groups and has a detection limit of 10–100 CFUs/ml compared to Pace 2 which requires 1000–10,000 CFUs/ml.[52]

4.5.5   *Identification and culture confirmation of* N. gonorrhoeae

Culture plates should be incubated between 48–72 h and examined on a daily basis.[26,41] Presumptive identification of *N. gonorrhoeae* from bacteriologic media requires the recognition of typical colony morphology, determination of positive oxidase reaction, and Gram stain demonstrating Gram-negative diplococci. On any chocolate-based medium, colonies are small, (0.5–1.0 mm in diameter) transparent to grayish-white with smooth glistening surfaces. AUH auxtrophs may be smaller (0.25 mm in diameter). Oxidase test is best performed by selecting a single colony on a sterile plastic or platinum bacteriologic loop. The colony is then inoculated onto a piece of filter paper impregnated with oxidase reagent or by selecting a colony on a swab and impregnating the swab with oxidase reagent. Oxidase positive colonies will turn purple within 10 s. A single colony should be used to prepare the Gram stain. Careful attention to the morphology should demonstrate a pure field of Gram-negative diplococci usually in pairs with flattened ends. Because *Kingella denitrificans* can grow on selective media and appear as diplococci and coccobacilli, careful attention to the Gram stain is necessary. *K. denitrificans* should not produce false-positive results with the confirmation tests.

Confirmation tests are broadly divided into growth dependent carbohydrate utilization tests and growth independent tests, e.g., rapid carbohydrate degradation, chromogenic substrates, combination biochemical tests, and immunologic and nucleic acid probes.[26,41] Most of the current tests are rapid and can be done on the same day an organism is presumptively identified. Accordingly, there is little need to issue preliminary reports and most *N. gonorrhoeae* isolates can be confirmed the same day they are isolated. These tests are discussed in detail in several references and it is important for laboratorians and clinicians to decide which tests should be used on specific specimens.[26,41] In our laboratory uncomplicated gonorrhea in adults involving the urogential tract or rectum are confirmed using a coagglutination technique. We have found that this technique is rapid, reliable, and cost effective and kits are available from several vendors. Fluorescent antibody techniques may be slightly more specific in comparison to coagglutination, but they require a fluorescent microscope and false-negative results have been reported.[53,54] Coagglutination specificity is reduced by cross reactions with *Neisseria lactamica*, but this problem is reduced when pharyngeal isolates are confirmed by an alternate technique. Chromogenic substrate systems are probably the most susceptible to false-positive results. Most commercially available reagents perform excellently when compared in large scale proficiency tests.[43,55]

All *N. gonorrhoeae* isolates from pharyngeal, pediatric, and known medicolegal cases should be confirmed by two tests, one of which should be a carbohydrate utilization or degradation test.[26,56,57] This increases the reliability of results from low prevalence groups and anatomical sites known to harbor nonpathogenic *Neisseria*. Carbohydrate utilization tests, using CTA sugars, require subculture of the *N. gonorrhoeae* isolate from selective media to nonselective chocolate agar. Additionally CTA sugars are prone to contamination, require a heavy inoculum, and must be incubated in a non-CO_2 incubator. Several rapid carbohydrate degradation or combinations of carbohydrate and enzyme tests are available. These tests use heavy inocula of bacteria to test for pre-formed enzymes. Several kits are commercially available which provide rapid identifications from selective agars.[58-60] These tests reduce some of the problems experienced with CTA sugars and have become widely used. The AccuProbe *N. gonorrhoeae* DNA probe can be used for culture confirmation and has been shown to be as sensitive and specific as carbohydrate degradation.[61] Note that this test is significantly more expensive than the other confirmatory tests.

4.6 N. gonorrhoeae *antimicrobial resistance and antimicrobial susceptibility testing*

Antimicrobial agents for gonorrhea should rapidly achieve blood and tissue concentrations well above the MICs of resistant strains, should be safe (especially in pregnancy and for nursing mothers), have minimal adverse side effects, and should be inexpensive. It is also desirable for these agents to be given in a single dose and be effective for pharyngeal and rectal gonorrhea incubating syphilis and *C. trachomatis*. The current recommendations for treatment of uncomplicated gonorrhea are shown in Table 6. Centers for Disease Control (CDC) treatment recommendations for other forms of gonococcal infections have been clearly described.[62]

Successful treatment of *N. gonorrhoeae* infections mirror the development of antibiotics and our understanding of microbial drug resistance.[63] Sixty years of antigonococcal chemotherapy clearly shows that when an organism's MICs increase against an antimicrobial,

Table 6   Treatment Recommendations for
Uncomplicated Gonococcal Infections

Recommended Regimens
Ceftriaxone 125 mg IM in a single dose
or
Cefixime 400 mg orally in a single dose
or
Ciprofloxacin 500 mg orally in a single dose
or
Ofloxacin 400 mg orally in a single dose
Plus
A regimen effective against possible coinfection with *C. trachomatis,* such as doxycycline 100 mg orally 2 times a day for 7 days.

From Centers for Disease Control and Prevention. 1993 Sexually Transmitted Diseases Treatment Guidelines, *MMWR,* 42 (No RR-14), 56–67, 1993.

there is a concomitant increase in the treatment failure.[64] This has been most clearly shown for penicillin G, once the main treatment for gonorrhea, and points out the need to closely monitor gonococcal resistance. Ceftriaxone, ciprofloxacin, and cefixime have all been shown to rapidly eliminate *N. gonorrhoeae* from urine, mucosa, and semen in males.[65] Patients treated for uncomplicated gonorrhea with the recommended regimens and who have symptomatic relief, need not return for test-of-cure.[62] Patients with persistent urethritis, cervicitis, or proctitis following appropriate treatment, should be screened for the reinfection or the possibility of a resistant *N. gonorrhoeae* isolate. Persistent infection with chlamydia or another organism (*Trichomonas, Ureaplasma, Candida,* etc.) may also be responsible for their return.

4.6.1   Current epidemiology of antibiotic resistance

Monitoring of *N. gonorrhoeae* antimicrobial susceptibility is accomplished by two major routes. The first involves routine laboratory susceptibility testing following standardized techniques.[66,67] Until 1990 the only standardized susceptibility test was β-lactamase testing to detect penicillinase-producing *N. gonorrhoeae* (PPNG). Currently standardized minimum inhibitory concentrations and disk diffusion zone sizes are available for cephalosporins, penicillin, tetracyclines, spectinomycin, and the quinolones. The second route uses national surveys to determine gonococcal antimicrobial susceptibility. These surveys were begun in the 1970s and have now been formalized into the Gonococcal Isolate Surveillance Project (GISP; Figure 5).[64,68] This project collects strains across the country, monitors temporal and geographic trends in susceptibility patterns, correlates patient characteristics and behavior with acquisition of resistant isolates, and develops treatment recommendations.

The prevalence of chromosomal- and plasmid-mediated resistance of *N. gonorrhoeae* are monitored by tracking resistance to penicillin and tetracycline. Plasmid-mediated penicillin resistance is characterized by positive β-lactamase test and tetracycline <16 μg/ml. Plasmid-mediated tetracycline resistant strains (TRNG) do not produce β-lactamase and have a tetracycline MIC ≥ 16 μg/ml and the penicillin MIC was ≤8 μg/ml. A strain can be resistant to both (PPNG-TRNG) and will produce β-lactamase and have a tetracycline MIC ≥ 16 μg/ml. Plasmid-mediated resistance to penicillin has decreased, while tetracycline has remained constant.[6] Chromosomally mediated resistant *N. gonorrhoeae* (CMRNG) results from a variety of genetic mutations and can produce resistance

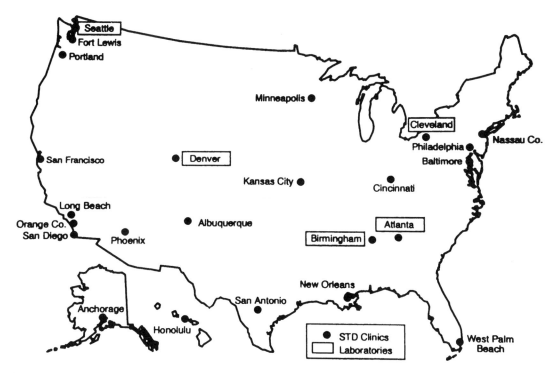

Figure 5   Gonococcal Isolate Surveillance Project [GISP] — location of participating clinics and regional laboratories. (From Division of STD prevention. *Sexually Transmitted Disease Surveillance, 1994.* U.S. Department of Health and Human Services, Public Health Service. Atlanta: Centers for Disease Control and Prevention, September 1995.)

to many different antibiotics.[68] CMRNGs are defined as strains which have penicillin, tetracycline, or cefoxitin MICs ≥ 2 µg/ml. Although this definition is somewhat arbitrary it has been observed that when MICs are ≥2 µg/ml, the treatment failure rate is in the 10–15% range. The presence of chromosomal resistance is not linked to plasmid-mediated resistance.[68]

In 1994, 30.5% of gonococcal strains were resistant to penicillin, tetracycline, or both. The percent of PPNG in the U.S. declined from 13.1% in 1991 to 7.8% in 1994, while TRNG has remained more stable (Figure 6). A similar pattern of changes was reported in NYC and indicates that reduced use of penicillin as treatment has had a profound effect in eradication of these strains. [69] Extremely high levels of PPNG are found in other countries where new inexpensive single-dose antimicrobial agents will be extremely important.[70] Nationally the percentage of chromosomally resistant isolates increased from 13.9% in 1990 to 16.2% in 1994 (Figure 7). Although no ceftriaxone-resistant *N. gonorrhoeae* have been recorded, it is important to monitor ceftriaxone MICs and treatment outcome.

4.6.2   Beta lactam antibiotics

The level of penicillin resistance has become large enough that the use of penicillin as a single-dose treatment without confirmation of susceptibility is no longer recommended for treating gonorrhea.[62] Nevertheless, penicillin had a major affect on treatment of gonorrhea because the treatment was so safe and effective. Review of the mechanisms of penicillin resistance is illustrative in two ways: first, it allows us to understand the mechanisms by which *N. gonorrhoeae* can acquire resistance and monitoring the spread of plasmid and chromosomal resistance will be helpful in monitoring gonococcal susceptibility to other antimicrobials.

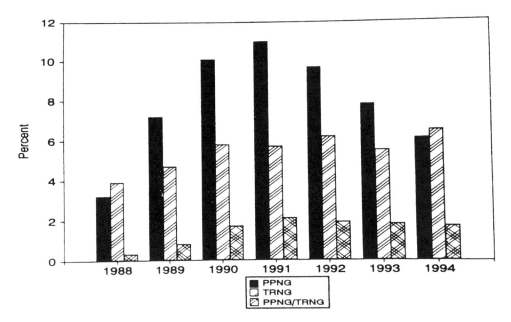

Figure 6   Trends in plasmid-mediated resistance, 1988–1994. (From Division of STD prevention. *Sexually Transmitted Disease Surveillance, 1994.* U.S. Department of Health and Human Services, Public Health Service. Atlanta: Centers for Disease Control and Prevention, September 1995.)

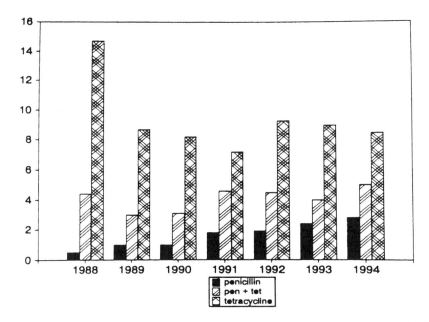

Figure 7   Trends in chromosomally mediated resistance, 1988–1994. (From Division of STD prevention. *Sexually Transmitted Disease Surveillance, 1994.* U.S. Department of Health and Human Services, Public Health Service. Atlanta: Centers for Disease Control and Prevention, September 1995.)

Chromosomal resistance is related to decreased cell permeability. The genes *mtr* and *env*, which are often found in rectal isolates, reduce permeability to toxic compounds and antibiotics.[13] The impact of CMRNG was described in a cluster of gonorrhea in North Carolina where all the isolates from 199 patients were found to have penicillin MIC of 2–4 µg/ml.[71] All the isolates were negative for β-lactamase, were similar by serotyping and antibiogram, and contained similar antibiotic loci (*pen* A, *pen* B, and *mtr*). Of these patients, 15 of the 16 failed treatment with 4.8×10^6 U penicillin with 1 g probenecid. Certain mutations that result in CMRNG also result in decreased *in vitro* susceptibility to other antimicrobial agents, including cefmetazole, cefuroxime, cefotetan, tetracycline, and erythromycin.[63] Interaction of the *pen*A, *pen*B mtr (multiple transformable resistance) produces a 16-fold increase in tetracycline MICs.[72]

Plasmid-mediated β-lactamase resistance to penicillin in *N. gonorrhoeae* (PPNG) was first reported in 1976 in the U.K. and North America. At least seven plasmids are responsible for β-lactamase activity of *N. gonorrhoeae*: a 4.2-kb pair cryptic plasmid, a large transfer plasmid, and five variations of a TEM-1 (5.1–7.2 kb). This latter plasmid produces a Richmond-Sykes class III enzyme that hydrolyzes penicillin and cephalosporins. The enzyme is inhibited by clavulonic acid and sulbactam and is common β-lactamase to *E.coli*, *Haemophilus* spp., *Neisseria* spp., *Salmonella* spp., *Shigella* spp., and *Pseudomonas* spp. European strains of PPNG were susceptible to tetracycline and linked to West Africa which had a 5.1 kb β-lactamase (African) plasmid and a 4.2-kb cryptic plasmid.[72] North American strains were linked to the Far East and were less susceptible to tetracyline and carried the 4.2-kb cryptic plasmid, a 7.2-kb β-lactamase plasmid (Asian) and the 39.2-kb transfer plasmid. The 7.2-kb plasmid can function in a wide host range and is homologous to other β-lactamase plasmids found in *Haemophilus spp.* The 39.2-kb transfer plasmid has now been recognized in North American and European strains. This plasmid also carries a tetracycline-resistant determinant (tetM) and can mobilize β-lactamase plasmid. Since 1976 the PPNG has spread worldwide, including many serotypes, auxotypes, and plasmid profiles. Chromosomal and plasmid resistance can be additive.[63] When a penicillin susceptible strain was transformed with a β-lactamase plasmid the MIC rose 32-fold, but when the same plasmid was inserted into a CMRNG the MIC rose 128-fold.

Cephalosporins have become the most important antibiotics for treating gonorrhea.[62,63] Ceftriaxone has been the main antibiotic used to treat gonorrhea because of its high intrinsic potency, long half life, good activity against urogenital, rectal, and pharyngeal gonorrhea, and no resistant isolates have been isolated. A single dose of oral cefixime is as effective as a 250 mg IM dose of ceftriaxone for uncomplicated gonococcal infections.[73] CMRNG may have ceftriaxone MICs in the 0.015–0.125 μg/ml vs. 0.0001–0.008 μg/ml for susceptible strains.[13] Routine doses of ceftriaxone still produce tissue levels over these higher MICs. No gonococcal resistance to ceftriaxone has been reported following 10 years of extensive study. The possibility that *N. gonorrhoeae* might acquire a β-lactamase active against ceftriaxone points out the need to systematically monitor susceptibility of *N. gonorrhoeae*.

4.6.3   Alternative antimicrobial agents active against N. gonorrhoeae

Tetracyclines were at once considered alternative gonococcal therapy when penicillin could not be used.[63] Successful treatment required multiple doses and in 1984 high level plasmid-borne resistance to tetracycline was recognized in the U.S. The spread of this plasmid, along with chromosomal resistance has made tetracyclines unreliable in the treatment of gonorrhea. Spectinomycin, an aminoglycoside, was developed and sold for treatment of gonorrhea. It is still considered an official alternative when patients cannot tolerate a cephalosporin or quinolone, but is likely to be less important if azithromycin is approved for use in uncomplicated gonococcal infections. Azithromycin, an oral macrolide with less gastrointestinal toxicity than erythromycin, is extremely active against *N. gonorrhoeae*. Although not yet recommended for use against gonorrhea, this drug has many ideal characteristics for treating gonorrhea, including activity against *C. trachomatis* and single-dose regimens. Susceptibility testing guidelines for azithromycin have recently been published and it is noteworthy that no azithromycin resistance was found.[74] Quinolones (ciprofloxacin and ofloxacin) have become important alternatives to cephalosporin therapy. Early studies in Africa demonstrated ciprofloxacin was safe and effective therapy for gonococcal urethritis for PPNG and CMRNG in HIV-infected men.[75] Unfortunately quinolone resistance has been reported in Asia[76,77] and now in the U.S.[78] In the U.S. documented treatment failures and transmission by commercial sex workers were also documented. This portents rapid spread of these resistant strains and the need to closely monitor quinolone susceptibility and treatment failures. The CDC has also recommended changes in susceptibility standards for ciprofloxacin and ofloxacin. Strains with MICs of ≥1.0 and ≥2.0, respectively, should be considered resistant. Previous disk diffusions standards had no breakpoints for resistant strains. The CDC also recommends that the standards include resistance breakpoints of ≤29 mm for ciprofloxacin and ≤24 mm for ofloxacin.

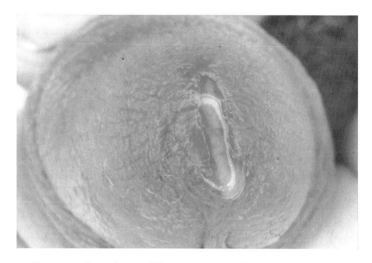

Gonococcal urethritis. (Photo courtesy of A.W. Hoke, M.D.)

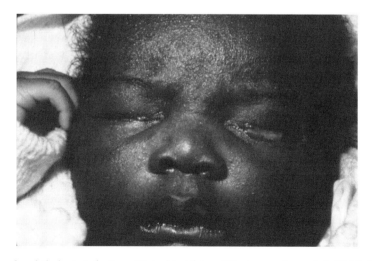

Gonococcal ophthalmic infection, Nairobi, Africa. (Photo courtesy of A.W. Hoke, M.D.)

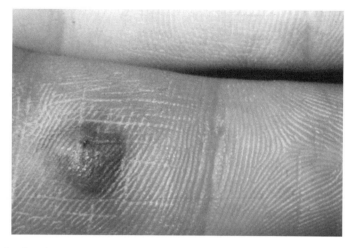

Lesion from gonococcemia. (Photo courtesy of A.W. Hoke, M.D.)

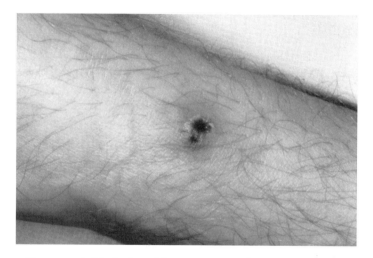

Gonococcal skin lesion. (Photo courtesy of A.W. Hoke, M.D.)

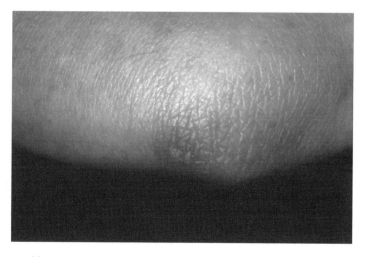

Gonococcal bacteremia and hemorrhage. (Photo courtesy of A.W. Hoke, M.D.)

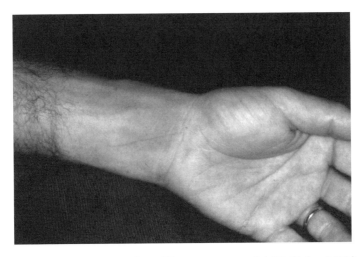

Tenosynovitis in gonorrhea. (Photo courtesy of A.W. Hoke, M.D.)

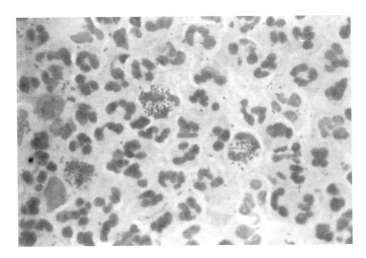

Urethral smear with gonococci. (Photo courtesy of K.A. Borchardt, Ph.D.)

References

1. Kampmeier, R.H., Identification of the gonococcus by Albert Neisser, *Sex. Trans. Dis.*, 5, 71, 1978.
2. Bøvre, K., Neisseriaceae, in *Bergey's Manual of Systematic Bacteriology*, Krieg, R.R. and Holt, J.G. Eds., Williams & Wilkins, Baltimore, 1984, page 288.
3. Knapp, J.S. and Rice, R.J., *Nesisseria* and *Branhamella*, in *Manual of Clinical Microbiology*, 6th ed., Murray, P.R. Editor-in-Chief, American Society for Microbiology, Washington, D.C., 1995, Chap. 26.
4. Vedros, N.A., *Neisseria*, in *Bergey's Manual of Systematic Bacteriology*, Krieg, R.R. and Holt, J.G. Eds., Williams & Wilkins, Baltimore, 1984, page 290.
5. Division of STD prevention, *Sexually Transmitted Disease Surveillance, 1994*. U.S. Department of Health and Human Services, Public Health Service. Atlanta: Centers for Disease Control and Prevention, September 1995.
6. Centers for Disease Control and Prevention, Recommendations of the International Task Force for disease eradication, *MMWR*, 42, RR-16, 1993.
7. Centers for Disease Control and Prevention, Summary of notifiable diseases, United States, 1994, *MMWR*, 43[53]: pages 29-31, 1995.

8. Rice, R.J., Roberst, P.L., Handsfield, H.H., Holmes, K.K., Sociodemographic distribution of gonorrhea incidence: implications for prevention and behavioral research., *Am. J. Public Health,* 81, 1252, 1991.

9. Gutman, L.T., Gonococcal infection, in *Infectious Diseases of the Fetus and Newborn Infant,* Remington, J.S. and Klein, J.O., Eds., W.B. Saunders, Philadelphia, 1995, Chap. 29.

10. Nassif, X., and So, M., Interaction of pathogenic Neisseriae with nonphagocytic cells, *Clin. Microbiol. Rev.,* 8:376-388, 1995.

11. Salyers, A.A. and Whitt, D.D., *Bacterial Pathogenesis: A Molecular Approach,* ASM Press, Washington, D.C., 1994, Chap. 20.

12. Seifert, H.S., Wright, C.J., Jerse, A.E., Cohen, M.S., Cannon, J.G., Multiple gonococcal pilin antigenic variants are produced during experimental human infections, *J. Clin. Invest.,* 93, 2744, 1994.

13. Handsfield, H.H. and Sparling, P.F., *Neisseria gonorrhoeae,* in *Principles and Practice of Infectious Diseases,* Mandell, G.L., Bennett, J.E., and Dolin, R., Churchill Livingstone, NY, 1995, Chap. 190.

14. Jerse, A.E., Cohen, M.S., Drown, P.M., Whicker, L.G., Isbey, S.F., Seifert, H.S., Cannon, J.G., Multiple gonococcal opacity proteins are expressed during experimental urethral infection in the male, *J. Exp. Med.* 179, 911, 1994.

15. Plummer, F.A., Chubb, H., Simonsen, J.N. et al., Antibody to Rmp [outer membrane protein 3] increases susceptibility to gonococcal infection, *J. Clin. Invest.,* 91, 339, 1993.

16. Sarafian, S.K. and Knapp, J.S., Molecular epidemiology of gonorrhea, *Clin. Microbiol. Rev.,* 2S, S49, 1989.

17. Knapp, J.S. and Holmes, K.K., Disseminated gonococcal infections caused by *Neisseria gonorrhoeae* with unique nutritional requirements, *J. Infect. Dis.,* 132, 204, 1975.

18. Bohnhoff, M., Morello, J.A., Lerner, S.A., Auxotypes, penicillin susceptibility and serogroups of *Neisseria gonorrhoeae* from disseminated and uncomplicated infections, *J. Infect. Dis.,* 154, 225, 1986.

19. Brunham, R.C., Plummer, F., Slaney, L., Rand, F., DeWitt, W., Correlation of auxotype and protein I type with expression of disease due to *Neisseria gonorrhoeae, J. Infect. Dis.,* 152, 339, 1985.

20. Camarena, J.J., Nogueira, J.M., Dasi, M.A., Moreno, F., Garcia, R., Ledesma, E., Llorca, J., Hernandez, J., DNA amplification fingerprinting for subtyping *Neisseria gonorrhoeae* strains, *Sex. Trans. Dis.,* 22, 128, 1995.

21. Poh, C.L., Ocampo, J.C., Sng, E.H., Bygdeman, S.M., Rapid *in situ* generation of DNA restriction endonuclease patterns for *Neisseria gonorrhoeae, J. Clin. Microbiol.,* 27, 2784, 1989.

22. Xia, M., Whittington, W.L., Holmes, K.K., Plummer, F.A., Roberts, M.C., Pulsed-field gel electrophoresis for genomic analysis of *Neisseria gonorrhoeae, J. Infect. Dis.,* 171, 455, 1995.

23. McCormack, W.M. and Rein, M.F., Urethritis, in *Principles and Practice of Infectious Diseases,* Mandell, G.L., Bennett, J.E., and Dolin, R., Eds., Churchill Livingstone, New York, 1995, Chap. 88.

24. Jacobs, N.F. and Kraus, S.J., Gonococcal and nongonococcal urethritis in men, *Ann. Intern. Med.,* 82, 7, 1975.

25. Gantz, N.M., Brown, R.B., Berk, S.L., Esposito, A.L., Gleckman, R.A., *Manual of Clinical Problems in Infectious Disease,* Little, Brown, Boston, 1994, Chap. 27.

26. Evangelista, A.T., Beilstein, H.R., Cumitech 4A, Laboratory diagnosis of gonorrhea, Abramson, C., Coordinating Ed., American Society for Microbiology, Washington, D.C., 1993.

27. Hook, E.W. and Handsfield, H.H., Gonococcal infections in the adult, in *Sexually Transmitted Diseases,* K.K. Holmes, P.-A. Mardh, P.F. Sparling, P.J Wiesner, W. Cates, S.M. Lemon, and W.E. Stamm, Eds., McGraw-Hill, New York, 1990, Chap. 14.

28. Bruins, S.C. and Tight, R.R., Laboratory-acquired gonococcal conjunctivitis, *JAMA,* 241, 274, 1979.

29. Karchmer, A., Sexually transmitted diseases, in *Scientific American, Medicine,* Rubenstein, E. and Federman, D.D., Eds., Scientific American, New York, New York, 1994, Chap. 22.

30. Curran, J.W., Rendtorff, R.C., Chandler, R.W., Wiser, W.L., Robinson, H., Female gonorrhea. Its relation to abnormal uterine bleeding, urinary tract symptoms and cervicitis, *Obstet. Gynecol.,* 45, 195, 1975.

31. Gutman, L.T. and Wilfert, C.M., Gonococcal diseases in infants and children, in *Sexually Transmitted Diseases,* K.K. Holmes, P.-A. Mardh, P.F. Sparling, P.J Wiesner, W. Cates, S.M. Lemon, and W.E. Stamm, Eds., McGraw-Hill, New York, 1990, Chap. 14.

32. Laga, M., Meheus, A., Piot, P., Epidemiology and control of gonococcal ophthalmia neonatorum, *Bull. WHO,* 67, 471–477, 1989.

33. Isenberg, S.J., Apt, L., Wood, M., A controlled trial of povidone-iodine as prophylaxis against ophthalmia neonatorum, *N. Eng. J. Med.,* 332, 562, 1995.

34. Schultz, J.M., Brown, G.R., Haley, C.E., Haley, R.W., Ferris, R., Green, H.G., Anderson, R.J., Initial STD visits by adolescent females, Dallas, County, Texas, *Tex. Med.,* 89, 56, 1993.

35. Whittington, W.L., Rice, R.J., Biddle, J.W., Knapp, J.S., Incorrect identification of *Neisseria gonorrhoeae* from infants and children, *Pediatr. Infect. Dis. J.,* 7, 3, 1988.

36. Jacoby, H.M and Mady, B.J., Acute gonocccal sepsis in an HIV-infected women, *Sex. Trans. Dis.,* 22, 380, 1995.

37. Case records of the Massachusetts General Hospital, # 44-1993, Gonococcemia, *N. Eng. J. Med.,* 329:1411, 1993.

38. Chapin-Robertson, K., Use of molecular diagnostics in sexually transmitted diseases, *Diag. Microbiol. Infect. Dis.,* 16, 173, 1993.

39. Galen, R.S. and Gambino, R.S., Screening for gonorrhea, how the model defines essential criteria for an efficient screening test, in *Beyond Normality*: The Predictive Value and Efficiency of Medical Diagnosis, News York, Wiley, 1975.

40. Zenilman, J.M., Gonorrhea: clinical and public health issues, *Hosp. Prac.,* 28, 29, 1993.

41. Knapp, J.S. and Rice, R.J., *Neisseria* and *Branhamella,* in *Manual of Clinical Microbiology,* 6th edition, Murray, P.R. Editor-in-Chief, American Society for Microbiology, Washington, D.C., 1995, Chap. 26.

42. Mardh, P.-A. and Danielsson, D., *Neisseria gonorrhoeae,* in *Sexually Transmitted Diseases,* K.K. Holmes, P.-A. Mardh, P.F. Sparling, P.J Wiesner, W. Cates, S.M. Lemon, and W.E. Stamm, Eds., McGraw-Hill, New York, 1990, Chap. 73.

43. College of American Pathologists, Bacteriology Survey Set D-A, Final Critique, pg. 5, 1994.

44. Goodhart, M.E., Ogden, J., Zaidi, A.A., Kraus, S.J., Factors affecting the performance of smear and culture test for the detection of *Neisseria gonorrhoeae, Sex. Trans. Dis.,* 9, 63, 1982.

45. Faur, Y.C., Weisburd, M.H., Wilson, M.E., May, P.S., Field evalutation of New York City medium in the biological environment-CO_2 chamber in recovery of *Neisseria gonorrhoeae* and urogenital mycoplasmas, *J. Clin. Microbiol.,* 5, 137, 1977.

46. Evans, G.L., Kopyta, D.L., Crouse, K., New selective medium for the isolation of *Neisseria gonorrhoeae, J. Clin. Microbiol.,* 27, 2471, 1989.

47. Martin, J.E. and Jackson, R.L., A biological environmental chamber for the culture of *Neisseria gonorrhoeae, Sex. Trans. Dis.,* 2, 28, 1975.

48. Kraus, S.J., Semiquantitation of urethral polymorphonuclear leukocytes as objective evidence of nongonococcal urethritis, *Sex. Trans. Dis.,* 9, 52, 1982.

49. Juchau, S.V., Nackman, R., Ruppart, D., Comparison of Gram stain with DNA probe for detection of *Neisseria gonorrhoeae* in urethras of symptomatic males, *J. Clin. Microbiol.,* 33, 3068, 1995.

50. Panke, E.S., Yang, L.I., Leist, P.A., Magevney, P., Fry, R.J., Lee, R.F., Comparison of Gen-Probe DNA probe test and culture for the detection of *Neisseria gonorrhoeae* in endocervical specimens, *J. Clin. Microbiol.,* 29, 883, 1991.

51. Iwen, P.C., Walker, R.A., Warren, K.L., Kelly, D.M., Hinrichs, S.H., Linder, J., Evaluation of the nuleic acid-based test (PACE 2C) for simultaneous detection of *Chlamydia trachomatis* and *Neisseria gonorrhoeae* in endocervical specimens, *J. Clin Microbiol.,* 33, 2587, 1995.

52. Ching, S., Lee, H., Hook III, E.W., Jacobs, M.R., Zenilman, J., Ligase chain reaction for detection of *Neisseria gonorrhoeae* in urogenital swabs, *J. Clin. Microbiol.,* 33, 3111, 1995.

53. Dillon, J.R., Carballo, M., Pauze, M., Evaluation of eight methods for identification of pathogenic *Neisseria* species: Neisseria-Kwik, RIM-N, Gonobio-test, Minitek, GonoGen, Phadebact monoclonal GC OMNI test and Syva MicroTrak test, *J. Clin. Microbiol.,* 26, 493, 1988.

54. Mohan, S.K., Monoclonal fluorescent antibody negative, non betalactamase-producing *Neisseria gonorrhoeae, Clin. Microbiol. Nwsl.,* 14, 24, 1992.

55. New York State Bacteriology Proficiency Survey, Bacteriology survey September 1995, Final Critque, pg. 13, 1995.

56. College of American Pathologists, Rapid microbial detection survey Set ID-B, Final Critique, pg. 2 1994.

57. College of American Pathologists, Rapid microbial detection survey Set ID-B, Final Critique, pg. 4 1995.

58. Phillip, A. Garton, G.C., Comparative evaluation of five commercial systems for the rapid identification of pathogenic *Neisseria* sp., *J. Clin. Microbiol.*, 22, 101, 1985.

59. Janda, W.M., Malloy, P.J., Schreckenberger, P.C., Clinical evaluation of the Vitek *Neisseria-Haemophilus* identification card, *J. Clin. Microbiol.*, 25, 37, 1987.

60. Janda, W.M., Branda, J.J., Ruther, P., Identification of *Neisseria* spp., *Haemophilus* spp. and other fastidious Gram-negative bacteria with the MicroScan *Haemophilus-Neisseria* Identification panel, *J. Clin. Microbiol.*, 27, 869, 1989.

61. Lewis, J.S., Kranig-Brown, D., Trainor, D.A., DNA probe confirmatory test for *Neisseria gonorrhoeae*, *J. Clin. Microbiol.*, 28, 2349, 1990.

62. Centers for Disease Control and Prevention, Sexually transmitted diseases treatment guidelines, *MMWR*, 42, (No. rr-14), 1993.

63. Fekete, T., Antimicrobial susceptibility testing of *Neisseria gonorrhoeae* and implications for epidemiology and therapy, *Clin. Microbiol. Rev.*, 6, 22, 1993.

64. Jaffe, H.W., Biddle, J.W., Thornsberry, C., Johnson, R.E., Kaufman, R.E., Reynolds, G.H., Wiesner, P.J., the cooperative study group, National gonorrhea therapy monitoring study, *in vitro* antibiotic susceptibility and its correlation with treatment results, *N. Eng. J. Med.*, 294, 5, 1976.

65. Haizlip, J., Isbey, S.F., Hamilton, H.A., Jerse, A.E., Leone, P.A., Davis, R.H., Cohen, M.S., Time required for elimination of *Neisseria gonorrhoeae* from the urogenital tract in men with symptomatic urethritis: comparison of oral and intramuscular single-dose therapy, *Sex. Trans. Dis.*, 22, 145, 1995.

66. Jones, R.N., Gavan, T.L., Thronsberry, C., Fuchs, P.C., Gerlach, E.H., Knapp, J.S., Murray, P., Washington, J.A., Standardization of disk diffusion and agar dilution susceptibility tests for *Neisseria gonorrhoeae*: ionterpretive criteria and quality control guidelines for ceftriaxone, penicillin, spectinomycin, and tetracycline, *J. Clin. Microbiol.*, 27, 2758, 1989.

67. National Committee for clinical laboratory standards, Performance standards for antimicrobial susceptibility testing, M100-S6, Vol 15, No. 14, National Committee for clinical laboratory standards, Villanova, PA, 1995.

68. Schwarcz, S.K., Zenilman, J.M, Schnell, D., Knapp, J.S., Hook, E.W., Thompson, S., Judson, F.N., Holmes, K.K., National surveillance of antimicrobial resistance in *Neisseria gonorrhoeae*, *JAMA*, 264, 1413, 1990.

69. Cummings, M.C., Covino, J.M., Smith, B.L., Ratiu, E.S., Draft, K., McCormack, W.M., Susceptibility of isolates of *Neisseria gonorrhoeae* to penicillin and tetracycline in Brooklyn, 1988–1992, *Sex. Trans. Dis.*, 22, 110, 1995.

70. Knapp, J.S., Brathwaite, A.R., Hinds, A., Duncan, W., Rice, R.J., Plasmid-mediated antimcirobial resistance in *Neisseria gonorrhoeae* in Kingston, Jamaica: 1990–1991, *Sex. Trans. Dis.*, 22, 155, 1995.

71. Faruki, H., Kohmescher, J.R.N., McKinney, W.P., Sparling, P.F., A community-based outbreak of infection with penicillin-resistant *Neisseria gonorrhoeae* not producing penicillinase (chromosomally mediated resistance), *N. Eng. J. Med.*, 313, 607, 1985.

72. Mortensen, J.E., Antimicrobial resistance mechanisms in *Neisseria* spp. and *Moraxella* spp., *Clin. Microbiol. Nwsl.*, 17, 57, 1995.

73. Handsfield, H.H., McCormack, W.M., Hook, E.W., Douglas, J.M., Covino, J.M., Verdon, M.S., Reichart, C.A., Ehret, J.M., gonorrhea treatment study group, A comparison of single-dose cefixime with ceftriaxone as treatment for uncomplicated gonorrhea, *N. Eng. J. Med.*, 325, 1337, 1991.

74. Mehaffey, P.C., Putnam, S.D., Barret, M.S., Jones, R.N., Evaluation of *in vitro* spectra of activity of azithromycin, clarithromycin, and erythromycin tested against strains of *Neisseria gonorrhoeae* by reference agar dilution disk diffusion and E-test methods, *J. Clin. Microbiol.*, 34, 479, 1996.

75. Bryan, J.P., Hira, S.K., Brady, W., Luo, N., Mwale, C., Mpoko, G., Krieg, R., Siwiwaliondo, E., Reichart, C., Waters, C., Perine, P.L., Oral ciprofloxacin versus ceftriaxone for the treatment of urethritis from resistant *Neisseria gonorrhoeae* in Zambia, *Antimicrob. Agent Chemother.*, 34, 819,1990.

76. Tanaka, M., Matsumoto, T., Kobayashi, I., Uchino, U., Kumazawa, J. Emergence of *in vitro* resistance to fluoroquinolones in *Neisseria gonorrhoeae* isolated in Japan, *Antimicrob. Agents Chemother.*, 39, 2367, 1995.

77. Tapsall, J.W., Limnios, E.A., Thacker, C., Donovan, B., Lynch, S.D., Kirby, L.J., Wise, K.A., Carmody, C.J., High level quinolone resistance in *Neisseria gonorrhoeae*: a report of two cases, *Sex. Trans. Dis.*, 22, 310, 1995.

78. Centers for Disease Control and Prevention, Fluoroquinolone resistance in *Neisseria gonorrhoeae* — Colorado and Washington, 1995, *MMWR*, 44, 761, 1995.

chapter five

Donovanosis

Mauro Romero Leal Passos, José Trindade Filho, and Nero Araújo Barreto

5.1   Introduction..103
5.2   History 103
5.3   Etiology...104
5.4   Epidemiology..106
5.5   Clinical picture...107
5.6   Clinical classification 108
5.7   Laboratorial diagnosis...108
      5.7.1   Collection, transportation, and conservation of clinical samples.................109
      5.7.2   Direct examination...109
      5.7.3   Culture 109
5.8   Histopathology 109
5.9   Differential diagnosis...110
5.10 Therapy 110
References...115

5.1   Introduction

A large bibliography revision (national and foreign) has been done with Donovanosis' actualization including information about history and recent therapeutics. Donovanosis is a bacterial disease of chronic evolution, not very contagious, characterized by ulcerated, painless, and autoinoculated granulomatous lesions, caused by *Calymmatobacterium granulomatis*. It mainly assails the skin and subcutaneous cell tissue of the genital and perianal areas and inguinal region, implicating with less frequency other regions of the skin, mucosa, or even the internal organs. Many denominations were proposed for this disease: inguinal granuloma, venereum granuloma, tropicum granuloma, pudendi tropicum granuloma, contagious granuloma, ulcerating granuloma, sclerosing granuloma, chronic venereum ulcer, and granuloma donovani.[17]

5.2   History

Donovanosis was described for the first time in 1882 by McLeod, in Madras, India, who named it serpiginous ulcer.[46]

In 1905, Donovan, mentioned by Trindade Filho, demonstrated the causative agent of the disease, and therefore considered it in the protozoa group. The disease then went by the name ulcerating granuloma of the pudenda.

In a very well established work, Aragão and Vianna, studying patients assisted by Domingos de Goes, Fernando Terra, Eduardo Rabello, Daniel de Almeida, and Werneck Machado in the Hospital da Misericordia do Rio de Janeiro, published in 1913 their conclusions about the etiological agent, also proposing the name *Calymmatobacterium granulomatis*.

At present, the etiological name of Donovanosis,[10] or granuloma inguinale, as many prefer, is accepted worldwide. Therefore, the articles that mention the researchers who in 1913 proposed this terminology are very rare.

In 1926, McIntosh, in a study about the etiology of Donovanosis, tried experimentally to reproduce the disease in a volunteer through the subcutaneous inoculation of the granulation tissue infected by corpuscle of Donovan.

In 1939, Greenblatt inoculated the pus of a pseudobubo of a patient with Donovanosis into a volunteer, obtaining in this lesion and posterior, a demonstration of the parasite.

Anderson, mentioned by Trindade Filho, in 1943, established the bacterial nature of Donovan's bodies, when he cultivated the microorganism in the vitelline embryonic yolk sac.

In 1950, Marmell and Santora created the term Donovanosis, in homage to Donovan.

5.3   Etiology

The *Calymmatobacterium granulomatis* was described for the first time by Donovan in 1905, when he performed many studies of morphology and coloration, demonstrating the intracellular parasitism of small rods, thick and halter shaped. Observing his patients, he admitted the possibility of the microorganism being a protozoa.

In 1913, in their studies, Aragão and Vianna mention the following:

> The aspect of the granuloma's microbe is very special. It sometimes presents itself in the shape of small cocci (coccuses) of 2–3 tenths of a diameter, surrounded by a capsule, and sometimes in the shape of rods, round extremities, measuring about 0.5–1 μ long, also surrounded by a very limited capsule or unprovided of it. Besides this shape in rods, other shapes with the halters or diplococo aspects is also always encapsulated according to the phase, more less advanced in the fission. The rods, halters, and diplococcus shapes belong to sequential phases of transversal bipartition of the germ. In the advanced phases of the segmentation of the microbe, the capsule also divided, straightening itself in the central part. The repose shapes of the germs are round and measure, with the capsule, 1–1.5 μ, and the ones in the fission phase are oval and measure 2–2.5 μ. The repose shapes of the germs are usually less numerous than the ones in segmentation period. Because of the special morphology of the germ of the granuloma and specially because of the particular and proper process of its fission, different from what we observe in other bacterias, we thought it would be proper to put the microbe of the granuloma in a special gender of bacterias denomination for which we proposed the name *kalymmabaterium* (from Kalymma manto) which must be amended to *Calymmatobacterium* and the species which occupies us will be denominated *Calymmatobacterium granulomatis*.

The structure of the germ, as we described, appears clearly only in the stained preparation by Giemsa and when a supercoloration is not done, neither is the preparation less stained.

Other researchers besides Donovan, around 1931, tried, and were not able to reproduce the disease in various laboratory animals, inoculating material rich in "corpuscles of Donovan." Therefore, they rejected the hypothesis of it being a protozoa and yes a Gram-negative, incapsuled bacteria, which could be also found in excrements of some patients.

Although it is traditional to accept the *Calymmatobacterium granulomatis* as the causative agent of Donovanosis, we know very little about the determinant of the disease and the responsible factors for the pathogenic expression of this bacteria. Even with the possibility of the disease being produced with human contaminated material with certain regularity, frequently the microorganisms that develop in appropriate culture media do not reproduce the same clinical manifestation when inoculated in human volunteers.

The case published by McIntosh is reported as the first experimental reproduction of the disease, which inoculated in human volunteer, granulation tissue of patient infected with Donovanosis.

In 1939, Greenblatt and colleagues, repeating McIntosh's experience, were able to reproduce the disease in four volunteers using material from pseudobuboes, without obtaining the growth of any microorganism from the coriollantoid membrane of chick embryos.

In 1943, Anderson obtained the growth of the bacteria in the chick embryonic yolk sac. Therefore, he did not obtain the reproduction of the disease in laboratory animals or human beings with this material.

During this century, the microorganism received other names, such as *Donovania granulomatis* and *Klebsiella granulomatis* despite the research of Brazilians Aragão and Vianna. After detailed bacteriological, clinical, and therapeutic studies, the bacteria was called *Calymmatobacterium granulomatis*.

They are Gram-negative rods, sometimes coccobacillis, measuring 0.5–1.5 µ wide by 1.0–2.0 µ long, presenting round extremities. They are steadfast and have a polysaccharide and fibrous capsule. Curiously, they demonstrate a chromatin condensation in one or both extremities, proposing characteristic shapes in "halters" or "safety pins" when stained by Giemsa or Wright. The microorganism stains with greater intensity in the extremities than in the center, varying from deep blue to black, and its capsule, red.

They appear isolated or form bunches in the interior of big mononuclear macrophages, being found also in extracellular space. The cellular wall is Gram-negative, similar to the *Klebsiella's* wall, although, it has not yet demonstrated any correlation to this bacteria.

Through electronic microscopy it was possible to observe that in its intracytoplasmatic parasitism, the bacteria presented a momogeneous capsule, limiting the cellular membrane constituted by three layers.[8]

The determination of intracytoplasmatic glandules is interpreted by some as bacteriophages[8,9,11] and by Monif as important structures in the origin of the disease; without them the infection would not occur.

Kuberski gives a different interpretation to the mentioned structures, affirming that they would result as a simple invagination of bacterial cell wall and not as bacteriophage particles adherent to the cellular wall.

The demonstration of viral material inside the *C. granulomatis* is very significant, suggesting the possibility of Donovanosis being a bacterium modified by phagocytosis, which occurs with the *Corynebacterium diphiteriae*. The modification by phago may be the necessary prerequisite to transform the fecal bacterial contamination to state of disease.[33]

Antigenetically, the *Calymmatobacterium granulomatis* demonstrates cross-reactivity with species of the *Klebsiella* gender, of which the *K. rhinocleromatis*, agent of the rhinoscleroma, is the best example.[9]

5.4 Epidemiology

The sexually transmitted nature of Donovanosis is controversial, seeming to be, by clinical and epidemiological observations, that it is not only transmitted by sexual intercourse. Strong arguments indicate the importance of sexual contact: (1) the lesions are more frequent in the genital or anal region; (2) the disease is more frequent at the most sexually active age rate of people; and (3) the anal localization of the disease in male homosexuals.[46]

Other arguments, however, indicate the possibility of transmission of the disease without sexual intercourse, such as: (1) the existence of lesions in children who are not sexually active; (2) the lack of lesion on a conjugal partner, while the other spouse presents the disease, sometimes even with an exuberant characteristic; (3) the evidence of no assailant of the disease, even in endemic areas (India, China) among people with multiple sexual relations, such as prostitutes; (4) the emergence of extragenital lesions localized in areas of the body which apparently have very little participation in sexual intercourse.

Authors such as Dienst and colleagues mentioned by Jardim, affirm that contact with bearers of Donovanosis does not always result in infection in a normal person, and that the skin, healthy or scraped, does not seem to enhance the transmission of the disease. The authors also point out that the experiences with infection are only positive when pieces from the sick tissue or pus aspirated from pseudobuboes were implanted or inoculated on subcutaneous tissue of human volunteers.

The disease is often frequent in tropical regions, but there are some endemic areas in other countries, such as India, China, Sri Lanka, Malaysia, Australia, New Guinea, South Africa, Zambia, Morocco, Madagascar, and French Guyana.[46]

Ramachander believes that the agent of Donovanosis is a germ, resident in the intestines, passing over to the genital, anal, and inguinal areas, where the emergence of the lesions would be determined. The transmission of the disease would be done through anal intercourse or by the lack of hygiene.

Despite Donovanosis being known worldwide as "tropical disease," we are of the opinion that this probable racial and/or geographical predisposition would be closely connected to socioeconomical and hygieniel factors. In habitational models of megacities, where it is possible to find "ghettos" of subhuman lives, even in rich countries, associated with the emergence of AIDS, it is now possible to verify that the disease known as "tropical," are happening worldwide. To use, it has very little to do directly with race and geographical localization of the sick people, but with the conditions in which these people live.

Although many authors affirm that the disease attacks more individuals of the male sex, the tendency today is to consider that it affects both men and women. Some authors, such as Lal (1970), Lynchg (1978), and Kubersky (1980), observed more cases among men, while Bhagwandeen (1977), Passos (1986), and Benzaken and Sardinha (1995) reported that the majority of their cases belonged to the female sex.

Other authors refer that the disease is more frequent among male homosexuals. Marmell, in 1958, mentioned by Goldberg, presents ten cases of Donovanosis, of which nine were homosexuals.[9] Reviewing the literature, he found a report of 48 cases with anal lesions, of which 44 revealed the practice of pederasty.

As for the age, all of them say that the absolute majority of the cases assailed young adults (20–40 years of age) which constitutes the age rate that presents greater sexual activity.

The reports of assailment on children and aged people are rare.

5.5   Clinical picture

The incubation period is variable according to many authors. To Rajam and Rangiah the period is 2 weeks to 1 month; Greenblatt and colleagues, 42 to 50 days; and Lal and Nicholas, 3 days to 6 months.

The disease begins as single or multiple subcutaneous nodules which erode through the skin, producing very well-defined ulceration that grows slowly and bleeds readily on contact. From this point, the manifestations are directly linked to the tissue responses of the host, originating localized or extensive forms and, may even be visceral lesions through hematogenic dissemination.[19]

In the male sex the lesions occur more often on the penis (prepare, glans, and balanoprepucial sulcus) and scrotum. In the female sex they are more likely to assail the labia minora, vulva, vagina, cervix, and pubis.

In most of the cases of Donovanosis registered in literature localization is restricted to cutaneous areas and mucosa of the genitalia and anal, perianal, and inguinal regions, where the lesion generally initiates as a small papule or painless nodule that ulcerates and grows as it develops. Through autoinoculation, satellite lesions emerge and join, reaching great areas.

The bottom of the lesion is soft and beefy red. The edges are irregular, elevated, well defined, and indurated. In recent lesions, the bottom is filled with serobloody secretion, while in old lesions, the surface of the lesions becomes granulated and the secretion is seropurulent and has a fetid odor. The occurrence of general symptoms or adenopathies is very rare.

The lesion can be present as a vegetating mass or tends to form fibrous or keloid tissues, sometimes leading to deformity of the genitalia, paraphimosis, or elephantiasis. Subramanian registers a case of granuloma inguinale and sclerosing granuloma inguinale on the penis of a 21-year-old heterosexual patient.

The long developing lesions can suffer secondary contamination through other microorganisms. Likely to occur are extensive and deep ulceration and necrosis of the soft tissues with subsequent fistulas and mutilation.

The inguinal localization (pseudobubo) can lead to a mix diagnosing the adenitis with that occurring in lymphogranuloma venereum, syphilis, and chancroid.

The extragenital Donovanosis represents a casualty in 3–6% of cases, almost all of them proceeding from endemic areas.[39]

The localization of the disease out of the anogenital site can be explained, according to Brigden, by the following: (1) hematogenous dissemination to organs, such as the liver, lungs, bones, and spleen; (2) continuity or contiguity to adjacent pelvic organs; (3) lymphatic dissemination; (4) autoinoculation.

Packer relates a case of Donovanosis with secondary osseous lesions of the tibia to distal extremity of the second metacarpal in which the primary lesion, similar to neoplasia, was localized in the vagina, cervix, and bladder.

Ishida, defending a master thesis at Universidade Federal do Rio de Janeiro, presents a case of systemic Donovanosis, also with osseous lesions. The patient reported homosexual behavior. Testing for anti-HIV antibodies was positive. A few years later, the patient developed AIDS, opportunistic infections, and death.

Endicott reports a case of Donovanosis of orbital localization with osseous implication.

Kirkpatrick and Brigden also emphasize the assailment of secondary osteological lesions.

Sehgal published a Donovanosis case which he considers an example of non-venereum transmission in adults, since the lesions were restricted to arms, face, and neck, without any evidence of lesions on the genital, inguinal, or oral regions.

Some publications emphasize the implication of the cervix, fallopian tubes, and ovary through Donovanosis.[7,30,36,38]

On men, the lesion can, through contiguity, assail the epididymis, as in the case reported by Marmell, in which the primary lesion was localized on the penis of a patient who also had pulmonary tuberculosis.

Brigden's publication mentions two cases of extragenital lesions. A case of a 41-year-old woman, with a history of fever, night sweats, and weight loss associated with edema on the inferior extremity of the legs. The examination of the genitalia evidenced a primary lesion of Donovanosis, which was localized in the vaginal introitus. The other case was a 47-year-old man who presented with lesions on the inferior abdominal wall and four fistulas, of which two of them were linked to the intestines. The primary lesion of the patient was localized on the glans and in the inside of the prepuce. The clinical picture got worse and the patient died.

Murugan reports a case of a 33-year-old patient with vaginal bleeding in which the lesion was localized on the cervix and in the inside of the vagina.

Scrimgeour published a case of an 18-year-old patient, in New Guinea who presented with a primary localization of Donovanosis on the endometrium and endocervix, parametrium, fallopian tubes, and ovary, complicated by an obstruction of the ureter and bilateral hydronephrosis. Lesions of the cervix, labia, and anus emerged after curettage of the endometrium for diagnostic purposes.

The localization of the oral cavity is not common, with very few reported cases.[13,39]

Hematogeneous dissemination occurs when conditions of the host are favorable for the formation of microorganisms, almost always in serious cases proceeding from endemic areas, as in the case published by Kalstone, in female patients, with destructive lesions of the vertebral body.

Attempting a new didatic systematization, Jardim proposed a clinical classification which we find interesting.[10]

5.6   Clinical classification

1. Genitals and perigenitals
   1.1. Ulcerous
   1.2. With hypertrophic edges
   1.3. With plane edges
   1.4. Ulcerovegetating
   1.5 Vegetating
   1.6 Elephantiasic
   1.7 Extragenital
   1.8 Systemic

Despite all the clinical information presented before, currently we know that the granuloma inguinale, as any other infectious disease, in HIV-positive patients and mainly in patients with AIDS, can assume a completely abnormal clinical development. This situation can complicate both diagnosis and treatment.

5.7   Laboratorial diagnosis

The correct diagnosis can be performed if appropriately selected laboratorial techniques are used to confirm the presumptive clinical aspects.

5.7.1 Collection, transportation, and conservation of clinical samples

The nonexistence of the *C. granulomatis* available in culture collections complicates the knowledge of its relation with the environment and hosts, phylogenetic studies with composition of bases C+G, nutritional demands, as well as repetition for transportation and conservation of samples.

It has been confirmed that the tissue is an excellent transportation and conservation medium of viable bacteria for a certain time, especially for those that need a low potential for oxidation-reduction. For this reason, the most adequate clinical material are fragments of subsuperficial tissue of an active granulation area. For a better exploitation, it is suggested to collect five to six tissue samples of different areas, radially, right below the edges of the lesions. The biopsy should be obtained before cleaning the lesion and removing necrotic tissue with saline solution and sterilized gauze, to finish contamination. Scrapings from the base of the lesion or exudate aspirated from pseudobuboes can also be used.[11]

5.7.2 Direct examination

From smears, scrapings, or lesions distended in lamina, dried or fixed with methyl alcohol, colored with Giemsa or Wright stains, one can observe in the interior of rods histocytes gathered in bunches, inside vacuoles or not, in "halters" or "safety pin" shapes because of the condensed chromatin in its extremities — corpuscles of Donovan. These metachromatic chromatin traces vary from deep blue to purple, and sometimes black. Stained this way, a thick and red capsule revesting the microorganism can be identified.

5.7.3 Culture

The *C. granulomatis* is difficult to cultivate and demands special growth nutrients and factors for its development. It can be cultivated *in vivo* in the chick embryonic yolk sac and *in vitro* in culture means enriched with egg yolk. Either way, it is always arduous, expensive, and of low reproducibility. For its growth, an environment with low potential for oxidation reduction, pH between 7.2–7.4, temperature at 35–37°C, and incubation period varying from 48–72 h is necessary.

5.8 Histopathology

The granulation picture is the histopathological picture. The epidermis is absent or atrophic, mainly in the center of the lesion. The biopsy must be done, preferentially on the edge of the lesion, where the pathological modifications are more substantial. Then the epidermis gets hypertrophic, sometimes reaching a state of pseudoepitheliomatous hyperplasia.

On the dermis there is a dense infiltration with the predominance of histocytes or macrophages and plasmocytes having inwardly, abscesses formed by neutrophils and a few lymphocytes.

The coloration usually made by hematoxylin eosin is not ideal for demonstration of Donovan's bodies in the interior of histocytes or macrophages.

Lever suggests, for better evidence of Donovan's bodies, make histological cuts with a density of 0.5 μ and stain them with toluidine blue. The Donovan's bodies appear as dark oval structures localized inside vacuoles. These structures can also exist outside the cells.

The differential histological diagnosis can be done with rhinoscleroma, histoplasmosis, leishmaniosis, and carcinoma of squamous cells.

5.9   Differential diagnosis

Many pathologies can be clinically assimilated to Donovanosis: primary syphilis, chancroid, lymphogranuloma venereum, neoplasia, condyloma acuminatum, leishmaniosis, deep mycosis, cutaneous tuberculisis, atypical myobacteriosis, and cutaneous amebiasis. The differentiation can be obtained through demonstration the specific casual agent or histopathological examination.[38]

The clinical similarity with carcinoma[38] can sometimes lead to confusion of diagnosis and therapy conduct, although real carcinoma can emerge, secondarily, from lesions of Donovanosis or can coexist with the disease.[1,38,42]

Goldberg tested the serum of a patient with carcinoma on the penis, with histological diagnosis, to determine antibodies against *C. granulomatis,* concluded by the April 23, 1996, activity of the agent.

In our experience we have examined both male and female patients for sexually transmitted diseases (STD) who had chronic and ulcerated lesions. The major clinical suspicion in males was of cancer of the penis and not a STD. Most lesions were of more than two years duration in patients more than sixty years of age.

Once more our attention is drawn to HIV-positive patients or AIDS patients, in whom the genital lesions of STD can assume a variety of clinical conformations. As a common example we can mention genital herpes, which in these situations, is usually presented as extensive, very painful, ulcerated lesions of long evolution.

5.10   Therapy

Even with various antimicrobial medications available today, it is still very difficult to treat bacterial diseases.

In a significant work in the beginning of the century, Aragão and Vianna reported difficulties treating granuloma inguinale. At the time the use of local, antiseptic, or caustic applications, general treatments with mercury, potassium iodide, 606, and others was very common. Surgery recommended was complete extirpation of the lesion whenever possible. Only one treatment was effective, the use of X-rays. This method was not often used because it depended on complicated equipment which was not always available, along with the inconvenience and time required to produce the cure of the granuloma.

This way, these two researchers tested the vaccine therapy with the microorganism they isolated from the granuloma, but they did not obtain the coveted success.

Because Vianna had already succeeded in treating cutaneous ulcerations caused by *Leishmania* with intraveneous injections of tarter emetic (tartrate of antimony and potassium), Aragão and Vianna decided to test such a product in eight cases of granuloma inguinale. In all cases there was a complete cure of the lesions.

McIntosh mentions other products, such as lithium thyomalate, antimony, and gentian violet.

The emergence of modern antimicrobials, sulfas (1930s), and penicillin (1940s), brought greater possibilities of obtaining quicker and more efficacious cures with less collateral effects. Therefore, even with today's huge therapeutic arsenal, various patients in many situations still suffer and present with a complete cicatrization of the lesions. For many reasons, some patients die before successful treatment.

To have the medications in existence does not mean to have the medications in every region, in every health service, or to have it for all cases (dosage and duration of the treatment).

In our experience, patients who presented with granuloma inguinale, in particular, are difficult to manage and assist, maybe because the lesions in general do not present pain and have a slow evolution, which may propitiate a more tolerable cohabitation between the parasite and the host. Another important fact is that patients are frequently people of low socioeconomical, cultural, intellectual, and hygiene status.

In cases that we studied, more than 80% of sexual partners examined did not present any suspicion of infection.

Therefore, as with Aragão and Vianna, the majority of patients assisted by us were hospitalized. For many, it may seen absurd nowadays to hospitalize a patient with granuloma inguinale, therefore, we believe that if such a procedure is possible, the cure can be obtained more frequently. That is because it will be possible to control the correct use of medications and assure adequate nourishment and hygiene.

There is a varied therapeutic arsenal for the treatment of granuloma inguinale. The medications can be used alone or in associations:

- Streptomycin: 1 g/day, Im, 20–30 days.
- Sulfametoxazole: 800 mg + trimethoprim 160 mg, 12/12 h, orally 20–30 days.
- Tetracycline: 500 mg, 6/6 h, orally 30–60 days.
- Doxycycline: 100 mg, 12/12 h, orally 30–60 days.
- Erythromycin: 500 mg, 6/6 h, orally 30–60 days.
- Chloramphenicol: 500 mg, 6/6 h, orally 15 days.
- Tianfenicol: 500 mg, 8/8 h, orally 15–20 days.
- Gentamycin: 30 mg, 12/12 h, IM 15 days.
- Ampicillin: 500 mg, 6/6 h, orally 20–30 days.
- Amoxicillin: 500 mg, 8/8 h, orally 20–30 days.
- Lincomycin: 500 mg, 6/6 h, orally 20–30 days.

The association of lincomycin with amoxicillin may be very effective.

Passos (1986) and Jardim (1990) obtained good results by treating Donovanosis with granulated Tianfenicol.

With the recent emergence of new macrolides, drugs of low toxicity which are very well tolerated, mainly Azithromycin which has excellent permanency on the tissues, are being tested. The therapeutic results were encouraging.[4]

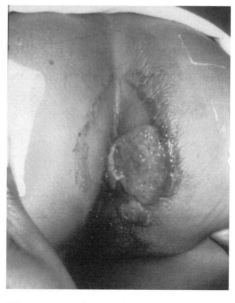

Figure 1 Perianal lesion — Donovanosis.

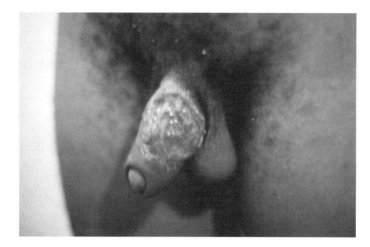

Figure 2 Donovanosis.

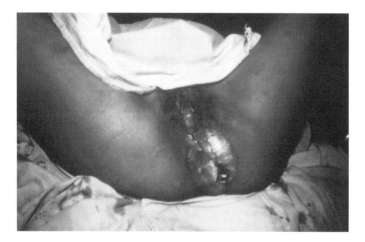

Figure 3 Perineal and perianal lesions — Donovanosis.

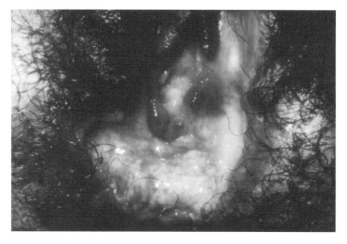

Figure 4 Perineal localization — Donovanosis.

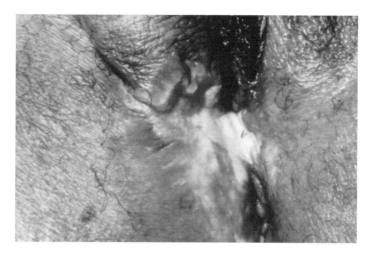

Figure 5 Perineal Donovanosis.

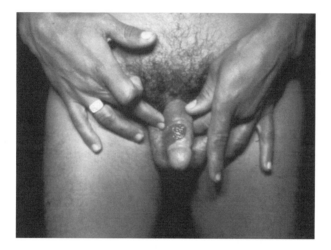

Figure 6 Donovanosis.

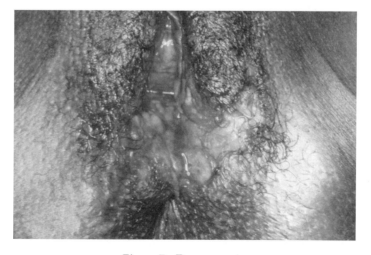

Figure 7 Donovanosis.

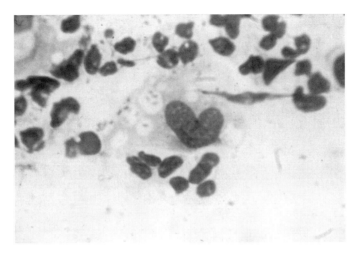

Figure 8   Donovan corpuscles.

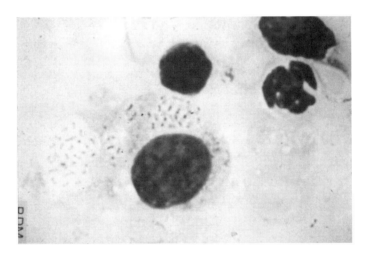

Figure 9   Donovan corpuscles.

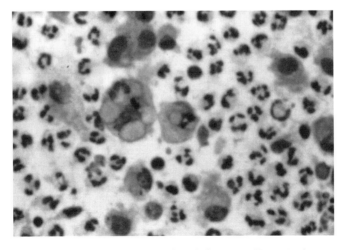

Figure 10   Donovan corpuscles. Coloration: Papanicolaou.

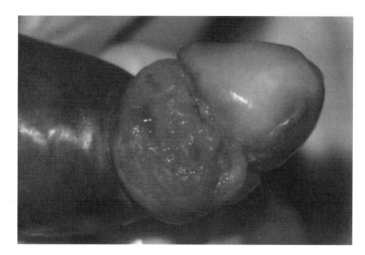

Figure 11   Penis cancer in 78-year-old man; an important differential diagnosis with Donovanosis.

References

1. Alexander, L.J. Squamous cell carcinoma of the vulva secondary to granuloma inguinale. *Arch. Derm. Syph.* 67:395–402, 1953.

2. Anderson, W.A.D. *Pathology.* St. Louis: C.V. Mosby, 1948, p. 313.

3. Aragão, H.B. and Vianna, G. Pesquisas sobre o Granuloma venéreo. Mem Inst. Oswaldo Cruz, Tomo V: 211–38, 1913.

4. Arevelo, C., Hernandez, I., and Ferreiro, M.C. Donovanosis (Granuloma Inguinale, Granuloma Venereum) Treated With Azitromycin. Eleventh Meeting of the International Society For STD Research. Abstract Monograph, no. 371 p. 208. New Orleans, 1995.

5. Benzaken, A.S. and Sardinha, J.C.S. Donovanosis in Women: A Retrospective Ten Year Study in Manaus, Amazonas, Brazil. Eleventh Meeting of the International Society For STD Research. Abstract Monograph, no. 370, p. 207, 1995.

6. Bhagwandeen, B.S. and Nailk, K.G. Granuloma venereum (granuloma inguinale) in Zambia, *East Afr. Med. J.V.* v. 54, no. 11 p. 637–42, 1977.

7. Brigden M. and Guard R. Extragenital granuloma inguinale in North Queensland, *Med. J. Aust.* 2:565–7, 1980.

8. Davis, C.M. and Collins, C. Granuloma inguinale: An ultrastructural study of Calymmatobacterium granulomatis. *J. Invest. Dermatol.* 53 (5): 315–21, 1969.

9. Davis, C.M. Granuloma inguinale. *JAMA.* 211(4): 623–36, 1970.

10. Dienst, R.B. and Brownell, G.H. Genus Calymmatobacterium Aragão & Vianna 1913. In: Krieg, N.R. and Holt, J.C. editors. *Bergery's Manual of Systematic Bacteriology,* v. 1. Williams & Wilkins, Baltimore, p. 585–87, 1984.

11. Dodson, R.F. Donovanosis: A morphologic study. *J. Invest. Dermatol.* 62(6): 611–4, 1974.

12. Endicott, J.N., Kirkconnell, W.S., and Beam, D. Granuloma inguinale of the orbit with bony involvement. *Arch. Otolarynol.* 96:457, 1972.

13. Garg, B.R., Lal, S., Bedi, B.M.S., Ratnam, D.V., and Maik, D.N. Donovanosis (Granuloma Inguinale) of the oral cavity. *Br. J. Vener. Dis.* 51:136–7, 1975.

14. Goldberg, J. and Bernstein, R. Studies of Granuloma Inguinale. VI. Two cases of perianal Granuloma Inguinale in male homosexuals. *Br. J. Vener. Dis.* 40:137, 1964.

15. Goldberg, J. and Annamunthodo, H. Studies on granuloma inguinale. VIII. Serological reactivity of sera from patients with carcinoma of penis when tested with Donovania antigens. *Br. J. Vener. Dis.* 42:205, 1966.

16. Greenblatt, R.B., Dient, R.B., and Torpin, R. Experimental and clinical granuloma inguinale. *JAMA,* 113(12):1109–16, 1939.

17. Hart, G. *Donovanosis in Sexually Transmitted Diseases Holmes.* In: March P.A., Sparling, P.F. and Wiesner, P.J., McGraw-Hill, New York, 1984.

18. Ishida, C.E. *Donovanose,* Rio de Janeiro, UFRJ, CCS, Tese, 1988.

19. Jardin, M.L. Donovanose. In: Naud, P. *Doencas Sexualmente Transmissíveis e AIDS*, Artes Médicas, Porto Alegre, 1993.
20. Jardin, M.L. Donovanose. Proposta de classificacão clinica. *An. Bras. Dermatol.* 62(3):169–72, 1987.
21. Jardin, M.L. Tratamento da Donovanose com tiafenicol. *An. Bras. Dermatol.* 65(2):93–4, 1990.
22. Joseph, A.K. and Rosen, T. Laboratory techniques used in the diagnosis of chancroid, granuloma inguinale and lymphogranuloma venereum. *Dermatol. Clin.* 12(1):1–8, 1994.
23. Kalstone, B.M., Howell, J.A. Jr., and Cline, F.X. Jr. Granuloma inguinale with hematogenous dissemination to the spine. *JAMA,* 176(6):530–2, 1961.
24. Kirkpatrick, D.J. Donovanosis (Granuloma inguinale). A rare case of osteoytic bone lesions. *Clin. Radiol.* 21:101, 1970.
25. Kuberski, T., Papadimitriou, J.M., and Philips, P. Ultrastructure of *Calymmatobacterium granulomatis* in lesions of granuloma inguinale. *J. Infect. Dis.* 142(5):744–9, 1980.
26. Lal, S. and Nicholas, C. Epidemiological and clinical features in 165 cases of granuloma inguinale. *Br. J. Vener. Dis.* 46:461, 1970.
27. Lever, W.F. and Schaumburg-Lever, G. *Histopathology of the Skin.* 5th ed. Philadelphia, J.B. Lippincott Company, 1975.
28. Lynchg, P.J. Sexually transmitted disease: granuloma inguinale lymphogranuloma venerium, chancroid and infectious syphilis. *Clin. Obstet. Gynecol.* v. 21, no. 4, p. 1041–52, 1978.
29. Marmell, M. and Santora, E. Donvanosis — granuloma inguinale. Incidence, nonmenclature, diagnosis. *Am. J. Syph. Gonor. Vener. Dis.* 34:83, 1950.
30. Marmell, M., Fielding, W.I., and Weintraub, S. Danovanosis — Granuloma of tubes and ovary treated with Aureomycin and surgery. *J. Obstet. Gynecol.* 63(4):893–5, 1952.
31. Marmell, M., Ultmann, R., and Weintraub, S. Donovanosis of the Epididymis complicating tuberculous infection. *J. Urol.* 70(5):776–80, 1953.
32. McIntosh, J.A. The etiology of granuloma inguinale. *JAMA* 87(13):996–1002, 1926.
33. Monif, G.R.G. Doencas Infecciosas em Obstetricia e Ginecologia. IV. Bactérias 76–82, Ed. Guanabara-Koogan, Rio de Janeiro, 1974.
34. Murugan, S., Venkatran, K., and Renganatham, P.S. Vaginal bleeding in granuloma inguinale. *Br. J. Vener. Dis.* 58:200–1, 1982.
35. Packer, H., Tuner, H.B., and Dulaney, A.D. Granuloma inguinale of the vagina, and cervix uteri with bone metastases. *JAMA* 136(5):327–9, 1948.
36. Pariser, R.J. Tetracycline — Resistant Granuloma Inguinale. *Arch. Dermatol.* 113:988, 1977.
37. Passos, M.R.L. et al. Donovanose: Um novo tratamento. II Congresso Mundial de DST. junho, Paris, 1986.
38. Pereira, A.C. Jr., Almeida, B.B., and Nascimento, L.V. Donovanose. *An. Bras. Dermat.* 2(3):305–12, 1977.
39. Rabello, F.E. and Fraga, S. Atlas de Dermatologia. Fundamentos da Medicina Cutânea. Rio de Janeiro. Ed. Guanabara-Koogan, 1970.
40. Rajam, R.V. and Rangiah, P.N. Donovanosis. World Health Orgnization Monograph 24, Geneva, 1954.
41. Ramachander, M. and Tulasi, V.R. Granuloma venereum and ABO blood groups. *Ind. J. Dermatol. Venerol.* 38(4): 176–8, 1972.
42. Schwartz, R.H. Chancroid Granuloma inguinale. *Obstet. Gynecol.* 26(1):138–42, 1983.
43. Scrimgeour, E.M., Semgrupta, S.K. and McGoldrick, I.A. Primary endometrial and endocervical granuloma inguinale (Donovanosis). *Br. J. Vener. Dis.* 59:198–201, 1983.
44. Sehgal, V.N., Sharma, N.L., Bhargava, N.C., Nayar, M., and Chandra, M. Primary extragenital disseminated cutaneous Donovanosis *Br. J. Dermatol.* 101:353–6, 1979.
45. Subramanian, S. Sclerosing granuloma inguinale. *Br. J. Vener. Dis.* 57:210–2, 1981.
46. Trindade Filho, J. Donovanose. In: Passos, M.R.L. DST-Doencas Sexualmente Transmissíveis, 4 ed. Cultura Médica, Rio de Janeiro, 1995.

chapter six

Lymphogranuloma venereum

René Garrido Neves and Omar Lupi da Rosa Santos

6.1   Introduction..117
6.2   History 117
6.3   Etiopathological aspects...118
6.4   Epidemiology...118
6.5   Clinical manifestations 119
6.6   Diagnosis 122
6.7   Treatment 124
    6.7.1   Antibiotics 124
    6.7.2   Surgery 124
6.8   Prognosis...124
References...126

6.1   Introduction

Lymphogranuloma venereum (LGV) is an acute to chronic sexually transmitted infectious disease with transient genital lesions followed by significant regional lymphadenopathy as well as systemic manifestations. LGV may progress to late fibrosis and tissue destruction in untreated cases. The causative organism is *Chlamydia trachomatis*. It is more frequent in tropical and subtropical climates, in areas of low socioeconomic development, or great sexual promiscuity. The disease was given numerous names and it has been known since antiquity by the Romans, which called it *struma* and it was called *althaun* by the Arabians.[1] The more modern denominations always tried to point out its main characteristics: regional adenopathy, almost always inguinal; subacute evolution; suppuration in multiple focus; and a possible climatic influence. The designations for LGV or Nicolas-Favre-Durand disease are pointed out as tropical bubo, climatic bubo, d´emblé bubo, scrofulous bubo, benign suppurative inguinal paradenitis, epidemic inguinal lymphadenopathy, sub-acute inguinal lymphogranulomatosis, and inguinal lymphogranuloma.[2,3]

6.2   History

The first description of LGV is attributed to Wallace who, in 1833, described the disease in the subtropical and tropical regions of Africa and Asia. The importance of adenitis was admitted by Chassaigne (1859) and Valpeau (1865), but the perfect individualization of the disease was effected by Nelaton (1890). Leyers proposed that LGV was a clinical variant of tuberculosis (1894). Marion and Gandy proposed the same etiology due to the LGV histopathological picture (1901). Only in 1913, did Durand, Nicolas, and Favre definitely establish a conception of the disease, rejecting the etiology of tuberculosis and identifying the venereum origin.

In 1905, Frei carried out the intradermal test with the antigen prepared with the pus from the lymph nodes. Grace (1930) obtained the antigen of the LGV after intracerebral inoculation of mice and Rake et al. (1940) produced the antigen after a culture performed in the yolk sacs of embryonated eggs. Page (1968) characterized two species of chlamydias.

6.3   Etiopathological aspects

Chlamydias are Gram-negative intracellular obligatory parasites, measuring 0.3 to 1.0 μ. Infection occurs by so-called elementary bodies which undergo reorganization to form metabolically active reticular bodies present in the fifth hour of infection. Their cycle of development is unique among the prokaryotes with a total disability to synthesize high-energy compounds such as ATP. In the cytoplasm of the host cell, they multiply by binary fission in microcolonies or inclusions that involve the nucleus and produce the cellular lysis in 48–72 h.[4] Many authors have demonstrated a high rate of spontaneous genomic recombination among the chlamydias.[5,6]

The *Chlamydia* genus belongs to the *Chlamydiales* order, Chlamydiaceae family, and consists of two species: *trachomatis* and *psittaci*. Chlamydias produce infection in man and fowl (psittacosis, ornithosis) with a remarkable tropism for ganglionar and ocular structures, lungs, and the genitourinary and gastrointestinal tract.

The causative organism is *C. trachomatis* (serotypes L1, L2, and L3). Other serotypes cause the trachoma, inclusion conjunctivitis, and ophthalmia of neonates (serotypes A-C), along with urethritis and exocervitis (serotypes D-K). The latter group is implicated in postvenereal Reiter syndrome, characterized by the classic triad of conjunctivitis, urethritis, and polyarthritis. The different manifestations of these serotypes depend on the diversity of the molecular structure of the DNA, also capable of giving an immunopathogenic identity to each strain of the *C. trachomatis*.[7,8]

The chlamydias have already been considered great viruses or rickettsias, visible in optical microscopy. The receptors for heparin and heparan sulfate, present in the eukaryotic cells, are essential in the infectiousness of the *C. trachomatis*.[9] Monoclonal antibodies against heparan sulfate block the infectiousness of elementary bodies. The lymphocytes CD4+ and CD8+ have an active participation in the immunological reaction against the chlamydias,[10-11] despite the absence of blastic transformation of the cells CD4+ induced by specific antigens for *C. trachomatis*.[12]

6.4   Epidemiology

LGV is more usual in the tropical and subtropical regions but does occur in relatively low incidence throughout the Western world.[13] The disease is almost always transmitted by sexual contact. The main age of onset is 25 years, but the disease can be seen in any age group from adolescents to adults. Highest prevalence was found in young single persons of low socioeconomic and educational status, probably because these factors correlate positively with sexual promiscuity. LGV is more common among men. Prostitutes and male homosexuals used to have a major role in the transmission of the disease.[14] Currently, greater sexual liberation and the acknowledgment that LGV organisms have been isolated from the cervix of asymptomatic female contacts modified this concept, making it more difficult to control and effect the prophylaxis of the LGV.

The serological screenings with the LGV complement fixation test performed in apparently healthy European populations revealed a low rate of LGV; however, this may merely reflect cross-reactions between antibodies directed against the sorotypes D-K and the LGV serotypes L1, L2, and L3. Panizza et al.[15] examined 6 cases of the disease in 1 year of serological screening of the population in Sicily, Italy. In Paris, Scieux et al.[16] detected 27 cases in 6 years.

An evaluation effected in a clinic for sexually transmitted diseases in Rwanda, studied 210 cases of genital ulcers. The LGV was the least frequent venereum disease, totaling 23 cases (11%). Other detected diseases were syphilis (40%), chancroid (24%), and genital herpes (17%); 59% of the patients presented positive serology for HIV.[17] The concomitance of venereum diseases can be better evaluated in the study performed by Sischy et al.[18] in 1170 African patients, where 34% of the patients with LGV presented positive serology for syphilis.

Epidemiological inquiry performed in Niteroi (Brazil), between 1948 and 1978, identified 361 cases of LGV, composing 0.26% of all 21,860 seeking dermatological assistance performed and 2.41% patients evaluated in the section of sexually transmitted diseases. About 91% of the cases of LGV occurred among men, 63% were single and there was no significant difference as to the ethnic group. The main complaint was inguinal adenopathy. The primary ulcerous lesion was referred by 19.4% of the patients and fever was observed in 8.3% of the cases. The incidence was higher among servants and merchants. A similar study performed in Rio de Janeiro (Brazil), between 1973 and 1979, identified 44 cases of LGV, 0.004% of the total of those seeking dermatological assistance. The epidemiological evaluations performed in these two Brazilian cities identified gradual decline of the LGV, maintaining itself as the fourth most frequent sexually transmitted disease succeeding gonococcal urethritis, syphilis, and chancroid.

6.5   Clinical manifestations

The incubation period is uncertain but has been estimated to be anywhere from 1 to 2 weeks. Some predisponent conditions of other sexually transmitted diseases are also accepted for LGV such as phimosis, intertrigo, eczema, balanitis, balanoposthitis, urethritis, vulvovaginitis, and proctitis.

The site of primary chancre is almost never noticed. In approximately one fourth of patients an evanescent and painless lesion, with a proteiform aspect, can be observed at the site of inoculation. This transient primary lesion usually appears as a vesicle, small erosion, erosed papule, or an exulcerated area (Figure 1). The coronal sulcus, glans, and the internal face of the labia minora are the habitual localizations.[19] The site of primary lesion is usually around the genitals but may be anal, rectal, or oral, mainly in male homosexuals. Occasionally patients may have symptoms of nonspecific urethritis but, in most patients, no primary lesion is clinically evident.[6,20] The primary lesion will last only 2–3 days. Recent reports of LGV situated in uncommon sites such as the tonsillar lymph tissues,[21] nasolabial folds, and submammary and umbilical regions[2,22] emphasize the need for a detailed history.

Adenopathy represents the most important objective element of the clinical exam and is unilateral in two thirds of these cases. It usually occurs 1–3 weeks after the initial lesion. In its earlier stages the adenopathy syndrome is manifested by discrete tender movable nodes. After several days they become matted, with a firm lobulated swelling not attached to the deep tissues. The overlying skin is often slightly reddened and edematous, but it later may become thickened and develop a purple hue. In a short time the lymph nodes become tender and fluctuant and are referred to as buboes (Figure 2). In the natural evolution of LGV, the nodes may undergo necrosis and spontaneous fistula tracts may develop.[2,22] These nodes may also become fluctuant and discharge purulent material (Figure 3). The emergence of many fistulous orifices explains the comparison made with

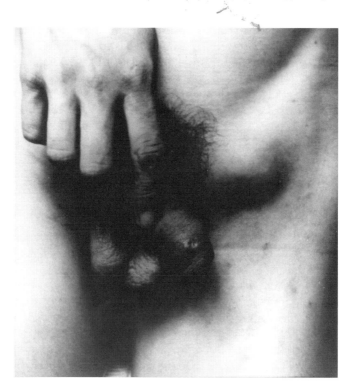

Figure 1   The primary chancre is inconspicuous and may escape notice. It consists of small painless erosion that heals in a short time without scarring. Lymphadenopathy is the main physical sign. (Photo courtesy of A.B. Lima, M.D., Ph.D.)

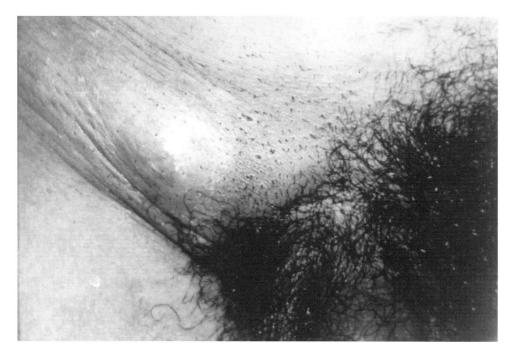

Figure 2   Unilateral inguinal tender lymphadenopathy of LGV. (Photo courtesy of A.B. Lima, M.D., Ph.D.)

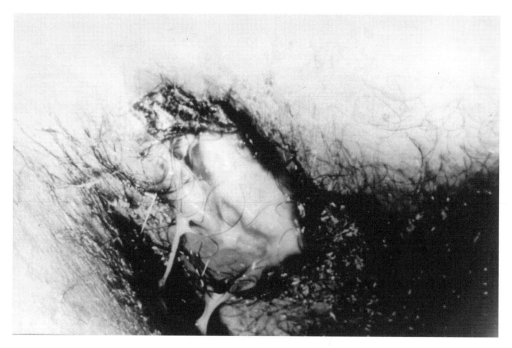

Figure 3   In a short time the lymph nodes quickly become fluctuant and are referred to as buboes when they ulcerate and discharge purulent material. (Photo courtesy of A.B. Lima, M.D., Ph.D.)

"watering-can." Painful elongated sausage-shaped swellings may occur in the inguinal area above and below Poupart's ligament. The linear depressions parallel to the inguinal ligament are the so-called "groove sign."[2]

There may be fever and chills during this stage of LGV, associated with other non-specific systemic symptoms such as headache, nausea, anorexia, weight loss, and myalgia. Infrequently, there are arthralgias, atypical pneumonia, erythema nodosum, scarlatiniform eruption, meningitis, meningoencephalitis, and keratoconjunctivitis.[22,23] In untreated cases, the lymphadenopathy usually subsides spontaneously in 8–12 weeks.

Anal coitus propitiates the implantation of the micorganism directly to the rectal mucosa. The lymph nodes rupture, causing hemorrhage and friability of the anorectal mucosa, with rectitis, tenesmus, mucosanguinous rectal discharge, and constipation.[6,20] Later, as healing occurs, there is formation of strictures, fistulas, and abscesses with destruction of anal and rectal structures.[6,20] The strictures may be bandlike or may involve extensive areas of the lower large bowel. This genitoanorectal syndrome occurs after late fibrosis and tissue destruction in untreated cases.

Elephantiasis of the vulva or penis and scrotum represents late manifestations which are rare today. "Saxophone penis" is the chronic and massive edema of the penis (Figure 4).[1,6] The esthiomenic syndrome, composed by vulvar ulceration followed by sclerosis and tegumentar hypertrophy, can occur in patients with LGV, but also in tuberculosis and syphilis. Inadequate treatment is the most important cause of the anorectal syndrome described by Gersild showing pararectal abscess, fistulas, rectovaginal fistulas, ulceration, strictures, and sclerosis of the skin (Figure 5).[24] Stenosing rectitis can produce complete intestinal occlusion, simulating anorectal neoplasia. This type of complication is more common in women and male homosexuals, but is now fortunately rare. Primary infection of the female genital tract or rectum results in primary perirectal or pelvic adenopathy, whereas infection of the male genital tract results in inguinal adenopathy. O'Farrell et al.[25] observed that the accuracy of the clinical diagnosis of LGV among men is of 66%, superior

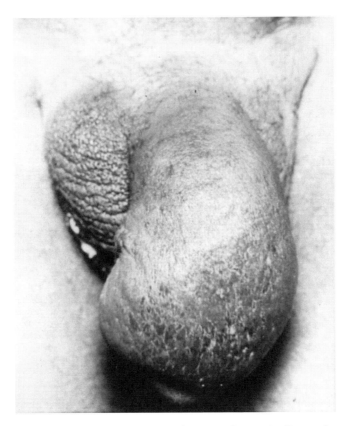

Figure 4 Sometimes there is massive edema deforming the penis ("saxophone penis"). (Photo courtesy of A.B. Lima, M.D., Ph.D.)

to the accuracy observed in other sexually transmitted diseases. The same analysis performed in females demonstrated that LGV is the most difficult diagnosis among the sexually transmitted ulcerative diseases.

6.6   Diagnosis

The diagnosis is established by careful history taking and clinical examination, emphasizing the painful adenopathy. Some specific laboratory methods are helpful but must be judiciously analyzed, establishing with confidence the concomitance of the illnesses.

The differential diagnosis should include reactive nodes, chancroid, syphilis, ganglionar tuberculosis (scrofuloderma), cat-scratch disease, and Hodgkin's disease. Syphilis and chancroid present ulcerated lesions and adenopathy with distinct clinical and evolutionary characteristics. The presence of *Treponema pallidum* or of *Haemophilus ducreyi* on touch preparation smears is a helpful adjunct in differential diagnosis.

Scrofuloderma of the inguinal or inguinocrural lymph nodes is an important differential diagnosis. The adenitis is torpid, dragged, and painless. The history of pulmonar tuberculosis among contacts, the tuberculinic test, the histopathological exam, culture for the *Mycobacterium tuberculosis*, and the inoculation in guinea pigs allow the diagnosis of tuberculosis. Cat-scratch disease is an acute disease preceded by trauma from the animal's nails. Hodgkin's disease is a systemic disease that affects many ganglionar lymph nodes.

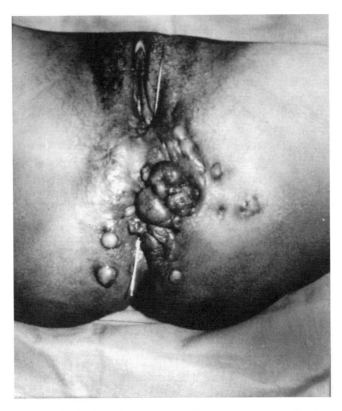

Figure 5 Chronic stage with thickened cutaneous plaques, numerous fistulae, massive lymphoedema of the vulva (esthiomene), and proliferating lesions of the rectum and anus. (Photo courtesy of S. Serpa, M.D.)

Late manifestations must be distinguished from neoplastic skin disease, filariasis, rectal cancer, inflammatory bowel disease, and hidradenitis suppurativa.

The diagnosis of the LGV can be complemented by the following exams:

1. Direct bacteriological exam and culture
2. Serological exams: complement fixation test and immunofluerescence test
3. Frei's test
4. Histopathological exam

Material may be obtained for direct bacteriological exam and culture from affected lymph nodes by inserting a needle into the area of fluctuance. Staining of the smear with Giemsa stain or fuscin stain reveals the intracellular corpuscles of Gamma-Miyagawa, which occur in some chlamydial infections.[26] The electron microscopy is not used in laboratorial routine. The culture of the C. *trachomatis* can be performed inoculating material derived from the node in yolk sac of embryonated eggs or in tissue cell culture previously treated with cytochalasina B (McCoy, Hela 229, L 929).[27]

A complement fixation test, using group-specific antigens, is reactive within one month of onset of infection. A titer of greater than or equal to 1:16, in the presence of a compatible clinical syndrome, is suggestive of LGV.[28] Serial samples with a 15-day interval frequently show a fourfold increment in titer in the acute stage of the disease. Indirect immunofluorescence represents a sensitive method but is not widely available. The enzyme-linked immunosorbent assay (ELISA) is also helpful for the identification of *C. trachomatis*. Monoclonal antibodies are an extremely sensitive method and of high specification in the diagnosis of the LGV, capable of preventing serological cross-reactivity among the causative serotypes L1, L2, and L3 and other serotypes of *C. trachomatis*.

Frei's intradermal test can be carried out with the pus collected from the bubo, through the material derived from simians (Pasteur Institute), and with the material proceeding from the culture performed in embryonic yolk sacs of embryonated eggs. The preparation is of simple execution, being only necessary to saline solution in the proportion of 1/5 and fenic acid at 0.5%. The test is read 48 h after intradermal injection of 0.1 ml of the solution. Induration measuring 5 mm or more in diameter or an erythematous halo is considered positive. The sensitivity and specificity of this test have been seriously questioned and Frei's test is now of historic interest only and the antigen is no longer commercially available.[26,28]

The histopathological exam of the lymphnodal mass is nonspecific but may help to exclude other disorders. The characteristic changes consist of an infectious granuloma with the formation of stellate abscesses. There is an outer zone of epithelioid cells with a central necrotic core composed of debris of lymphocytes, endothelial cells, and leukocytes. Marked hyperglobulinemia occurs, particularly in patients with chronic complications.[28]

6.7   Treatment

6.7.1   Antibiotics[29-32]

- Tetracyclines: 500 mg p.o. every 6 hours, during 2 to 4 weeks
- Doxycycline: 100 mg p.o. every 12 hours, for 3 weeks
- Erythromycin: 500 mg every 6 hours, for 2 to 3 weeks
- Tianfenicol: 500 mg (2 capsules) p.o. every 8 hours, during 2 to 3 weeks
- Sulfadiazine: 500 mg p.o. every 6 hours, during 2 to 3 weeks
- Sulfisoxazole: beginning dose of 4 g p.o. and then 2 g during 2 to 3 weeks

After an initial course of treatment, patients should be seen at least every three months for one year, and the titer of the LGV complement fixation test should be followed. Retreatment should be given if there is a fourfold increase in serologic titer or if there is clinical evidence of relapse. Sexual contacts should be treated similarly.

6.7.2   Surgery

Tense and fluctuant nodules should be aspirated, rather than incised and drained, with a thick needle through healthy adjacent normal skin to prevent rupture and formation of fistulous tracts. Dilation and partial amputation of the rectum are measures occasionally indicated to correct rectal stricture.[11,20] Vulvectomy and colostomy are seldom necessary.

6.8   Prognosis

The prognosis is excellent for acute infections treated with appropriate antibiotics. The late disease becomes rare each day, but severe lymphatic involvement is frequently irreversible. The malignant transformation of the genital lesions of elephantiasis and anorectal syndrome, more common in females, is considered exceptional.[33]

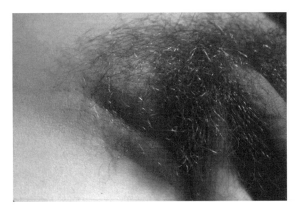

Patient contacted LGV three weeks before in Columbia. (Photo courtesy of A.W. Hoke, M.D.)

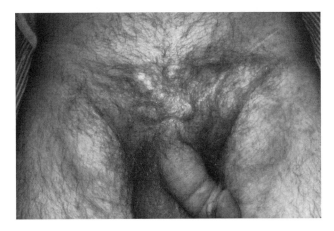

LGV "groove sign." (Photo courtesy of A.W. Hoke, M.D.)

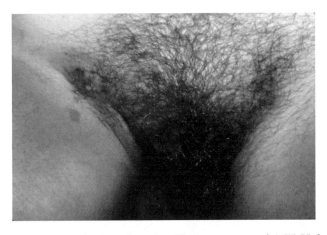

Spontaneous rupture of a lymph node. (Photo courtesy of A.W. Hoke, M.D.)

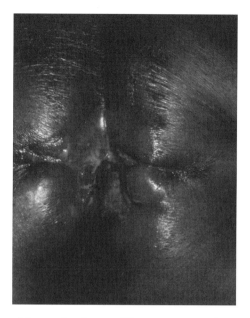

Late infection with rectal stricture. (Photo courtesy of A.W. Hoke, M.D.)

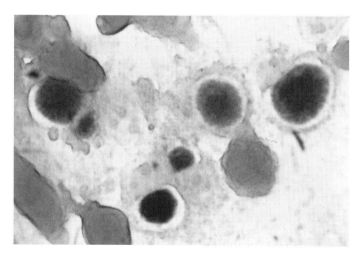

LGV culture at 48 h with Lugol's iodine stain. (Photo courtesy of J. Schacter, Ph.D.)

References

1. Oehme A, Musholt PB, Dreesbach K. Chlamydiae as pathogen — an overview of diagnostic techniques, clinical features, and therapy of human infection. *Klin. Wochenschr.*, 69: 463, 1991.
2. Hayes LJ, Yearsley P, Treharne JD, et al. Evidence for naturally occurring recombination in the gene encoding the major outer membrane protein of lymphogranuloma venereum isolates of *Chlamydia trachomatis. Infect. Immun.*, 62: 5659, 1994.
3. Bauwens JE, Lampe MF, Suchland RJ, et al. Infection with *Chlamydia trachomatis* lymphogranuloma venereum serovar L1 in homosexual men with proctitis: molecular analysis of an unusual case cluster. *Clin. Infect. Dis.*, 20: 576, 1995.

4. de le Maza LM, Fielder TJ, Carlson EJ, et al. Sequence diversity of the 60-kilodalton protein and of a putative 15-kilodalton protein between the trachoma and lymphogranuloma venereum biovars of *Chlamydia trachomatis. Infect. Immun.,* 59: 1196, 1991.

5. Watson MW, Lambden PR, Ward ME, et al. *Chlamydia trachomatis* 60 Kda cysteine rich outer membrane protein: sequence homology between trachoma and LGV biovars. *FEMS Microbiol. Lett.,* 53: 293, 1989.

6. Chen JC, Stephens RS. Trachoma and LGV biovars of *Chlamydia trachomatis* share the same glycosaminoglycan-dependent mechanism for infection of eukaryotic cells. *Mol. Microbiol.,* 11: 501, 1994.

7. Igietseme JU, Magee DM, Williams DM, et al. Role for CD8+ cells in antichlamydial immunity defined by Chlamydia-specific T-lymphocyte clones. *Infect. Immun.,* 62: 5195, 1994.

8. James SP, Graeff AS, Zeitz M, et al. Cytotoxic and immunoregulatory function of intestinal lymphocytes in *Chlamydia trachomatis* proctitis of nonhuman primates. *Infect. Immun.,* 55: 1137, 1987.

9. Zeitz M, Quinn TC, Graeff AS, et al. Mucosal T cell provide helper function but do not proliferate when stimulated by specific antigen in lymphogranuloma venereum proctitis in nonhuman primates. *Gastroenterology,* 94: 353, 1988.

10. King A, Nicol C, Rodin P. *Venereal Diseases,* 4th ed., Baillière Tindall, London, 1980, 231.

11. Bechelli LM, Curban GV. *Comp. Dermatol.,* 6th ed., Atheneu S.A., São Paulo, 1988, 195.

12. Azulay RD. Doença de Nicolas-Favre-Durand. Clínica e experimentação. *Rev. Flum. Med.,* 8: 7, 1943.

13. Eichmann A. Sexually transmissible diseases following travel in tropical countries. *Schweiz. Med. Wochenschr.,* 123: 1250, 1993.

14. Sales JB. Doença de Nicolas-Favre e sua incidência entre meretrizes de Fortaleza. *Rev. Bras. Med.,* 10: 269, 1953.

15. Panizza E, Nigro M, Pasquale R, et al. Epidemiologic considerations apropos of 6 cases of lymphogranuloma venereum recorded in Sicily in a 1-year period. *G. Ital. Dermatol. Venereol.,* 122: 11, 1987.

16. Scieux C, Barnes R, Bianchi A, et al. Lymphogranuloma venereum: 27 cases in Paris. *J. Infect. Dis.,* 160: 662, 1989.

17. Bogaerts J, Ricart CA, Van Dick E, et al. The etiology of genital ulceration in Rwanda. *Sex. Trans. Dis.,* 16: 123, 1989.

18. Sischy A, L'Exposto F, Dangor Y, et al. Syphilis serology in patients with primary syphilis and non-treponemal sexually transmitted diseases in southern Africa. *Genitourin. Med.,* 67: 129, 1991.

19. Elgart ML. Sexually transmitted diseases of the vulva. In: *Vulvar Diseases,* Turner MLC, Mariniff SC, Eds. W.B. Saunders, Philadelphia, 1992, 387.

20. Ghinsberg RC, Firsteter-Gilburd E, Mates A, et al. Rectal lymphogranuloma venereum in a bisexual patient. *Microbiologica,* 14: 161, 1991.

21. Watson DJ, Parker AJ, Macleod TI. Lymphogranuloma venereum of the tonsil. *J. Laryngol. Otol.,* 104: 331, 1990.

22. Burgoyne RA. Lymphogranuloma venereum. *Prim. Care,* 17: 153, 1990.

23. Buus DR, Pflugfelder SC, Schachter J, et al. Lymphogranuloma venereum conjunctivitis with a marginal corneal perforation. *Ophthalmology,* 95: 799, 1988.

24. Jeanpretre M, Harms M, Saurat JH. Stenosing anal mass and veneral lymphogranuloma. *Schweiz. Med. Wochenschr.,* 124: 1587, 1994.

25. O'Farrell N, Hoosen AA, Coetzee KD, et al. Genital ulcer disease: accuracy of clinical diagnosis and strategies to improve control in Durban, South Africa. *Genitourin. Med.,* 70: 7, 1994.

26. Paris-Hamelin A, Catalan F. Techniques de laboratoires applicables aux diagnostics des M.S.T. Librairie le François. Paris, 1978, Chap. 6.

27. Mittal A, Sachdeva KG. Monoclonal antibody for the diagnosis of lymphogranuloma venereum: a preliminary report. *Br. J. Biomed. Sci.,* 50: 3, 1993.

28. Schachter J. Chlamydial infection. *N. Engl. J. Med.,* 298: 428, 1978.

29. Tavares W. *Manual de Antibióticos para o Estudante de Medicina*, 3rd ed., Atheneu S.A., Rio de Janeiro, 1988.
30. Cunha BA, Garabedian SM. Tetracyclines in urology: current concepts. *Urology*, 36: 548, 1990.
31. Agakishiev DD, Kuliev TG. The combined treatment with doxycycline and methyluracil of a patient with lymphogranuloma venereum. *Vestn. Dermatol. Venereol.*, 1: 77, 1990.
32. Linnemann CC, Heaton CL, Ritchey M. Treatment of *Chlamydia trachomatis* infections: comparision of 1 and 2 g doses of erythromycin for seven days. *Sex. Trans. Dis.*, 14: 102, 1987.
33. Chopda NM, Desai DC, Sawant PD, et al. Rectal lymphogranuloma venereum in association with rectal adenocarcinoma. *Ind. J. Gastroenterol.*, 13: 103, 1994.

Spirochete

chapter seven

Syphilis

Gerald J. Domingue

7.1   Introduction..131
7.2   Etiology, classification, and transmission...132
7.3   Epidemiology...132
      7.3.1   Interaction of HIV and syphilis..132
      7.3.2   Morphology and propagation..133
7.4   Molecular biology — antigenic and immunogenic characteristics...........133
7.5   Pathogenesis and pathology 134
      7.5.1   Immunity...134
7.6   Hypothesis for a dormant bacterial phase of *T. pallidum* resulting in
      spirochetal persistence in syphilis: an analog? 135
7.7   Collection of specimens and diagnostic laboratory tests.............................135
      7.7.1   Direct examination...135
      7.7.2   Nontreponemal serologic tests..135
      7.7.3   Treponemal tests..136
      7.7.4   Other emerging diagnostic tests..136
              7.7.4.1   Polymerase chain reaction (PCR) 136
              7.7.4.2   Enzyme-linked immunosorbent assay (ELISA)..................137
7.8   Clinical manifestations 137
7.9   Treatment..138
7.10 Prevention...138
References..145

7.1   Introduction

There is no real agreement among scholars as to the origin of syphilis. It is generally considered that it got its start as a disease in the Americas and became widespread in Europe shortly after the return of Columbus in 1493. A leading Chinese paleoanthropologist, Xinhua-Zhang Shemblao, on the other hand, claims that syphilis existed in China 2000 years ago. Whatever its actual origins, syphilis was a plague that spread rapidly throughout Europe at the end of the fifteenth century. In the sixteenth century, syphilis carried many of the same social stigmas as acquired immune deficiency syndrome (AIDS) does today.

Syphilis is a complex and variable sexually transmitted disease. According to the 1995 World Health Organization executive report, there were 19 million cases of syphilis during the year. Syphilis, therefore, is a major public health problem. There has been an increase in the prevalence of human immune deficiency virus (HIV) infection among individuals with syphilis. It has been hypothesized, therefore, that asymptomatic syphilis may be a potent cofactor in the progression of HIV-related immune deficiency.

7.2   Etiology, classification, and transmission

Syphilis is a bacterial infection caused by the spirochete *Treponema pallidum*. *Treponema* is one of five genera in the family Spirochaetaceae. Thirteen species of *Treponema* are currently recognized, but only three are considered to be human pathogens. Besides *T. pallidum*, two other species are pathogenic, *T. pertenue* (causative agent of yaws) and *T. carateum* (causative agent of pinta). This chapter, however, will concentrate entirely on *T. pallidum* and syphilis.

Humans are believed to be the only natural host of *T. pallidum*. In addition to being the host, humans are also the vectors for this disease. In adults, syphilis is usually contracted through sexual activity when contact is made with infectious lesions. Syphilis occurs most commonly in persons between the ages of 15 and 40 years, which are usually the most sexually active years for individuals. The disease is rarely transmitted to health care personnel attending to patients with syphilis, other subjects who accidentally come in contact with infectious lesions, or laboratorians handling infected animals. Transmission of *T. pallidum* following transfusion of blood from a syphilitic donor has been recorded. An infant can be infected *in utero* by transplacental passage of *T. pallidum* from an infected mother. Infection may also occur in infants from contact with an infectious lesion during passage through the birth canal.

T. pallidum is very susceptible to heat, drying, a wide range of disinfectant agents, and soaps, and does not survive well outside the human host. It is inhibited by penicillin and low concentrations of tetracyclines, erythromycin, and other antimicrobials. Transmission by fomites is extremely rare.

7.3   Epidemiology

Table 1 shows reported cases of syphilis in the U.S. (including Guam, Puerto Rico, and the Virgin Islands) from 1990–1994. There were 53,350 fewer cases reported in 1994 than in 1990. Whether this is a true reflection of a decrease in the incidence of syphilis is not clear. It has been estimated by some sources that, presently, there may be more than 500,000 cases (including all stages of the disease) of unreported, untreated, syphilis in the U.S. It is assumed that most of these cases are in the latent stage and can only be detected by blood tests.

Since 1985, there have been dramatic increases in congenital syphilis. Several factors may account for this changing epidemiology. Many individuals have limited access to health care, thereby delaying diagnosis of syphilis. This is especially true of residents of the inner cities where syphilis rates are highest. Illegal drug distribution and the exchange of sex for drugs or money have contributed to increasing rates of the disease. The risk of contracting syphilis rises as the number of sexual partners increases. There are difficulties in tracing contacts because subjects with syphilis who are drug users often have partners who cannot be found.[1]

7.3.1   Interaction of HIV and syphilis

Hook and Marra[2] have delineated a number of levels where syphilis and HIV infection interact. The acquisition and transmission of HIV may be enhanced by syphilitic genital ulcers, and the natural course of syphilis may be altered in patients coinfected with HIV. Laboratory diagnosis of syphilis may be different with HIV-infected individuals also.

Table 1 Reported Cases of Syphilis in the U.S. and Outlying Areas (Guam, Puerto Rico, and Virgin Islands) 1990–1994

	1990	1991	1992	1993	1994
Number of cases	137,101	130,716	114,815	103,859	83,751

From Centers for Disease Control and Prevention. Sexually Transmitted Disease Surveillance 1994, Division of STD Prevention, September 1995, U.S. Department of Health and Human Services, Public Health Services.

Finally, current therapeutic modalities may be less effective for patients who are coinfected with HIV. Overall, the interactions between the diseases probably depend on the extent of immunosuppression in the HIV-infected patient at the time of infection with these pathogenic spirochetes.

7.3.2 Morphology and propagation

T. pallidum is a spiral bacterium that is highly motile. It has an average diameter of 0.13 to 0.15 μ and is 10 to 13 μ in length. The cells are tightly coiled, and three periplasmic flagella (also called axial fibrils) are inserted at the end of each cell. Lying beneath the cytoplasmic membrane are 6 to 8 cytoplasmic tubules. These tubules originate at each cell end. Because of its narrowness, the organism is below the resolution of the light microscope. Darkfield microscopy is most often used to visualize the organisms in specimens containing the bacteria. It has long been hypothesized that *T. pallidum* has a slime layer that prevents phagocytosis and early antigen processing. *T. pallidum* has not been successfully cultured on artificial culture media *in vitro*. It has, however, been maintained in animal hosts by inoculation. It is often propagated by intratesticular injection of rabbits that are free of *T. paralius-cunniculi*, the etiologic agent of rabbit syphilis.

7.4 Molecular biology — antigenic and immunogenic characteristics

Recent data suggest that the vast majority of *T. pallidum's* membrane proteins are lipoproteins. These lipoproteins are immunogenic and are anchored in the cytoplasmic membrane. The outer membrane contains only a limited number of surface-exposed transmembrane proteins. Several studies emanating from the laboratory of M. V. Norgard have resulted in a unique model of *T. pallidum's* molecular architecture based on the bacterium's integral membrane proteins.[3-5] The reasoning of these scientists is provocative and may have clinical significance. These investigators have developed a strategy for refining the model by demonstrating that the physiological functions of treponemal membrane proteins are consistent with their proposed cellular locations. They used an ampicillin digoxigenin conjugate to demonstrate by chemiluminescence that the 47-kDa lipoprotein immunogen of *T. pallidum* (Tpp47) is a penicillin-binding protein. Reexamination of the Tpp47 primary sequence revealed the three amino acid motifs characteristic of penicillin-binding proteins. A recombinant, nonlipidated, soluble form of Tpp47 was used to demonstrate that Tpp47 is a zinc-dependent carboxypeptidase. *Escherichia coli* expressing Tpp47 was characterized by cell wall abnormalities. The presence of such abnormalities was consistent with altered peptidoglycan biosynthesis.

Treponemal research has been impeded by the inability to cultivate *T. pallidum in vitro* as well as the lack of genetic exchange systems. However, the data and hypotheses of Norgard et al. advance strategies for utilizing *E. coli* molecular genetics as a means of elucidating the complex relationship between syphilis pathogenesis and the basic membrane biology of *T. pallidum*.[3-5] Additionally, their molecular model may partly help to explain the organism's remarkable ability to evade host immune defenses and establish persistent infection. The availability of the recombinant 47-kDa immunogen has provided an opportunity for biochemical analysis of the protein, structure-function studies, examination of its role in spirochetal pathogenesis, and assessment of its diagnostic value and vaccine potential for the prevention of syphilis.

Although the 47-kDa lipoprotein has attracted the most attention as a potential immunogen and might indeed have the greatest clinical relevance, other lipoproteins have also been identified. A 34-kDa molecule has been described[6] which, in both the native and recombinant states, displays hydrophobic biochemical characteristics. This proteolipid was localized in both the inner and outer membranes of a recombinant host.

7.5   Pathogenesis and pathology[7-9]

It is presumed that *T. pallidum* enters through tiny breaks in squamous or mucous epithelium as a result of sexual contact. After a 14- to 21-day incubation period, a red, painless papule may appear at the site of inoculation within a few days. The organism propagates in the dermis. The papule ulcerates, and the lesion is typical of the syphilitic chancre. The organism may enter the bloodstream once the bacterium has been established and dissemination occurs.

The histology of the papule shows a relatively acellular central area abundant in mucopolysaccharides and is surrounded by an infiltrate of degranulated polymorphonuclear leukocytes and lymphocytes. Progression of the lesion results in a necrotic central area with plasma cells and macrophages predominating at the periphery. There is a characteristic endothelial proliferation with perivascular infiltration by lymphocytes and plasma cells. The chancre heals spontaneously within approximately three to six weeks. It has been postulated that local immunity may be operative in the healing mechanism when the primary lesion is regressing and disseminated secondary lesions appear. The disseminated lesions are a result of the spirochetemia occurring during the incubation or pretreatment stage of syphilis. A period of three or more weeks elapses between departure of the organisms from the dermis and emergence of secondary lesions. Despite the presence of specific antitreponemal antibodies, the infection progresses. The secondary lesions do not ulcerate, possibly due to some type of local immunity. Tertiary or late syphilis produces granulomatous lesions often with giant cells; palisading cells are infrequently seen at the periphery. It is difficult to demonstrate the presence of *T. pallidum* in the lesions in late syphilis. Although a number of theories have been proposed for the pathogenesis of late syphilis, none have been conclusively proven. There is evidence to suggest that delayed hypersensitivity appears in late secondary syphilis prior to the onset of latency. Delayed hypersensitivity is uniformly present in tertiary syphilis. There is, however, no uniform retention of antigen in all areas, which complicates invoking delayed hypersensitivity as a primary factor in pathogenesis.

The exact mechanisms by which *T. pallidum* damages the host are unclear. No specific endotoxins or exotoxins have yet been identified; however, immune complexes and hypersensitivities could play a role. The ability of the organism to evade the immune system may be due to the limited number of surface-exposed transmembrane proteins.

7.5.1   Immunity

It is thought that immunity to syphilis is short lived if the patient is successfully treated in the early stages of the disease. The immune status alone (whether humoral or cell-mediated) does not seem to be sufficient to eradicate established disease. In immunocompromised patients, syphilis may present with aberrant manifestations and aggressive disease.

7.6   Hypothesis for a dormant bacterial phase of T. pallidum resulting in spirochetal persistence in syphilis: an analog?

I hypothesize that *T. pallidum* may develop a dormant bacterial phase evading immune recognition in a manner similar to that which has been observed for cell wall-aberrant Gram-positive bacteria involved in the pathogenesis of idiopathic hematuria and other chronic, dormant infections of the urinary tract.

Observations in my laboratory[10-14] of electron dense cytoplasmic particles within cell wall-defective enterococci and from other Gram-positive bacteria as well as findings by Margulis et al.[15] on the presence of 2 to 12 protoplasmic cylinders inside a single common membrane of free-living spirochetes might suggest that symptom reappearance in certain chronic bacterial infections, including spirochetoses, may be related to bacterial differentiation into resistant "propagules" that persist in tissues. The above similarities may be compelling in syphilis and research may be warranted to search for a persistent, morphologically aberrant, dormant phase of *T. pallidum*. Such "propagules" or persistent dense forms, if found to be associated with *T. pallidum*, might account for the unpredictable appearance of spirochetes in the tissues of syphilitic patients.

7.7   Collection of specimens and diagnostic laboratory tests

7.7.1   Direct examination[1]

Serous fluid from a syphilitic chancre in primary syphilis can be examined by darkfield microscopy. The lesion should be gently abraded with dry, sterile gauze until serous fluid appears (with minimal bleeding because erythrocytes interfere with the darkfield examination). Wipe off the initial fluid that appears and then touch the fluid exudate with a glass slide, coverslip, and examine it under the darkfield microscope. Gloves should be worn to procure the specimen because the lesions are infectious. Special precautions should be taken while handling the specimen in the laboratory and in discarding waste materials. Laboratory practices for handling hazardous specimens in the laboratory should be strictly followed. The slide specimen should be immediately examined under the microscope for the presence of spirochetes.

7.7.2   Nontreponemal serologic tests[1]

There are two widely accepted serologic tests for the presence of nontreponemal antibodies in syphilitic patients: (1) VDRL (Venereal Disease Research Laboratory) and (2) Rapid Plasma Reagin (RPR) card test or Automated Reagin Test (ART).

Both of these tests measure nontreponemal antibodies (also known as "reaginic" or Wasserman antibodies) reacting with a cardiolipin-lecithin antigen (a normal tissue constituent). The term reaginic is no longer used because of confusion arising with IgE antibodies that mediate hypersensitivity reactions. The tests have exquisite sensitivity but are not totally specific for syphilis. The tests are also inexpensive and serve a useful purpose for screening. Any positive test must be confirmed with specific treponemal tests that detect antibodies specifically to *T. pallidum* antigens.

The VDRL is reactive in approximately 75% of patients with primary syphilis. This test may be useful in evaluating the effectiveness of antibiotic therapy. The nontreponemal tests usually decline in titer over 6 to 8 months following adequate treatment. In secondary and late syphilis VDRL is 100 and 96% sensitive, respectively. The test has a 98% specificity for nonsyphilis. The VDRL may be positive (generally in low dilution) in patients with viral (infectious mononucleosis and hepatitis), mycoplasma, or protozoal infections.

Heroin addicts, geriatric subjects, patients with cirrhosis, malignancies, and autoimmune diseases may react positively to the VDRL test.

The RPR test is 86, 100, and 98% sensitive in primary, secondary, and late syphilis, respectively, with a 98% specificity for nonsyphilis.

Both VDRL and RPR are performed on human serum but can also be performed on cerebrospinal fluid in neurosyphilis.

7.7.3   Treponemal tests[1]

These serologic tests react specifically with *T. pallidum* antigens. The most widely recognized and used tests are:

1. FTA-ABS (fluorescent treponemal antibody absorption test)
2. FTA-ABS 19S IgM (fluorescent treponemal antibody absorption 19S IgM test)
3. MHA-TP (*T. pallidum* microhemagglutination test)
4. TPI (*T. pallidum* immobilization test)

The FTA-ABS is the most widely used test. Cross-reacting antibodies are first removed from the patient's serum by absorption with a nonpathogenic treponemal antigen (*T. phagedenis*, biotype Reiter). The absorbed serum is placed on a slide containing a preparation of *T. pallidum* (Nichol's strain) and incubated in a moist chamber at 37°C. The slide is then washed, then fluorescein-labeled antihuman globulin conjugate is added to the slide, reincubated, washed, and examined under a fluorescent microscope for the presence of fluorescent treponemes. The presence of fluorescent treponemes indicates a positive test for antibodies in the patient's serum to *T. pallidum*.

A modification of the FTA-ABS test is the FTA-ABS 19S IgM procedure for diagnosing congenital syphilis. Because IgM does not cross the placenta (but IgG does), a positive reaction in this test indicates that anti-*T. pallidum* antibodies have been formed by the neonate. Serum obtained from the blood of a newborn suspected of having syphilis is used to perform this test. The technical procedure is identical to that of the FTA-ABS test. Recently, a Western immunoblot has been developed for detection of fetal IgM antibodies against *T. pallidum* antigens. This test may help to improve serodiagnosis of congenital syphilis.

Although the *T. pallidum* immobilization test (TPI) was one of the first specific treponemal tests devised for diagnosing syphilis, it has been replaced with tests that are less cumbersome, technically difficult, and expensive. This procedure is mainly used in research laboratories and not in the routine clinical microbiological diagnosis of syphilis.

7.7.4   Other emerging diagnostic tests

7.7.4.1   Polymerase chain reaction (PCR)

This sensitive and specific method for detecting bacterial genomes in clinical specimens is beginning to show promise in diagnostic microbiology. For *T. pallidum* infections, studies have been performed that suggest the sensitive detection of spirochetes. Burstain et al.[16] have reported that a 658-bp portion of the gene encoding the 47-kDa membrane immogen could be amplified. The PCR products were probed by DNA-DNA hybridization with a 496-bp fragment internal to the amplified DNA. The assay detected approximately 0.01 pg of purified *T. pallidum* DNA. Positive results were obtained routinely from suspensions of treponemes calculated to contain 10 or more organisms and from some suspensions calculated to contain a single organism. Specific PCR products were obtained for the closely related agent of yaws, *T. pallidum* subspecies *pertenue*, but not with human DNA or DNAs from other spirochetes (including *Borrelia burgdoferi*), skin microorganisms, sexually transmitted disease pathogens, and central nervous system pathogens. *T. pallidum* DNA was detected in serum, cerebrospinal fluids, and amniotic fluids from syphilitic patients, but not in nonsyphilitic controls. *T. pallidum* DNA was amplified from paraffin-embedded tissue. The diagnosis of syphilis using PCR may become a significant addition to the diagnostic armamentarium and serve as a worthwhile technique for the investigation of syphilis pathogenesis.

Noordhoek et al.[17] have reported on the use of PCR in patients with neurosyphilis, employing nested primer pairs based on the DNA sequence of the 39-kDa bmp gene of T. *pallidum* subspecies *pallidum*. Their method allowed the detection of purified *T. pallidum* DNA equivalent to the amount of DNA in a single bacterium and was specific for T. *pallidum* subspecies. After a concentration of DNA, using diatomaceous earth, it was possible to detect about 100 treponemes in 1 ml of cerebrospinal fluid. Cerebrospinal fluid samples from a total of 29 symptomatic and asymptomatic patients with neurosyphilis were tested for the presence of treponemal DNA before and at various intervals after intravenous treatment with penicillin. Prior to the penicillin treatment, Noordhoek and colleagues detected *T. pallidum* DNA in 5 of 7 patients with acute symptomatic neurosyphilis, in 0 of the 4 patients with chronic symptomatic neurosyphilis tested before treatment, and in 2 of 16 patients with asymptomatic neurosyphilis. They unexpectedly found that *T. pallidum* DNA was also often detected in cerebrospinal fluid long after intravenous treatment with penicillin, sometimes up to 3 years after therapy. The authors conclude from the results of their study, that the presence of *T. pallidum* DNA in cerebrospinal fluid does not necessarily mean that these patients were treated inadequately, because none of the patients had a clinical relapse 2 to 9 years after treatment. It is important to determine whether the treponemal DNA detected by PCR originates from treponemes that are viable at the time of sampling or from killed or lysed spirochetes. DNA is a very stable biopolymer, and the data of these investigators suggest that it might remain present in cerebrospinal fluid for prolonged periods of time after assumed effective treatment (and possible killing of *T. pallidum*) by intravenous penicillin treatment. I speculate that it is also possible that the persistence of *T. pallidum* DNA (despite the absence of symptoms) represents nucleic acid derived from dormant, viable persistent forms of the organism (as described previously in this chapter) that do not elicit clinical symptoms, yet maintain the dormant presence of the microbe in tissues and body fluids and contribute to spirochetal persistence and relapse. Noordhoek et al.[17] conclude that the detection of T. *pallidum* DNA by PCR seems to be of limited use when checking the efficacy of antibiotic treatment of patients with neurosyphilis. Studies on the stability of DNA from killed T. *pallidum* in cerebrospinal fluid are needed for complete assessment of the diagnostic potential of these findings.

7.7.4.2   *Enzyme-linked immunosorbent assay (ELISA)*[1]

This test is presently commercially available as a diagnostic test for syphilis. Specific monoclonal antibodies directed against the 47-kDa protein may have diagnostic potential. Serologic assays employing several purified recombinant DNA-derived *T. pallidum* antigens seem to compare favorably with the conventional serologic tests. The diagnosis of congenital infection and untreated acquired disease in adults may well be aided by emerging immunoblot and antibody-capture assays for detection of *T. pallidum*-specific IgM.[8]

7.8   *Clinical manifestations*[1,7,9]

The clinical features of syphilis (several having been previously described under pathogenesis and pathology) involve primary, secondary, latent (detected only by the presence of a reactive serologic test), and tertiary (late) syphilis. The characteristic lesion in primary syphilis is the chancre. If syphilis is untreated, it progresses to a secondary phase. In this stage, the lesions are widespread and contain many spirochetes. The mucous membranes and skin (including the palms of the hands and soles of feet) are most commonly affected. Complete dissemination may occur, and any organ could be infected. The secondary lesions disappear in 2 to 4 weeks, and the disease appears to be in a latent phase. Approximately one third of the patients with latent secondary syphilis recover, one third develop latent infection with the presence of specific treponemal antibodies without symptoms, and the other one third develop the most serious consequence of *T. pallidum* infection, tertiary (late) syphilis. Tertiary syphilis may occur 3 to 20 years after initial infection. Granulomatous lesions are widespread and are referred to as gummata. The skin, soft tissue, mucous membranes, bone, central nervous system, eyes, and cardiovascular system may be involved. Neurosyphilis may lead to general paralysis as well as to aortic aneurysms.

Often neurosyphilis may be asymptomatic. Symptomatic neurosyphilis involves several clinical syndromes: meningeal syphilis, meningovascular syphilis, and paretic neurosyphilis described as chronic progressive and dementing (may develop many years after initial infection). Tabes dorsalis symptoms include autonomic dysfunction, sensory ataxia, optic atrophy, and shooting pains.

Congenital syphilis develops when there is transplacental transmission of *T. pallidum* into the fetal circulation. The consequences of this infection could result in spontaneous abortion or stillbirth. Newborns exhibit flu-like symptoms that could result in meningitis, malformation of long bones, iritis, lymphadenopathy, hepatosplenomegaly, and maculopapular lesions.

7.9 Treatment[7,8,18]

Penicillin remains the drug of choice for all stages of acquired syphilis. Parenteral administration of benzathine penicillin G, penicillin aluminum monostearate (PAM), or aqueous procaine penicillin G are effective in all stages of the disease. For patients with penicillin allergies, patients may be desensitized, then treated with penicillin. Alternatively, doxycycline or tetracycline may be used for penicillin allergic patients. The usual dosage of benzathine penicillin G is 2.4 million units IM. A patient with latent syphilis, HIV infection, and a normal CSF examination can be treated with benzathine penicillin G 7.2 million units (as 3 weekly doses of 2.4 million units each). Therapeutic guidelines for syphilis have been extensively published.[8] Fortunately, *T. pallidum* does not seem to have developed resistance to chemotherapeutics useful in treatment.

7.10 Prevention[7]

The most effective means of prevention would be to have a universal vaccine. To date, there is no available vaccine for the prevention of syphilis. The membrane lipoproteins of *T. pallidum* that have received extensive molecular investigation (biochemical, physiologic, antigenic, and immunogenic properties) may hold promise as vaccine candidates. Protective sexual activity (use of condoms) can be highly effective, but condoms are underutilized and are often improperly used by many persons. Improving the identification of infected individuals in the population through serologic screening would greatly aid in preventing the spread of the disease in the population. Epidemiologic treatment of contacts would undoubtedly prevent thousands of new cases of syphilis. Epidemiologists should devise methods for interacting with physicians and syphilitic patients to assure that all cases of infectious syphilis are identified and reported to public health authorities. This methodology should stress:

1. Inteviewing and re-interviewing all reported cases of early syphilis to identify sexual contacts
2. Offer of a medical examination within a minimal period to prevent further spread of the disease
3. Counseling and performing blood tests of individuals who may be involved in an infectious chain (cluster procedure)
4. Treatment of all sexual contacts of individuals with infectious syphilis.

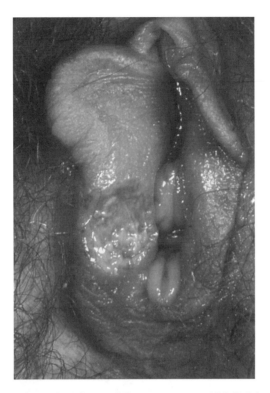

Primary syphilis on the labium. (Photo courtesy of M. Sulzberger, M.D.)

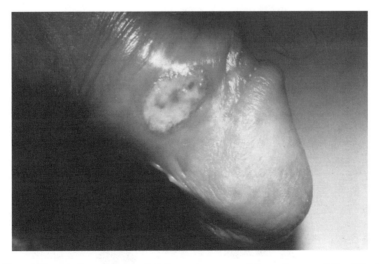

Primary syphilis on the penis, with a painful erosion caused by a human bite. (Photo courtesy of A.W. Hoke, M.D.)

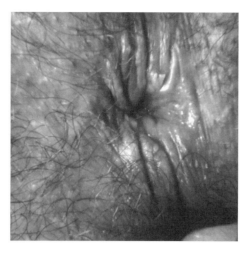

Primary syphilis in the anus with a small anal wart. (Photo courtesy of A.W. Hoke, M.D.)

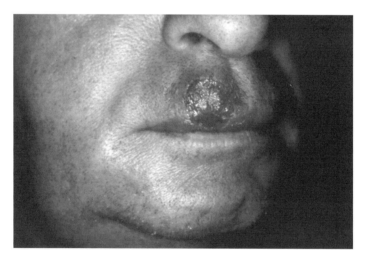

Primary syphilis with chancre on the patient's upper lip that was initially diagnosed as herpes. Note the cervical adenopathy on the patient's right side. (Photo courtesy of A.W. Hoke, M.D.)

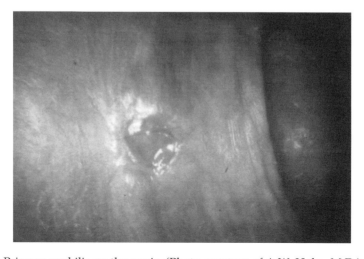

Primary syphilis on the penis. (Photo courtesy of A.W. Hoke, M.D.)

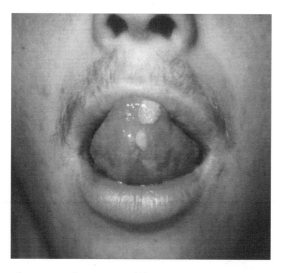

Condyloma latum on the tongue. (Photo courtesy of A.W. Hoke, M.D.)

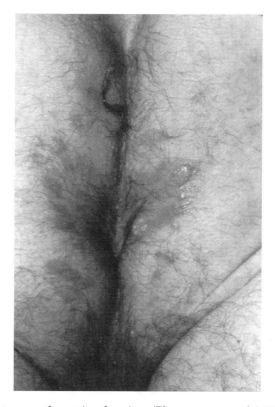

Condyloma latum on the perianal region. (Photo courtesy of A.W. Hoke, M.D.)

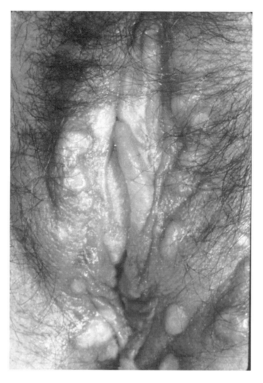

Condyloma latum on the labium. (Photo courtesy of Professor Degos.)

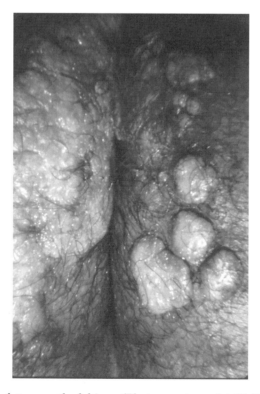

Condyloma latum on the labium. (Photo courtesy of A.W. Hoke, M.D.)

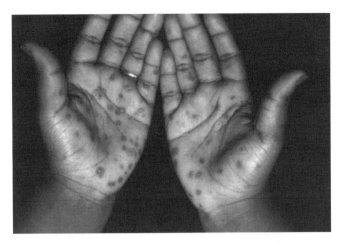

Secondary syphilis showing scaling papular eruptions on the palms. (Photo courtesy of A.W. Hoke, M.D.)

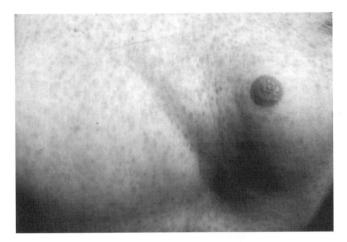

Papular lesions of secondary syphilis on the chest and abdomen. (Photo courtesy of A.W. Hoke, M.D.)

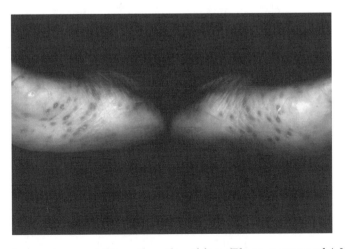

Papular lesions of secondary syphilis on the soles of feet. (Photo courtesy of A.W. Hoke, M.D.)

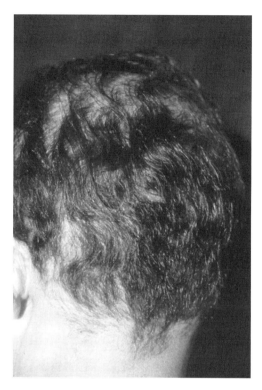

Moth-eaten alopecia in secondary syphilis. (Photo courtesy of A.W. Hoke, M.D.)

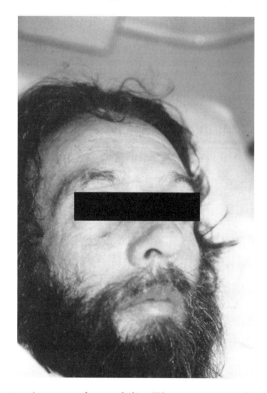

Late secondary meningovascular syphilis. (Photo courtesy of A.W. Hoke, M.D.)

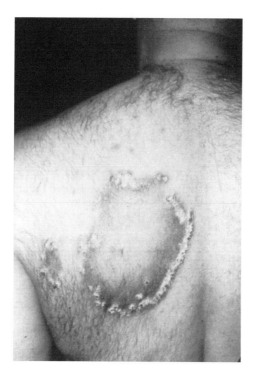

Nodular tertiary syphilis. (Photo courtesy of CDC.)

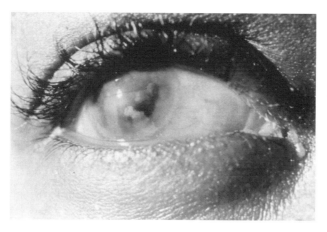

Congenital syphilis with ocular scarring. (Photo courtesy of CDC.)

References

1. Johnson, R.C. and Norton Hughes, C.A., Spirochetes, in *Clinical and Pathogenic Microbiology,* Howard, B. J., Ed., second edition, Mosby, St. Louis, 1994, pp. 532–535.
2. Hook, E.W. III and Marra, C.M., Acquired syphilis in adults. *N. Engl. J. Med.,* 326, 1060, 1992.
3. Weigel, L.M., Radolf, J.D., and Norgard, M.V., The 47-kDa major lipoprotein immunogen of *Treponema pallidum* is a penicillin-binding protein with carboxypeptidase activity. *Proc. Natl. Acad. Sci.,* 91, 11611, 1994.
4. Weigel, L.M., Brandt, M.E., and Norgard, M.V., Analysis of the N-terminal region of the 47 kilodalton integral membrane lipoprotein of *Treponema pallidum. Infect. Immun.,* 60, 1568, 1992.

5. Radolf, J.D., Chamberlain, N.R., Clausell, A., and Norgard, M.V., Genetic and physiochemical characterization of the recombinant DNA-derived 47-kilodalton surface immunogen *Treponema pallidum* subsp. *pallidum. Infect. Immun.,* 56, 71, 1998.

6. Swancutt, M.A., Riley, B.X., Radolf, J.D., and Norgard, M.V., Molecular characterization of the pathogen-specific, 34-kilodalton membrane immunogen of *Treponema pallidum. Infect. Immun.,* 57, 3314, 1989.

7. Musher, D.M., Syphilis of the genital tract, in *Infectious Diseases and Medical Microbiology,* Braude, A.I. Ed., W.B. Saunders Company, Philadelphia, 1986, pp 1225–1231.

8. Chiu, M.J. and Radolf, J.D., Syphilis, in *Infectious Diseases,* fifth edition, Hoeprich, P.D., Jordan, M.C., and Ronald, A.R., Eds., 1977, pp. 694–714.

9. Murray, P.R., Koyabashi, G.S., Pfaller, M.A., and Rosenthal, K.S., *Medical Microbiology,* Mosby, St. Louis, 1994, p. 334.

10. Green, M.T., Heidger, P.M., and Domingue, G.J., Demonstration of the phenomena of microbial persistence and reversion with bacterial L-forms in human embryonic kidney cells. *Infect. Immun.,* 10, 889, 1974.

11. Green, M.T., Heidger, P.M., and Domingue, G.J., A proposed life cycle for a relatively stable L-phase variant of *Streptococcus faecalis. Infect. Immun.,* 10, 915, 1974.

12. Domingue, G.J., Thomas, R., Walters, F., Serrano, A., and Heidger, P.M., Cell wall-deficient bacteria as a cause of "idiopathic hematuria." *J. Urol.,* 150, 483, 1993.

13. Domingue, G.J., Ghoniem, G.M., Bost, K., Fermin, C., and Human, L., Dormant bacteria in interstitial cystitis. *J. Urol.,* 153, 1321, 1995.

14. Domingue, G.J., Electron dense cytoplasmic particles and chronic infection: A bacterial pleomorphy hypothesis. *Endocytob. Cell Res.,* 11, 19, 1995.

15. Margulis, L., Ashen, J.B., Sole, M., and Guerrero, R., Composite, large spirochetes from microbial mats: spirochete structure review. *Proc. Natl. Acad Sci.,* 90, 6966, 1993.

16. Burstain, J.M., Grimprel, E., Lukehart, S.A., Norgard, M.V., and Radolf, J.D., Sensitive detection of *Treponema pallidum* by using the polymerase chain reaction. *J. Clin. Microbiol.,* 19, 62, 1991.

17. Noordhoek, G.T., Wolters, E.C., DeJonge, M.E.J., and Van Embden, J.D.A., Detection by polymerase chain reaction of *Treponema pallidum* DNA in cerebrospinal fluid from neurosyphilis patients before and after antibiotic treatment. *J. Clin. Microbiol.,* 29, 1976, 1991.

18. Centers for Disease Control and Prevention. 1993 Sexually transmitted diseases treatment guidelines. *MMWR,* 1993, 42 (no. RR-14).

Fungal

chapter eight

Candidiasis

Nancy G. Warren and Barbara A. Body

8.1 Candidiasis 149
    8.1.1 Ecology and epidemiology 149
        8.1.1.1 Occurrence, carriage, and species distribution 149
        8.1.1.2 Subtyping and strain identification 150
        8.1.1.3 Routes of spread 152
    8.1.2 Laboratory aspects 154
        8.1.2.1 Specimen collection and transport 154
        8.1.2.2 Detection and isolation of yeasts 154
        8.1.2.3 Identification of yeasts 154
        8.1.2.4 The role of serologic diagnosis in vaginitis 155
    8.1.3 Clinical disease 155
        8.1.3.1 Predisposing conditions 155
        8.1.3.2 Vaginitis 155
        8.1.3.3 Balanitis 156
    8.1.4 Antifungal drugs, susceptibility testing, and therapy 156
        8.1.4.1 Antifungal drugs — description and mode of action 156
        8.1.4.2 Treatment options 156
            8.1.4.2.1 Topical therapy 156
            8.1.4.2.2 Oral therapy 157
            8.1.4.2.3 Therapy for recurrent vulvovaginal candidiasis 157
        8.1.4.3 Susceptibility testing 158
References 160

8.1 Candidiasis

8.1.1 Ecology and epidemiology

8.1.1.1 Occurrence, carriage, and species distribution

Yeasts are ubiquitously distributed in soil and aquatic habitats and in association with both warm and cold blooded animals, insects, and a variety of plants. *Candida* species have been reported often, with *Candida albicans* being reported most commonly.[1] However, it is important to remember that the lack of a report of any particular *Candida* species from a particular host species may reflect the bias introduced by sampling error. Lack of sampling or sampling only a subset of a population (i.e., sampling only those people/animals/plants with a particular symptom) may not truly reflect the species or anatomic site distributions. Given the increasing interest in nontraditional animals as pets (snakes, birds, rodents, amphibians) it seems likely that there will be an incentive for better documentation of the routine microflora of these animals and the occurrence of *Candida* species as pathogen and commensal will be extended to additional hosts.

In addition to bias introduced by sampling, methods used for cultivation and identification can also affect the recovery rates and lead to disparities in rates of carriage from various sources. Another factor that contributes to our understanding of candidiasis is the public health reportability, or lack thereof, for specific types of candidal infections. For instance, surveillance for nosocomial infections in the United States has led to good documentation of the increasing incidence of bloodstream infections due to *Candida* species, but vulvovaginal candidiasis is not reportable so there is little study of prevalence in the U.S.[2] Alternately, in Great Britain and other countries where data from genitourinary clinics is compiled, there is excellent documentation of the incidence of vulvovaginal candidiasis.[3-6] Finally, the population sampled and circumstances at the time of sampling can also have a significant effect on carriage rates that are determined. Hooton and coworkers[7] showed that sexual intercourse did not affect rates of carriage of candida, but intercourse with use of a diaphragm and spermicides did. In this study, the prevalence of *C. parapsilosis* increased from about 2 to 35% and lactobacilli decreased. Mild symptoms of vaginitis were associated with about 20% of these cases. Intercourse alone was not associated with increased carriage or symptoms.[7] Not examined in this study was the time it took for vaginal flora to "normalize."

Table 1 summarizes selected carriage data compiled from Odds.[1] In this summary, most subsets of populations such as those listed as "patients" consistently have yeast, predominantly *C. albicans*, as part of their flora at certain sites. Notable, but not unexpected, is increased oral carriage by adults who are "patients" compared to "normal" adult groups and both of these groups compared to "infants." Alternately, rates of carriage on skin, in the gastrointestinal tract, and in feces are not so different among these populations except for pregnant women who have increased rates of carriage at several sites compared to other groups. The reports of Hurley and others clearly indicate that there have been sharp increases in candida vulvovaginitis (CVV) during the last two decades.[3-5] They estimate that 75% of women have experienced CVV, that about 50% of these women will have a second episode, and about 5% suffer from repeated recurrent CVV.[3-5]

Species distribution of *Candida* is summarized in Table 2.[1] The consistent trend is *C. albicans* as the most prevalent isolate, with *C. glabrata* and *C. tropicalis* consistently ranked a distant second and third. More recent studies are showing increases in *C. glabrata, C. tropicalis*, and *C. parapsilosis* among certain groups of patients (e.g., HIV-positive patients).[8]

8.1.1.2   Subtyping and strain identification

Initial attempts at subtyping *C. albicans* demonstrated A and B serotypes.[9] Most studies on serotyping performed outside of the U.S. indicated a predominance of serotype A, whereas the two studies done in the U.S. indicate substantially higher proportions of the B serotype generally and specifically among vaginal isolates. Two of the relevant associations with serotypes are increased incidence of flucytosine resistance among serotype B (49–89%) compared to type A (1–11%) and studies that implicate expression of the A antigen with pathologic conditions.[10,11]

As investigators became interested in whether there were associations of particular strains or subtypes of *Candida* species more or less commonly associated with disease, other methods for subtyping candida were developed. These included physiologic biotyping, resistograms, biotyping by resistance to yeast killer factors, and colony morphotyping.[1,12-15] As candida became increasingly important as a nosocomial pathogen, interest grew in applying typing schemes to epidemiologic investigations in attempts to demonstrate the extent of an outbreak and the mode(s) of transmission and to monitor areas

Table 1 Summary of Carriage[a]

Site subgroup studied	Number of individuals tested	Yeast isolated (%)	*C. albicans* isolated (%)	% Of yeast that were *C. albicans*
Oral				
Normal infants[b]	864	75 (8.7)	53 (6.1)	70.8
Normal children	144	34 (23.6)	23 (16.0)	67.5
Normal adults	1012	270 (26.7)	156 (15.4)	57.6
Patients 1960s[c]	1499	813 (54.2)	634 (42.3)	78.0
Patients 1970s	2225	1013 (45.5)	777 (34.9)	76.7
Patients 1980s	555	358 (64.5)	215 (38.7)	60.0
Total patients	4279	2184 (51.0)	1626 (38.0)	74.4
Skin				
Normals	1275	111 (8.7)	12 (0.9)	10.9
Patients	1492	160 (10.7)	54 (3.6)	33.8
GI tract[d]				
Normals	46	35 (76.1)	25 (54.3)	71.4
Patients	202	128 (63.3)	67 (33.2)	52.4
Feces				
Normal children	824	172 (20.9)	101 (12.3)	58.5
Normal adults	325	66 (20.3)	62 (19.1)	93.9
Patients (children)	381	63 (16.5)	33 (8.7)	52.7
Patients (adults)	1378	407 (29.5)	270 (19.6)	66.4
Patients (pregnant)	274	202 (73.7)	94 (34.4)	46.6
Vagina				
Normal	3699	380 (10.3)	268 (7.2)	70.4
Patients (non-gyn)	2962	602 (20.3)	282 (9.5)	46.7
Patients (gyn)	8715	2295 (26.3)	1786 (20.5)	77.8
Patients (vaginitis)	4667	1604 (34.4)	1604 (23.9)	69.9
Penis				
Males in G/u clinic[e]	310	41 (13.2)	Not given	Not given

[a] Data selected from Reference 1 Tables 7.3, 7.4, 7.6, 7.7, 7.9–7.12, and 7.14–7.16.

[b,c] Classification as normal subject or patient subjects according to Reference 1, as above.

[d] GI tract sites included the stomach, duodenum, jejunum, and ileum.

[e] Men were attending a genitourinary clinic.

Table 2 Summary of Distribution of *Candida* Species

Candida species	Percent of *Candida* from					
	Oral cavity	GI	Anorectal	Vagina (without vaginitis)	Vagina (with vaginitis)	Blood cultures
Candida albicans	69.6	56.5	50.9	69.7	84.2	50.4
C. glabrata	6.6	16.1	9.1	11.7	5.5	9.7
C. guilliermondii	0.4	0.5	0.7	0.5	0.5	0.9
C. kefyr	1.0	0.7	0.1	0.4	0.4	0.2
C. krusei	1.7	2.6	2.9	2.6	1.7	1.1
C. parapsilosis	1.9	6.1	5.4	1.9	1.2	12.1
C. tropicalis	6.9	9.7	2.3	4.7	5.3	8.5
C. species	7.0	1.4	7.1	21.0	0.5	2.0
Other yeast	4.5	6.4	21.7	6.4	0.7	4.9

such as wards or units where infection is prevalent. Lack of standardization, inter- and intralaboratory reproducibility, stability, or power of differentiation eliminated these methods as suitable for the strain typing.

Table 3   Summary of Molecular Typing Methods

Typing method	Method
DNA typing[19,24,50,51]	Treat DNA with restriction enzymes, electrophoretically separate by polyacrylamide gel electrophoresis (PAGE), stain with ethidium bromide. Analyze different banding patterns.
RFLP and Southern blot hybridization analysis[17,22,50]	As above, but rather than staining with ethidium bromide, the DNA is transferred to nitrocellulose membranes and then specific DNA probes or cloned DNA fragments corresponding to repeated sequences in the DNA are hybridized with the digested DNA
Electrophoretic karyotyping[23]	Separate chromosome size pieces of DNA by one of several different methods (orthogonal-field alternation gel electrophoresis, OFAGE; contour clamp homogeneous field gel electrophoresis, CHEF; field inversion gel electrophoresis, FIGE). This can be combined with southern blot hybridization to various DNA probes
Electrophoretic analysis of cellular proteins[24,52]	Using PAGE, proteins are separated in one or two dimensions and patterns are visualized by labeling with ^{35}S and autoradiography, staining, or immunoblotting
Multilocus enzyme electrophoresis (isoenzyme analysis)[54]	Proteins from cell lysates are separated by PAGE and then isoenzymes are identified for comparison by histochemical staining with specific substrates

Building on the successes in typing bacterial pathogens in epidemiological investigations, a number of mycologists have recently applied analogous molecular methods for subtyping yeast isolates. The systems used are summarized in Table 3. Molecular methods of subtyping have been used to demonstrate the relationship of sequential *Candida* spp. isolates from patients with candidiemia, oropharyngeal infection, vulvovaginal isolates from women with recurrent infection and isolates carried by sexual partners, and to demonstrate the selection of resistant strains in patients on fluconazole therapy.[16-24]

8.1.1.3   *Routes of spread*

Endogenous spread is the primary source of vulvovaginal candidiasis, with the gastrointestinal tract the likely source from which the vagina acquires yeast. Thin and co-workers demonstrated through statistical analysis that as much as 40% of vulvovaginal candidiasis may be sexually transmitted.[25] Other studies using biotyping and resistogram typing have also implicated sexual transmission in vulvovaginal candidiasis.[14]

The source of the candida strain in recurrent vulvovaginal candidiasis has been the subject of a number of molecular epidemiologic studies. These studies have defined three

Table 3 Summary of Molecular Typing Methods (continued)

Advantages	Disadvantages
• Relatively simple	• Lack of standardization
• Enzymes are readily available	• Differences in DNA extraction can cause
• Rapid turn around time (48–72 hr)	variability in patterns
• Intralaboratory reproducibility and stability	• Use of multiple restriction enzymes may be
of patterns	necessary to show differences
• Large number of polymorphisms allow	• It is not possible to predict which enzyme(s) will
ability to differentiate various species as	be best
well as strains of the same species	• Patterns are complex, difficult to interpret
• Has been successfully employed in	• Lack of standardization
epidemiologic investigations	• Labor intensive, highly technical
• Fingerprint patterns are not so complex so	• Limited probe availability
interpretation can be easier	• Most commonly uses radioisotopes for detection
	• May lack discriminatory power, may be necessary
	to use several combinations of enzymes and
	probes to insure differential power
• High degree of strain discrimination	• Specialized equipment
• Use of a single test to differentiate strains	• Different methods for electrophoresis give
• Combine with use of DNA probes	different types of patterns
	• Limited batch size
• Rapid	• Lack of standardization
• Simple and easy to perform	• Variation of fingerprints depending on how cell
	lysates are prepared
	• Variation in fingerprints depending on
	immunoblot antisera
	• Gel to gel variation
	• Excessive numbers of bands leading to a large
	number of "single" fingerprint isolates
• Ease of performance	• Lack of standardization
• Stable	• Variation of fingerprints depending on how cell
• Widely available reagents	lysates are prepared
• High level discrimination	• Not yet validated epidemiologically for *Candida*

scenarios for the genetic relatedness of strains from patients with recurrent vaginitis: (1) strain maintenance without genetic variation, (2) strain maintenance with minor genetic variation, and (3) strain replacement.[17,23,26] Vasquez used karyotyping to follow isolates obtained from 10 women with recurrent vulvovaginal candidiasis due to *C. albicans*.[23] The women were followed for an average of 35 months, with an average of 8 isolates per woman. In 8 of 10 women, only one karyotype was observed, whereas the other two women had two or three types, respectively. In one patient, one strain was observed during the first 16 months, another for 11 months, and then a third type. The other patient had two different types: one for the first 5 months, then another for the next 26 months. There were no data on isolates types from sexual partners of these women.[23] Alternately, Schröppel and colleagues[26] demonstrated that the strain isolated from the glans penis of the male partner of a woman with recurrent vulvovaginal candidiasis was the same as her vaginal isolate. A different strain was found in his mouth, and this strain subsequently replaced the original vulvovaginal isolate in a recurrent episode of vaginitis.[26] Most recently, Lockhart and co-workers[17] used fingerprinting and Southern blot hybridization with three different probes to follow 18 patients with recurrent vulvovaginal infections. They found that in most women, the same strain was responsible for successive infections, but in 56% of patients there were minor strain differences (referred to as strain shuffling). In eight cases, isolates were also obtained from male partners and these were shown to be identical or highly related to the infecting strain of the woman. Finally, these authors showed that oral and vaginal isolates were identical in 45%, highly related in 35%, and unrelated in 20% of the cases.[17] Whether women not suffering from recurrent infection and their partners also carry the same strains has yet to be studied.

8.1.2   Laboratory aspects

8.1.2.1   Specimen collection and transport

Ideally, the diagnosis of all types of candidal infections should involve the detection, isolation, and identification of the causative agents. The first step for the most sensitive yeast isolation method is the proper and careful collection of the specimen from the site of infection. Polyester swabs are the most commonly used collection devices for the recovery of yeasts from the genitalia and surrounding skin. Swabs should be sent to the laboratory as soon as possible after collection to prevent desiccation. *C. albicans* can survive at least 24 h on a moist swab without loss of viability; however, use of a transport medium can assure adequate hydration.[1]

8.1.2.2   Detection and isolation of yeasts

Candida are yeasts, that is, fungi that exist predominately in a unicellular form. They are usually small, oval cells that reproduce by budding. If the buds do not break off, but remain attached to the mother cell, then a string of buds is produced that is called a pseudohypha. Additionally, true hyphae can be produced (usually in tissue) and thickened, rounded cells, called chlamydospores will be formed by some species.

Microscopic examination of the clinical specimen is helpful for early detection of the presence of yeasts. Gram-stained or 20% KOH preparations of material expressed from the specimen swab will often result in a positive finding. The presence of oval budding yeasts, often with pseudohyphae and hyphae, are typically the structures associated with candidal infections. While microscopic examination is not definitive for the diagnosis of *C. albicans* infection, observation of the typical yeast forms is indicative of the presence of yeast.

The most commonly used media for the isolation of yeast are variations of Sabouraud dextrose agar (Sab). Sab has a pH of less than 6.0 and therefore retards the growth of many bacteria. Additionally, antibacterial agents are often incorporated into Sab when specimens from nonsterile sites are to be cultured. Sab with chloramphenicol or gentamicin are two such frequently used media. Sab with chloramphenicol and cycloheximide is also commonly used when the recovery of only *C. albicans* is desired as cycloheximide inhibits the growth of most other *Candida* spp., other yeasts, and many environmental molds. *Candida* spp. form smooth, creamy white, glistening colonies on these conventional media. More recently media containing chromogenic substrates are being evaluated for the isolation and the identification of various yeasts. Reports of media such as CHROMagar Candida (CHROMagar, Paris, France) and Albicans ID (BioMérieux Vitek, Hazelwood, MO) offer the advantages of better detection rates than the standard Sab-chloramphenicol medium and satisfactory identification capabilities.[27]

8.1.2.3   Identification of yeasts

Complete identification of *Candida* spp. requires a combination of morphologic and physiologic tests.[28] Temperature, presence or absence of certain enzymes, pseudohyphae, chlamydospores and hyphae, and utilization of nitrogen and carbon sources, all constitute a complete workup of an unknown yeast. Practically, however, most yeasts recovered from clinical sources can be identified with much less effort. One of the most valuable and simplest tests for the rapid identification of *C. albicans* is the germ tube test. While neither 100% sensitive nor specific, this test is the one most frequently used for rapid, presumptive identification. After inoculation of a colony into rabbit or other animal serum, *Candida* spp. produce hyphal initials that are called "germ tubes." Within 2–3 h after inoculation, *C. albicans* usually produces germ tubes that are not constricted below the blastoconidium. Other yeasts take longer to produce germ tubes, do not produce germ tubes, or produce germ tubes with constrictions. Additionally, *C. albicans* will produce budding yeasts, pseudohyphae, and chlamydospores when inoculated to cornmeal agar. Identification of other yeasts may require a more extensive workup and rapid biochemical test systems are available commercially for that purpose. Systems such as API 20 C (BioMérieux Vitek, Hazelwood, MO) and MicroScan Yeast Identification Panel (MicroScan, West Sacramento, CA) provide a rapid, convenient method for identification of common yeast species. There are more than 150 species of *Candida* but only a few are regarded as common pathogens: *C. albicans*, *C. glabrata*, *C. guilliermondii*, *C. krusei*, *C. parapsilosis*, *C. tropicalis*, *C. lusitaniae*, and *C. rugosa*. Because of variations in species pathogenicity and drug susceptibility, complete speciation is desirable.

8.1.2.4.   The role of serologic diagnosis in vaginitis

The clinical usefulness of antibody detection is limited by false-positive and false-negative testing depending on the population and type of infection. All investigators seem to agree that there is no role for serodiagnosis by antibody detection in candida vaginitis.[29,30] Newer serologic tests for *Candida* spp. have targeted antigen detection aimed at the diagnosis of systemic candidiasis by the detection of mannan or other antigens. Clinical experience with these tests for the diagnosis of systemic candidiasis has been mixed, but in no case are they recommended for use in the diagnosis of vaginitis.[30]

8.1.3   Clinical disease

8.1.3.1   Predisposing conditions

Candida spp. can be commensals, being present as normal flora on the human body. For these yeasts to become pathogens, interruption of normal defense mechanisms is necessary. Predisposing factors include diabetes mellitus, antibiotic therapy, pregnancy, and other immune system altering diseases such as AIDS. The ability of *Candida* spp. to adhere to vaginal and oral epithelial cells has been recognized, and, while the precise role of adherence in the pathogenesis of infection has not been completely defined, given the findings in bacterial systems, adherence will likely play an important part.[31] While estimates of candidal vaginitis are high, and some suggest that 75% of women will experience this disease, many women have no recognizable underlying predisposing factor. *Candida* is one of the most common causes of vaginitis today, and widespread use of antibiotic therapy may be the most important factor responsible for its emergence.[32]

8.1.3.2   Vaginitis

Presentation of candidal vaginitis encompasses the entire spectrum from rare to few symptoms, to scanty discharge, to the more typical thick, curd-like discharge. The thick discharge consists of epithelial cells and mats of hyphae, yeast cells, and pseudohyphae. Painful burning sensations can occur during urination or sexual intercourse and is often worse just before the onset of menstruation. Intense pruritus of the vulva is almost always present. The vagina and labia are usually erythematous and extension onto the vulva often occurs. Papular and granular lesions may be seen and spread to the perianal region and inner aspects of the thighs can occur.[1] Chronic, recurrent, vulvovaginal candidiasis is seen in women who have had at least 3 clinically and mycologically proven episodes of vaginal candidiasis within a 12-month period. The symptoms are similar to those observed in acute episodes; however, progress in control of recurrence is lacking.[33]

8.1.3.3. Balanitis

Clinical presentations of balanitis range from itching of the penis and redness of the glans to an erosive balanitis. The process usually begins as vesicles on the penis, next patches resembling thrush occur and finally, severe itching and burning. Papular lesions with edema of the prepuce may be present and extension to the thighs, gluteal folds, scrotum, and buttocks has been rarely reported.

Less than 20% of men cultured for the presence of yeasts have been shown to harbor the organisms and uncircumcised men are more likely to be positive than circumcised men. The presence of yeasts and symptomatic balanitis are found when female sex partners have vaginal thrush, suggesting that sexual transmission is often the route of infection in penile candidiasis.[25]

8.1.4 Antifungal drugs, susceptibility testing, and therapy

8.1.4.1 Antifungal drugs — description and mode of action

The topical azole drugs (Figure 1), particularly clotrimazole and miconazole are the mainstay of therapy for vulvovaginal candidiasis. More recently, there has been interest in use of oral azole drugs (Figure 2) for candidiasis, particularly for prophylaxis in recurrent vulvovaginal candidiasis. Just as physiologic conditions for susceptibility testing affect minimum inhibitory concentrations that are observed with azole antifungal drugs, so too do they affect the ability to demonstrate target effects of these agents. All azole derived drugs inhibit 14-demethylation in fungal sterol biosynthesis, the primary target of which is the demethylation of lanosterol, a cytochrome P-450. Additionally, azoles also affect membrane permeability. At concentrations higher than those that interfere with cytochrome P-450 (5 µg/ml), imidazoles (butoconazole, clotrimazole, ketoconazole, miconazole, tioconazole) but not triazoles (fluconazole, itraconazole, terconazole) can directly damage fungal membranes, causing a variety of deleterious effects (e.g., changes in transport systems, decrease in cellular ATP, K+ leakage, and others). Some azoles have also been shown to inhibit ATPase of fungal membranes.

8.1.4.2 Treatment options

8.1.4.2.1 Topical therapy. Topical agents are considered the first line of therapy.[34] Presently, butoconazole, clotrimazole, miconazole, tioconazole, and terconazole are FDA-approved for the topical treatment of vulvovaginal candidiasis. No regime is considered superior.[34] Systemic adsorption of these agents is typically quite low with negligible amounts of ticonzole detected, 1% for miconazole, 3–10% for clotrimazole, 5% for butoconazole, and 5–16% for terconazole.[35-37] All have been found to be safe and effective. However, because there is some absorption, none is recommended during the first trimester of pregnancy. Treatment with any of these agents during second or third trimesters is safe. Most agents come in several formulations and cost generally ranges from $12–$25. In comparative trials conducted in the 1970s, miconazole and clotrimazole, at doses of 100 mg/day for 10–14 days, demonstrated higher cure rates (80–90%) than nystatin (70–80%).[34,38] Subsequently, 3-day courses of therapy with 200 mg/day of these agents were shown to have acceptable cure rates. In the 1980s, butoconazole, tioconazole, and terconazole were approved for use with similar regimes. Most recently clotrimazole and

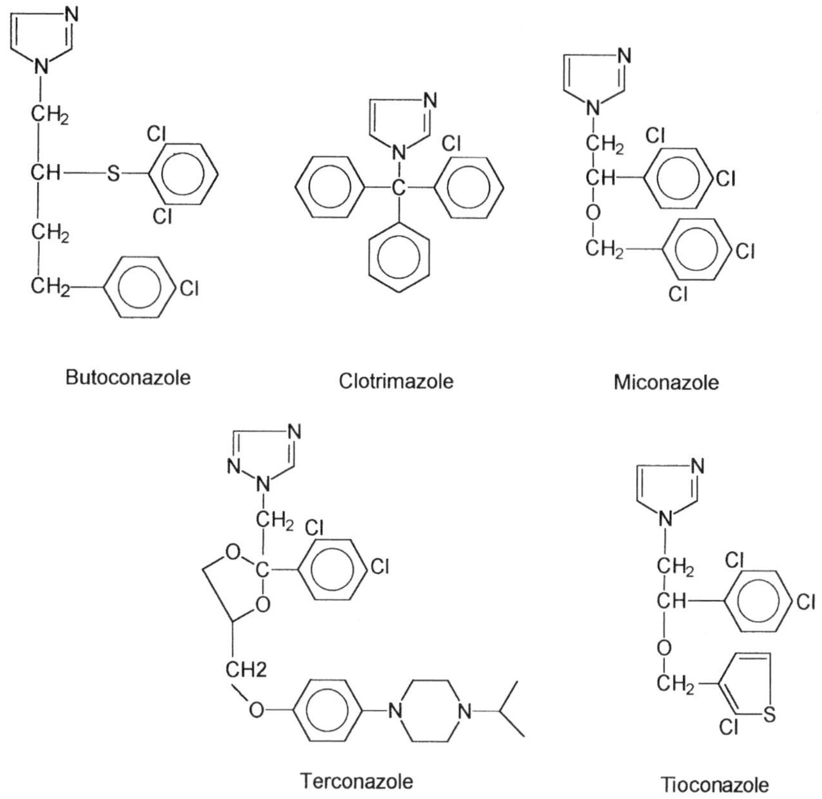

Figure 1 Topical azole drugs.

miconazole have become available in over-the-counter formulations. Over-the-counter formulations have half the potency of the prescription formulations, in 3 to 14 day dosing schedules. Although specific directions for use of these products are included, women treated previously with a different formulation may not adhere to the correct schedule and this may promote the emergence of drug resistance. Another concern regarding the use of self-diagnosis is its inaccuracy, since studies of patients referred to clinics for the treatment of recurrent vulvovaginal candidiasis have shown that as few as 25% of patients may really have recurrent infection.[39]

8.1.4.2.2 Oral therapy. Oral azole therapy has been used in Europe for some time, but concerns about toxicity and side effects delayed introduction in the U.S.[34] Results of studies with itraconazole and ketoconazole imply that these therapies are about as effective as topical therapies, but optimal regimes have not yet been established.[40] Fluconazole is an attractive alternative since it persists at levels above the usual minimum inhibitory concentrations for *C. albicans* for 72 h or more; treatment schedules may consist of a single dose or multiple doses at 4-7 day intervals. It is important to note, however, that high failure rates with non-*albicans* isolates, especially *C. glabrata*, may limit use of this drug.[39]

8.1.4.2.3 Therapy for recurrent vulvovaginal candidiasis. The optimal treatment for recurrent vulvovaginal candidiasis has not been established. In particular, there have been no studies published detailing experience in women with AIDS, where vulvovaginal

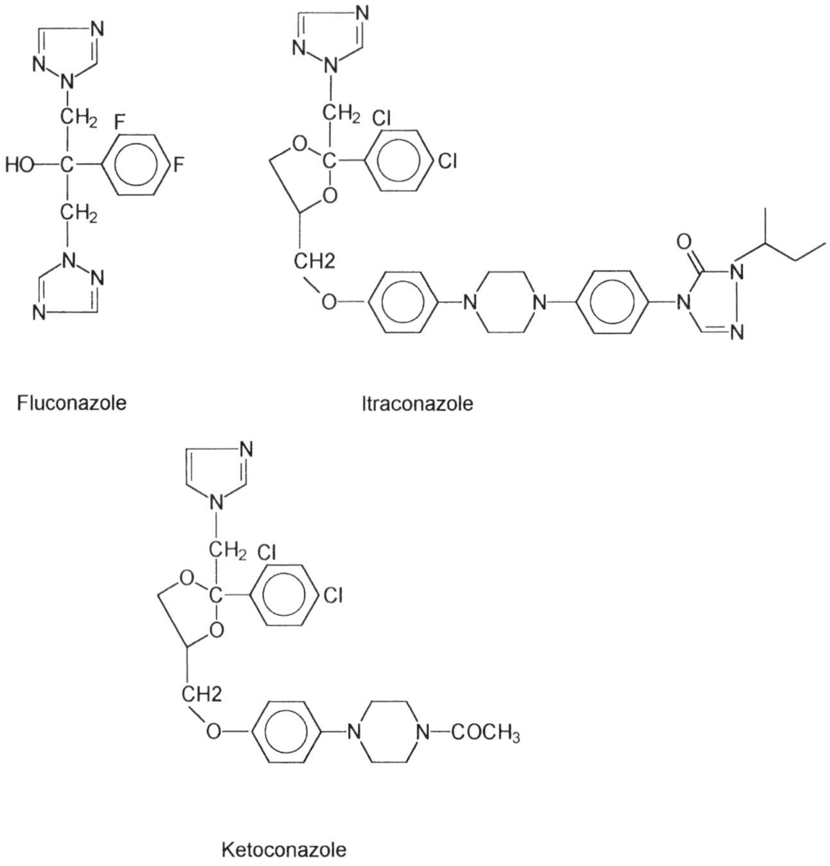

Fluconazole   Itraconazole

Ketoconazole

Figure 2 Oral azole drugs.

candidiasis is common. Treatment for an acute episode in a woman with a history of recurrent infection can be the same as an initial acute episode. Other alternatives that have been reported include a 14-day course of ketoconazole 400 mg daily and 200 mg fluconazole every 4 days for three doses followed by suppressive 200 mg doses of fluconazole weekly for 3 months.[39] There have been anecdotal reports of success using boric acid 600 mg twice daily intravaginally for two weeks.[32,39]

Prophylactic strategies for recurrent infection include both topical and oral therapy in maintenance dosages, but recurrence/relapse occurs with high frequency when maintenance is stopped. Regimes that have been reported to reduce the incidence of recurrent episodes include ketoconzole 100 mg/daily or 400 mg/daily for 5 days at the beginning of menses and clotrimazole intravaginally once weekly or monthly.[34,41] Monthly doses of 150 mg of fluconazole have not been as successful as daily ketoconazole; a weekly dose of 100 mg of fluconazole is under investigation.[34]

8.1.4.3 Susceptibility testing

The skyrocketing frequency of serious fungal infections has driven the development of numerous antifungal agents and these have, in turn, contributed to increasing interest in antifungal susceptibility tests (AFST) for both yeasts and molds.[42] The increased long-term

Table 4 Parameters Currently Specified by NCCLS M27-T
for Susceptibility Testing

Method	Macrobroth dilution
Inoculum size	$0.5–2.5 \times 10^3$ cfu/ml
Medium	RPMI
pH	7.0
buffer	MOPS[a]
Temperature of incubation	35°C
Duration of incubation	
Candida species	48 h
Cryptococcus species	72 h
Endpoint	Prominent decrease compared to control

[a] MOPS = Morpholinopropanesulfonic acid.

use of antifungal agents among the immunocompromised and normal women with recurrent vaginitis has led to numerous reports of resistance to antifungal agents and more recently, cross-resistance among imidazoles.[16,18,20,32] Clinicians would like to be guided in therapeutic choices by AFST results along with epidemiologic data on susceptibility patterns for their locale. Unfortunately, AFST is in its infancy and methods have not been well standardized. Often the *in vitro* susceptibility does not correlate with clinical outcome.[42] The variations of susceptibility test methods include macro- and microbroth dilutions, semisolid agar methods, agar-dilution methods, and adaptations using newer commercial systems, such as the Alamar or E test systems.[43,44] For each method, variations in inoculum size, method of inoculum preparation, media, buffer, pH, length and temperature of incubation, end point definition and solubilizing drugs lead to an exhaustive list of permutations that can create widely disparate results among methods or even when investigators use the same method but do not define all the variables exactly. Significant efforts have been made through the National Committee for Clinical Laboratory Standards (NCCLS) toward a standardized method for AFST for *Candida* species and *Cryptococcus neoformans,* and the proposed standard, M27-P, has just been revised to a tentative standard.[45-48] These collaborative studies have shown the conditions listed in Table 4 to yield acceptable reproducibility for inter- and intralaboratory tests for amphotericin B, ketoconazole, and amphotericin B and fluconazole.[45,49] Unlike amphotericin B, imidazole drugs and 5 fluocytosine are subject to what has been termed a "trailing endpoint." With these drugs there is typically a prominent drug effect, but small amounts of turbidity persist in the increasing concentrations that are routinely tested. A successful approach to deal with this endpoint is analogous to endpoint determinations used in antibacterial testing with sulfonamide drugs, namely the use of an 80% decrease compared to the growth control to quantitate the meaning of a "prominent decrease in turbidity."[49]

Clinical correlation of the results of susceptibility testing using the NCCLS format and clinical outcome have been disappointing.[42] Some encouraging results have been obtained in the case of oropharyngeal candidiasis, when sequential isolates were available for testing. In these studies, it has been possible to show that initial isolates were relatively susceptible and long-term therapy results in the selection of relatively resistant strains.[20] Somewhat disturbing are reports of resistance to fluconazole, both clinically and by susceptibility testing, among isolates from patients never treated with the drug.[32]

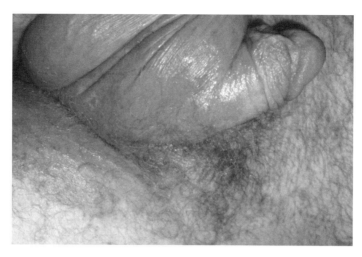

Genital candidiasis in an HIV patient. (Photo courtesy of A.W. Hoke, M.D.)

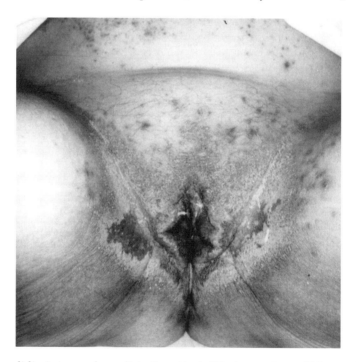

Severe genital candidiasis in an obese diabetic patient. (Photo courtesy of Mervyn L. Elgart, M.D.)

References

1. Odds, F.C., *Candida and Candidosis: A Review and Bibliography,* Second Edition Baillière Tindall, London, 1988, p. 68–92.
2. Jarvis, W.R., Epidemiology of nosocomial fungal infections, with emphasis on *Candida* species, *Clin. Infect. Dis.,* 20, 1526, 1995.
3. Hurley, R., Trends in candidal vaginitis, *Proc. R. Soc. Med.,* 70 (Suppl. 4), 1, 1977.
4. Hurley, R., De Louvois, J., *Candida* vaginitis, *Postgrad. Med. J.,* 55, 645, 1979.
5. Hurley, R., Recurrent Candida infection, *Clin. Obstet. Gynecol.,* 8, 209, 1981.
6. Bingham, J.S., Vulvovaginal candidosis — an overview, *Acta Dermatol. Venereol.,* (Suppl. 121), 125, 1986.

7. Hooton, T.M., Roberts, P.L., Stamm, W.E., Effects of recent sexual activity and use of a diaphragm/spermicide on the vaginal microflora, *Clin. Infect. Dis.*, 19, 274, 1994.

8. Spinillo, A., Michelone, G., Cavanna C., Colonna, L., Capuzzo, E., Nicola, S., Clinical and microbiological characteristics of symptomatic vulvovaginal candidiasis in HIV seropositive women. *Genitourin. Med.*, 70, 268, 1994.

9. Hasenclever, H.F., Mitchell, W.O., Antigenic studies of *Candida* I. Observations of two antigenic groups of *Candida albicans*, *J. Bacteriol.*, 82, 570, 1961.

10. Auger, P., Dumas, C., Joly J., A study of 666 strains of *Candida albicans:* Correlation between serotype and susceptibility to 5-fluorocytosine, *J. Infect. Dis.*, 139, 590, 1979.

11. Hasenclever, H.F., Mitchell, W.O., Antigenic studies of *Candida* IV. The relationships of the antigenic groups of *Candida albicans* to their isolation from various clinical specimens, *Sabouraudia*, 2, 201, 1963.

12. Odds, F.C., Abbott, A.B., Reed, T.A.G., Willmott, F.E., *Candida albicans* strain types from the genitalia of patients with and without *Candida* infection, *Eur. J. Obstet. Gynecol.*, 15, 37, 1983.

13. McCreight, M.C., Warnock, D.W., Enhanced differentiation of isolates of *Candida albicans* using a modified resistogram method, *Mykosen*, 25, 589, 1982.

14. Warnock, D.W., Speller, D.C.E., Milne, J.D., Hilton, A.L., Kershaw, P.I., Epidemiological investigation of patients with vulvovaginal candidosis. Application of resistogram method for strain differentiation of *Candida albicans*, *Br. J. Vener. Dis.*, 55, 357, 1979.

15. Polonelli, L., Castagnola, M., Rossetti, D.V., Morace, G., Use of killer toxins for computer-aided differentiation of *Candida albicans* strains, *Mycopathologia*, 91, 175, 1985.

16. Barchiesi, F., Hollis, R.J., McGough, D.A., Scalise, G., Rinaldi, M.G., Pfaller, M.A., DNA subtypes and fluconazole susceptibilities of *Candida albicans* isolates from the oral cavities of patients with AIDS, *Clin. Infect. Dis.*, 20, 634, 1995.

17. Lockhart, S.R., Reed, B.D., Pierson, C.L., Soll, D.R., Most frequent scenario for recurrent *Candida* vaginitis is strain maintenance with "substrain shuffling": demonstration by sequential DNA fingerprinting with probes Ca3, C1, and CARE2, *J. Clin. Microbiol.*, 34, 767, 1996.

18. Pfaller, M.A., Rhine-Chalberg, J., Redding, S.W., Smith, J., Farinacci, G., Fothergill, A.W., Rinaldi, M.G., Variations in fluconazole susceptibility and electrophoretic karyotype among oral isolates of *Candida albicans* from patients with AIDS and oral candidiasis, *J.Clin. Microbiol.*, 32, 59, 1994.

19. Reagan, D.R., Pfaller, M.A., Hollis, R.J., Wenzel, R., Characterization of the sequence of colonization and nosocomial candidiemia using DNA fingerprinting and a DNA probe, *J. Clin. Microbiol.*, 28, 2733, 1990.

20. Redding, S., Smith, S., Farinacci, G., Rinaldi, M., Fothergill, A., Rhine-Chalber, J., Pfaller, M., Resistance of *Candida albicans* to fluconazole during treatment of oropharyngeal candidiasis in a patient with AIDS: documentation by *in vitro* susceptibility testing and DNA subtype analysis, *Clin. Infect. Dis.*, 18, 240, 1994.

21. Schmid, J., Rotman, R., Reed. B., Pierson, C.L., Soll, D.R., Genetic similarity of *Candida albicans* strains from vaginitis patients and their partners, *J. Clin. Microbiol.*, 31, 39, 1993.

22. Soll, D.R., Staebell, M., Langtimm, C., Pfaller, M.A., Hicks, J., Gopala Rao, T.V., Multiple *Candida* strains in the course of a single systemic infection, *J. Clin. Microbiol.*, 26, 1448, 1988.

23. Vasquez, J.A., Sobel, J.D., Demitriou, R., Vaishampayan, J., Lynch, M., Zervos, M.J., Karyotyping of *Candida albicans* isolates obtained longitutinally in women with recurrent vulvovaginal candidiasis, *J. Infect. Dis.*, 170, 1566, 1994.

24. Vaudry, W.L., Tierney, A.J., Wenman, W.M., Investigation of a cluster of systemic *Candida albicans* infections in a neonatal intensive care unit, *J. Infect. Dis.*, 158, 1375, 1988.

25. Thin, R.N., Leighton, M., Dixon, M.J., How often is genital yeast infection sexually transmitted?, *Br. Med. J.*, 2, 93, 1977.

26. Schröppel, K., Rotman, M., Galask, R., Mac, K., Soll, D.R., Evolution and replacement of *Candida albicans* strains during recurrent vaginitis demonstrated by DNA fingerprinting, *J. Clin. Microbiol.*, 32, 2646, 1994.

27. Baumgartner, C., Freydiere, A.-E., Gille, Y., Direct identification and recognition of yeast species from clinical material by using Albicans ID and CHROMagar Candida plates, *J. Clin. Microbiol.*, 34, 454, 1996.

28. Warren, N.G., Hazen, K.C., *Candida, Cryptococcus* and other yeasts of medical importance, in *Manual of Clinical Microbiology*, 6th ed., Murray, P.R., Baron, E.J., Pfaller, M.A., Tenover, F.C., and Yolken, R.H., Eds., ASM Press, Washington, D.C., 1995, chap. 61.

29. Kaufman, L., Reiss, E., Serodiagnosis of fungal diseases, in Rose, N. R., Friedman, H., M*anual of Clinical Laboratory Immunology*, 4th ed., American Society for Microbiology, Washington, D. C., 1992, p. 506–528.

30. de Repentigny, L., Serodiagnosis of candidiasis, aspergillosis, and cryptococcosis, *Clin. Infect. Dis.*, 14 (Suppl. 1), S11, 1992.

31. Calderone, R.A., Braun, P.C. Adherence and receptor relationships of *Candida albicans*, *Microbiol. Rev.*, 55, 1, 1991.

32. Sobel, J.D., Vasquez, J.A., Symptomatic vulvovaginitis due to fluconazole- resistant *Candida albicans* in a female who was not infected with human immunodeficiency virus, *Clin. Infect. Dis.*, 22, 726, 1996.

33. O'Connor, M., Sobel, I.D., Epidemiology of recurrent vulvovaginal candidiasis: identification and strain differentiation of *Candida albicans*, *Clin. Infect. Dis.*, 154, 358, 1986.

34. Reef, S.E., Levine, W.C., McNeil, M.M., Fisher-Hosch, S., Holmberg, S.D., Duerr, A., Smith, D., Sobel, J.D., Pinner, R.W., Treatment options for vulvovaginal candidiasis, 1993, *Clin. Infect. Dis.*, 20 (Suppl. 1), S80–90, 1995.

35. Tatum, D.M., Eggleston, M., Butoconazolenitrate. *Infect. Con. Hosp. Epidemiol.*, 9, 122, 1988.

36. Abramowicz, M., Topical drugs for vaginal candidiasis, *Med. Lett. Drugs Ther.*, 33, 81, 1988.

37. Clissold, S.P., Heel, R.C., Ticoconazole: a review of its antimicrobial activity and therapeutic use in superficial mycoses, *Drugs*, 31, 29, 1986.

38. Bentley, S., Bourne, M.S., Powell, A., A comparative study of miconazole nitrate pessaries and nystatin vaginal tablets in the treatment of vaginal candidiasis, *Br. J. Clin. Prac.*, 32, 258, 1978.

39. Nyirjesy, P., Syeny, S.M., Terry Grody, M.H., Jordan, C.A., Buckely, H.R., Chronic fungal vaginitis, The value of cultures, *Am. J. Obstet. Gynecol.*, 173, 820, 1995.

40. van Heusdan, A.M., Merkus, J.M.W.M., Chronic recurrent vaginal candidosis: easy to treat, difficult to cure. Results of intermittent prophylactic treatment with a new oral antifungant?, *Eur. J. Obstet. Gynecol.*, 65, 435, 1985.

41. Roth, A.C., Milsom, I., Forsman, L., Wahlen, P., Intermittent prophylactic treatment of recurrent vaginal candidiasis by postmenstrual application of a 500 mg tablet of clotrimazole vaginal tablet, *Genitourin. Med.*, 66, 357, 1990.

42. Ghannoum M.A., Rex, J. H., Galgiani, J.N., Susceptibility testing of fungi: current status of correlation of in vitro data with clinical outcome, *J. Clin. Microbiol.*, 34, 489, 1996.

43. Columbo A.L., Barchiesi, F., McGough, D.A., Rinaldi, M.G., Comparison of Etest and National Committee for Clinical Laboratory Standards broth macrodilution method for azole antifungal susceptibility testing, *J. Clin. Microbiol.*, 33, 535, 1995.

44. Pfaller M.A., Barry A.L., Evaluation of a novel colorimetric broth microdilution method for antifungal susceptibility testing of yeast isolates, *J. Clin. Microbiol.*, 32, 1992, 1994.

45. Fromtling, R.A., Galgiani, J.N., Pfaller, M.A., Espinel-Ingroff, A., Bartizal, K.F., Bartlett, M.S., Body, B. A., Frey, C., Hall, G. Roberts, G.D., Nolte, F.B., Odds, F.C., Rinaldi M.G., Sugar, A.M., Villareal, K., Multicenter evaluation of macrobroth antifungal susceptibility test for yeasts, *Antimicrob. Agent Chemother.*, 37, 39, 1993.

46. Pfaller, M A., Rinaldi, M.G., Galgiani, J.N., Bartlett, M.S., Body, B.A., Espinel-Ingroff, A., Fromtling, R.A., Hall, G.H., Huges, C.A., Odds, F.C., Sugar, A.M., Collaborative investigation of variables in susceptibility testing of yeasts, *Antimicrob. Agent Chemother.*, 34, 1648, 1990.

47. National Committee for Clinical Laboratory Standards, *Reference Method for Broth Dilution Antifungal Susceptibility Testing of Yeasts*, Proposed standard M27-P, National Committee for Clinical Laboratory Standards, Villanova, PA, 1992.

48. National Committee for Clinical Laboratory Standards, *Reference Method for Broth Dilution Antifungal Susceptibility Testing of Yeasts*, Tentative standard M27-T, National Committee for Clinical Laboratory Standards, Villanova, PA, 1995.

49. Espinel-Ingroff, A., Kish, C.W., Kerkering, T.M., Fromtling, R.A., Bartizal, K., Galgiani, J.N., Villareal, K., Pfaller, M.A., Gerarden, T., Rinaldi, M.G., Fothergill, A., Collaborative comparison of broth macrodilution and microdilution antifungal susceptibility tests, *J. Clin. Microbiol.*, 30, 3138, 1992.

50. Pfaller, M. A., Strain variation among *Candida* species: application of various typing methods to study epidemiology and pathogenesis of candidiasis in hospitalized patients, *Infect. Control*, 8, 273, 1987.

51. Scherer, S., Stevens, D.A., Application of DNA typing methods to epidemiology and taxonomy of *Candida* species, *J. Clin. Microbiol.*, 25, 675, 1987.

52. Magee, B.B., D'Souza, T.M., Magee, P.T., Strain and species identification by restriction fragment length polymorphisms in the ribosomal DNA repeat of *Candida* species, *J. Bacteriol.*, 169, 1639, 1987.

53. Lee, W., Burnie, J., Matthews, R., Fingerprinting *Candida albicans*, *J. Immunol. Methods*, 93, 177, 1986.

54. Lehmann, P.K., Kemker, B.J., Hsaio, C.B., Dev, S., Isoenzyme biotypes of *Candida* species, *J. Clin. Microbiol.*, 27, 2514, 1989.

Protozoan

chapter nine

Amebiasis

Lynne S. Garcia

9.1. Introduction..167
    9.1.1 Historical information 167
    9.1.2 Pathogenicity...168
    9.1.3 Immunology...169
9.2. Epidemiology and prevention 171
    9.2.1 Overview 171
    9.2.2 Sexual transmission 171
    9.2.3 Vaccine development...172
9.3. Life cycle and morphology..172
    9.3.1 Morphology of trophozoite 172
    9.3.2 Morphology of cyst..173
    9.3.3 Initiation of infection 174
9.4. Clinical disease 175
    9.4.1 Asymptomatic infection...178
    9.4.2 Intestinal disease 178
    9.4.3 Hepatic disease 178
9.5. Diagnosis 179
    9.5.1 Immunodetection 180
    9.5.2 Antibody detection 181
    9.5.3 Histologic detection 182
    9.5.4 Review of laboratory diagnosis 183
    9.5.5 Differentiation of amebiasis and inflammatory bowel disease....185
9.6. Treatment...185
    9.6.1 Asymptomatic patient..185
    9.6.2 Mild to moderate disease 186
    9.6.3 Severe intestinal disease..186
    9.6.4 Hepatic disease 186
References..186

9.1 Introduction

9.1.1 Historical information

In 1875, *Entamoeba histolytica* was first described by Lösch, in Russia, from a patient with dysenteric stools.[1] Although he found the organisms in human colonic ulcers at autopsy and was able to induce dysentery in a dog which was inoculated rectally with the patient's stools, he failed to recognize the causal relationship. Another important finding in the history of amebic dysentery was the discovery of the cause of bacillary dysentery by Shiga in 1898 and confirmed by Flexner in 1900. Based on these findings, Brown in 1911 stated in his book, *Amebic or Tropical Dysentery*, "The discovery that dysentery itself is not a single disease may be regarded as one of the most remarkable advances in modern medical science."

In 1925, Brumpt noted two different clinical presentations in amebiasis; many patients were completely asymptomatic or had mild diarrhea, while in approximately 10% of the cases there would be colitis, dysentery, and potential dissemination to other body sites.[2] This organism was eventually more fully investigated and differentiated from *Entamoeba coli*, both in terms of morphology and pathogenesis. These studies are reviewed by Imperato.[3]

E. histolytica has been recovered worldwide and is more prevalent in the tropics and subtropics than in cooler climates. However, in unsanitary conditions in temperate and colder climates, infection rates have been found to equal that seen in the tropics.

9.1.2 Pathogenicity

Although a large number of people throughout the world are infected with this organism, only a small percentage will develop clinical symptoms. Depending on geographic area, organism strain, and the patient's immune status, morbidity and mortality due to *E. histolytica* vary. In the years since Brumpt published his monograph, the issue of pathogenicity has been very controversial with, essentially, two points of view. Some felt that what was called *E. histolytica* was really two separate species of *Entamoeba*, one being pathogenic causing invasive disease and the other being nonpathogenic causing mild or asymptomatic infections. Others felt that all organisms designated *E. histolytica* were potentially pathogenic, symptoms depending on the result of host or environmental factors, including intestinal flora.

In 1961, with the development by Diamond of successful axenic culture methods requiring no bacterial coculture, sufficient organisms could be obtained for additional studies.[4] Approximately 15 years later, work by Sargeaunt and his colleagues indicated that *E. histolytica* clinical isolates could be classified into groups using starch gel electrophoresis and review of banding patterns related to specific isoenzymes.[5-9] The four isoenzymes are glucophosphate isomerase (GPI), phosphoglucomutase (PGM), malate dehydrogenase (ME), and hexokinase (HK). Sargeaunt concluded from this work that there are pathogenic and nonpathogenic strains (zymodemes) of *E. histolytica* that can be differentiated by isoenzyme analysis. Based on analysis of thousands of clinical isolates, he also concluded that the zymodeme patterns were probably genetic, rather than phenotypic.

Others argued that bacterial flora present in the gut played a role in potential pathogenicity of *E. histolytica*.[10] Some of the *in vitro* culture studies indicated that bacteria were shown to enhance virulence.[10-12] During the 1980s and early 1990s, several publications reviewed these issues, with a number of questions still remaining unanswered.[13-16] More recent evidence supports the differentiation of the pathogenic *E. histolytica* from the non-pathogenic *E. dispar* as two distinct species,[17] while other reports indicate *E. histolytica* may be able to modulate its virulence, depending on culture conditions.[18]

According to Clark and Diamond,[13] after failing to obtain conversion of "nonpathogenic" *E. histolytica* isolates to the "pathogenic" form during axenization of the amebae, the most logical explanation was culture contamination. In reviewing this possibility, they used a method based on analysis of stable DNA polymorphisms that allows the identification of individual pathogenic isolates. The DNA patterns obtained using the "converted" amebae were identical to reference isolates present in the laboratory at the time of conversion.[17] They also found that transfer of very few pathogenic organisms was necessary to become established in a nonpathogenic culture. Within the context of this study, cross-contamination fully explained the conversion and the designation of specific pathogenic *E. histolytica* and nonpathogenic *E. dispar* was confirmed.[17]

Studies by Orozco and colleagues investigated the molecular basis underlying the variability of *E. histolytica* strains.[19] They detected, cloned, sequenced, and characterized a variable DNA region that is differentially transcribed in *E. histolytica* clones and strains. The significance of these studies is based on the use of genetically related trophozoites from the same strain, cultured under the same conditions, and belonging to the same pathogenic zymodeme II; however, they showed different degrees of virulence. A number of factors could be responsible for these differences: presence of highly variable genomic DNA regions or a high rate of mutation and recombination in specific regions of the genome.[19] The only thing that appears to be agreed upon is that the molecular basis of any variability that may exist is not completely understood.[20] However, based on current knowledge, pathogenic *E. histolytica* is considered to be the etiologic agent of amebic colitis and extraintestinal abscesses, while nonpathogenic *E. dispar* produces no intestinal symptoms and is not invasive in humans.[21]

There is evidence that *E. histolytica* trophozoites interact with the host through a series of steps: adhesion to the target cell, phagocytosis, and cytopathic effect.[22,23] Numerous other parasite factors may also play a role. From the perspective of the host, *E. histolytica* induces both humoral and cellular immune responses, with cell-mediated immunity representing the major human host defense against this complement-resistant cytolytic protozoan.

9.1.3   Immunology

With the development of axenic culture and antigen purification techniques, *E. histolytica* infections and subsequent host immune responses have been more thoroughly investigated. However, in spite of the fact that both humoral and cellular responses occur in amebiasis, the role of immunity is still not well understood.

In patients with amebic dysentery, coproantibodies can be detected in approximately 80% of patients, with a steady decline over a period of weeks to about 55%.[24] During this same time, an increase in serum antibodies can also be demonstrated. The information related to copro- and serum antibodies may indicate a transient secretory response followed by tissue invasion and penetration with production of circulating antibody. Once invasive amebiasis has been established, a serologic response can usually be detected within a week after the onset of symptoms. Titers are usually high and can persist for several years, even after invasive disease has healed or a subclinical infection has been controlled. Unfortunately, this humoral response during the invasive phase of the disease apparently has little impact on potential reinfections or in the healing process.

Immunoglobulin IgM is produced, although IgG is found at a higher concentration with the predominant subclass being IgG2.[25] The production of antiameba IgE is unclear. A cytotoxic effect is produced on the trophozoites; organisms lose motility when in contact with serum containing specific antibodies. Also, introduction of antibodies to cultures will inhibit growth and antibody-treated organisms will not induce liver abscess in susceptible animal models.

Sera from healthy individuals with no evidence of past or present amebiasis will also produce the same effects on organisms as immune sera. Even after absorption with *E. histolytica* trophozoites, the effects persist, suggesting that they are due to causes other than the presence of natural antibodies. Complement activation is involved, via both the classic and alternative pathways, and apparently does not require antibodies. Activation of these complement pathways results in trophozoite lysis. Because highly virulent strains of *E. histolytica* are more resistant to complement lysis, complement may also play a role in natural resistance to infection with a potential reduction in invasive capacity.[26] However, it is not known if reduced complement activity may play a role in the susceptibility of certain individuals to infection or whether it may be related to host defenses.

The majority of research in cell-mediated immunity in amebiasis has been conducted in animal models of amebic liver abscess. However, a number of different approaches have been taken to try and clarify the role of cellular immunity in humans. One example involved the use of skin test antigens obtained from *E. histolytica* culture. This procedure detects amebiasis long after the patient has recovered from the infection and has been used in epidemiologic studies. Patients with invasive amebiasis exhibit a typical delayed-type hypersensitivity reaction, although the reaction is usually negative during the acute phase of an untreated liver abscess.[25] Macrophage migration-inhibition assays have shown similar results to those obtained with skin test antigens during invasive disease. Results were negative during the early phases of liver abscess, but they became positive after therapy. A number of different animal model studies also confirm cell-mediated immunity plays an active role in the overall immune response to infection with *E. histolytica*.[25]

Lymphocyte transformation induced by concanavalin A (Con A) has been reported comparable with cells from both patients with amebic liver abscess and healthy controls; similar results have also been demonstrated with phytohemagglutinin (PHA). However, studies in infected hamsters indicated reduced reactivity to Con A and PHA, while other reports indicate *E. histolytica* extracts are mitogenic for murine lymphocytes. Induced blastogenesis in lymphocytes from patients with amebic liver abscess has been shown with aqueous *E. histolytica* extracts and using a subcellular antigenic fraction, thus indicating *in vivo* sensitization of T lymphocytes to amebic antigens.[25,27]

Most studies emphasize the importance of cell-mediated immunity as the main factor in acquired protective immunity.[28] A number of factors support this conclusion including: (1) cellular anergy that supports the initial *E. histolytica* invasion; (2) increased incidence of invasive amebiasis after T-cell suppression or splenectomy; (3) protective impact of T-cell stimulants; (4) after recovery from amebic liver abscess, appearance and persistence of a delayed-type hypersensitivity reaction to amebic antigens; (5) transfer to immunity via sensitized T cells; and (6) the lysis effect of cytotoxic T cells stimulated with antigen and activated macrophages.

It is well documented that anergy is seen during the course of amebic liver abscess and that animal models reveal tissue destruction with minimal inflammatory reaction surrounding these areas. One explanation for this anergy might be a temporary desensitization caused by circulating antigen; it is not thought to be due to decreased T-cell numbers since normal levels have been detected in amebic liver abscess cases.[25]

Reduction of phagocytosis by peripheral blood polymorphonuclear leukocytes (PMNs) and monocytes has been found in various circumstances related to amebiasis. Depressed phagocytic function in PMNs was seen in patients with amebic liver abscess, compared with other manifestations of *E. histolytica* infection or healthy controls. In evaluating the functional capacity of monocytes, phagocytosis was significantly depressed in both liver and intestinal amebiasis and bactericidal function was depressed even more in liver amebiasis.[29]

Studies on patients with amebic liver abscess who had been healed for at least 9 weeks indicated that the CD4+ (helper, inducer T cells) lymphocyte subpopulation was smaller and the CD8+ (suppressor, cytotoxic T cells) subpopulation was increased, resulting in a smaller cell ratio in patients with amebic liver abscess than in controls.[30] However, when this same group of patients was checked a year later, four out of five demonstrated an increased CD4+ cell percentage and three out of five showed an increased ratio of CD4+ to CD8+ cells. Because T lymphocytes from cured amebic liver abscess patients have been shown to destroy *E. histolytica* after activation with parasite antigens, this may have an impact on host resistance in these patients.

9.2 Epidemiology and prevention

9.2.1 Overview

Infections with *E. histolytica* are worldwide in distribution and generally more prevalent in the tropics. In 1984, 500 million people were estimated to be infected with *E. histolytica*, 40–50 million of whom had extensive symptoms including colitis or extraintestinal abscesses.[31] Prevalence figures for the U.S. in 1961 were estimated to be 3 to 7%. Recent data from the Centers for Disease Control, (CDC) indicate prevalence figures from public health laboratories in various regions of the U.S. from less than 2% of specimens examined (*E. histolytica*) in all but six states; 2 to 3.9% in California, Texas, Illinois, and Pennsylvania; 4 to 5.9% in Oklahoma and New York City; and 8% in Arizona. It has also been estimated that for every case of invasive disease diagnosed, there are at least 10 to 20 asymptomatic individuals excreting infective cysts.

In 1994, analysis of 216,275 stool specimens examined by state diagnostic laboratories in 1987 indicated an overall positive rate of 20%.[32] Percentages were highest for intestinal protozoa and included: *Giardia lamblia* (7.2%), *Entamoeba coli* and *Endolimax nana* (4.2% each), *Blastocystis hominis* (2.6%), and *E. histolytica* (0.9%). In this data from 1978, *E. histolytica* was identified in 45 states, although in only 0.9% of the specimens. California laboratories accounted for almost half of the *E. histolytica* identifications (45.6%) and the majority (55.8%) of the *Dientamoeba fragilis* identifications.

Population groups which have been found to have a higher incidence of amebiasis include recent immigrants and refugees from South and Central America and from Southeast Asia. Residents from southeastern and southwestern parts of the U.S. also tend to have more infections with intestinal parasites as do other groups, including patients in mental institutions. Some studies show that 33% of sexually active homosexuals carry *E. histolytica* and transmit the infection venereally. It has been estimated that the worldwide infection rate ranges from 3 to 10%.

There are certain urban areas within the world (Mexico City; Medellin, Columbia; and Durban, South Africa), where the incidence of invasive disease is considerably higher than the rest of the world. Although contributing factors are not well delineated, they may include poor nutrition, tropical climate, decreased immunologic competence of the host, stress, altered bacterial flora in the colon, traumatic injuries to the colonic mucosa, alcoholism, and genetic factors.

Man is the primary reservoir host for *E. histolytica* and can transmit the infection to other humans, primates, dogs, cats, and possibly pigs. The cyst stages are very resistant to environmental conditions and can remain viable in the soil for 8 days at 28 to 34°C, 40 days at 2 to 6°C, and for 60 days at 0°C.[33] Cysts are normally removed by sand filtration or destroyed by 200 ppm of iodine, 5 to 10% acetic acid, or boiling. The asymptomatic cyst passer who is a food handler is generally thought to play the most important role in transmission.

9.2.2 Sexual transmission

Following broad social changes seen in the late 1960s, open expression of homosexuality, increased numbers of sexual contacts, increased frequency of sexual activities, and anonymity of sexual partners contributed to dramatic increases in sexually transmitted organisms, including *E. histolytica*. Although infections with this organism are usually associated with poor sanitation and underdeveloped areas of the world, epidemiologic studies in both Europe and the U.S. in the 1970s documented that sexual transmission of amebiasis occurred mainly among urban homosexual men.[34] With the increase in sexually transmitted pathogens, a number of clinical syndromes have been recognized; these clinical presentations have been grouped together and referred to as "the gay bowel syndrome." Many published reports confirm that *E. histolytica* is one of the major pathogens in the gay bowel syndrome. It is also well known that the clinical presentations within the homosexual community often differ from those seen in the heterosexual population.

Epidemiologic evidence of sexual transmission of *E. histolytica* has grown significantly since the early 1970s, particularly in areas such New York City and San Francisco. In San Francisco, the incidence of reported symptomatic intestinal amebiasis has increased over 1000% during the last 10 years among homosexual men between 20 and 39 years of age.[34] Although percentages vary, it appears that approximately 30% of urban homosexual men may be infected with *E. histolytica*, a sharp increase over the estimated rate of less than 5% seen in the general population within the U.S.

Direct oral-anal contact (anilingus) is a common practice among homosexual men which leads to both fecal exposure and oral contact with a variety of intestinal pathogens. Although anilingus has often been listed as a key risk factor in potential exposure, transmission can also occur during oral-genital sex after anal intercourse has occurred. It has also been shown that active heterosexuals can acquire infection with *E. histolytica* through sexual activities that provide an opportunity for fecal-oral contamination. The key factor is not necessarily homosexuality, but the frequency of sexual activity and potential for fecal-oral contact.

Another factor within this population is the fact that there is a high prevalence rate of asymptomatic individuals who carry *E. histolytica*; almost half of all homosexual men found to be positive are asymptomatic. Various studies have confirmed the lack of correlation between symptoms and the presence of *E. histolytica* in this risk group.[35,36]

With the advent of the AIDS, and subsequent modifications in sexual practices within homosexual communities, the incidence of *E. histolytica* infection is thought to be much lower than before. In recent years, the recovery of coccidian parasites, *Isospora belli* and *Cryptosporidium parvum* and the microsporidia, *Enterocytozoon bieneusi* and *Encephalitozoon intestinalis* have become much more of a problem in patients with AIDS.[34,37]

9.2.3   Vaccine development

According to Petri et. al., a colonization-blocking vaccine could eliminate *E. histolytica* as a cause of human disease, particularly since humans serve as the only significant reservoir host.[21] The galactose-specific adhesin is a possible candidate for a vaccine. It is antigenically conserved and has a high-affinity interaction with galactose-terminal colonic mucin glycoproteins which are thought to be important prerequisites for colonization. A number of other potential protective antigens are being investigated; hopefully, one of these options will prove to be the key to the development of a cost-effective vaccine for the reduction or elimination of amebiasis as a human disease.

9.3   Life cycle and morphology

The life cycle is seen in Figure 1. The cyst form is the infective form for humans.

9.3.1   Morphology of trophozoite

Living trophozoites vary in size from about 10 to 60 μm in diameter and may be confused with other organisms (Table 1). Organisms recovered from diarrheic or dysenteric stools

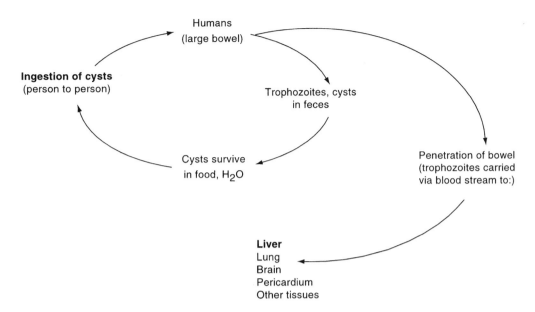

Figure 1   Life cycle of *Entamoeba histolytica*. (Adapted from Garcia, L.S. and D.A. Bruckner, *Diagnostic Medical Parasitology*, 3rd ed. American Society for Microbiology, ASM Press, Washington, D.C., 1997. With permission.)

are generally larger than those in a formed stool from an asymptomatic individual (Figures 2–4). The motility has been described as rapid and unidirectional with pseudopods forming quickly in response to the conditions around the organism. The motility may appear to be sporadic. Although this characteristic motility is often described, it is rare to diagnose amebiasis on the basis of motility seen in a direct wet mount. The cytoplasm is differentiated into a clear outer ectoplasm with a more granular inner endoplasm.

When the organism is examined on a permanent stained smear (trichrome or iron hematoxylin), the morphological characteristics are seen more easily. The nucleus is described as having evenly arranged chromatin on the nuclear membrane and the presence of a small, compact centrally located karyosome. The cytoplasm is usually described as finely granular with few ingested bacteria or debris in vacuoles. In a case with dysentery, red blood cells (RBCs) may be visible in the cytoplasm, and this feature is considered diagnostic for *E. histolytica*. Most often infection with *E. histolytica* will be diagnosed on the basis of organism morphology without the presence of RBCs.

9.3.2   Morphology of cyst

For reasons which are not specifically known, the trophozoites may condense into a round mass, (precyst), and a thin wall is secreted around the immature cyst (Figures 3 and 4). There may be two types of inclusions within this immature cyst, a glycogen mass and highly refractile chromatoidal bars with smooth, rounded edges. As the cysts mature (metacyst), there is nuclear division with the production of four nuclei (very rarely eight nuclei may be produced) and the cysts range in size from 10 to 20 μm (Table 2). Often, as the cyst matures, the glycogen completely disappears and the chromatoidals may also be absent in the mature cyst. Cyst formation occurs only within the intestinal tract; once the stool has left the body, cyst formation does not occur. The 1-, 2-, and 4-nucleated cysts are infective and represent the mode of transmission from one host to another (Figures 3 and 4).

Table 1 Trophozoites of Amebae in the Genus *Entamoeba*

Characteristic	*E. histolytica*	*E. hartmanni*	*E. coli*
Pathogenicity	Pathogenic[a]	Nonpathogenic	Nonpathogenic
Size[b] (diameter or length) **A**	12–60 µm; usual range: 15–20 µm; invasive forms may be over 20 µm	5–12 µm; usual range: 8–10 µm **B**	15–50 µm; usual range; 20–25 µm
Motility	Progressive, with hyaline, fingerlike pseudopodia; motility may be rapid	Usually nonprogressive	Sluggish nondirectional, with blunt, granular pseudopodia
Nucleus: number and visibility	Difficult to see in unstained preparations; 1 nucleus	Usually not seen in unstained preparations; 1 nucleus	Often visible in unstained preparation; 1 nucleus
Peripheral chromatin (stained) **C**	Fine granules, uniform in size and usually evenly distributed; may have beaded appearance	Nucleus may stain more darkly than *E. histolytica* although morphology is similar; chromatin **D** may appear as solid ring rather than beaded	May be clumped and unevenly arranged on the membrane; may also appear as solid, dark ring with no beads or clumps; may mimic *E. histolytica*
Karyosome (stained)	Small, usually compact; centrally located but may also be eccentric	Usually small and compact; usually centrally located or eccentric; often looks like "bull's eye"	Large, not compact; may or may not be eccentric; may be diffuse and darkly stained
Cytoplasm appearance (stained)	Finely granular, "ground glass" appearance; clear differentiation of ectoplasm and endoplasm; if present, vacuoles are usually small	Finely granular	Granular, with little differentiation into ectoplasm and endoplasm; usually vacuolated
Inclusions (stained) **E**	Noninvasive organism may contain bacteria; presence of red blood cells diagnostic	May contain bacteria; **F** no red blood cells; debris usually small and uniform	Bacteria, yeast, other debris

[a] The genus/species name *Entamoeba histolytica* actually includes two different species in the genus *Entamoeba*: *E. histolytica* (pathogenic) and *E. dispar* (nonpathogenic). Unless trophozoites of *E. histolytica* contain ingested red blood cells (RBCs), there is no way to morphologically distinguish *E. histolytica* from *E. dispar*. Most laboratories will continue to report "*Entamoeba histolytica*" when, in fact, the majority of these organisms may be *E. dispar*. (See text for additional information.)
[b] Wet preparation measurements (permanent stains; organisms usually measure 1–2 µm less).

9.3.3   Initiation of infection

After cyst ingestion, no changes occur in an acid environment; however, once the pH becomes neutral or slightly alkaline, the encysted organism becomes active, with the outcome being four separate trophozoites (small, metacystic trophozoites). These organisms develop into the normal trophozoites when they become established in the large intestine.

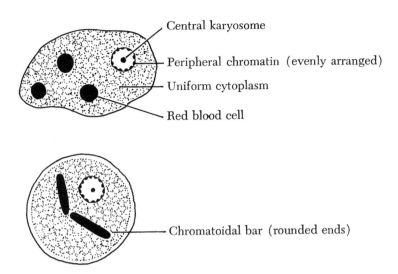

Figure 2 E. histolytica trophozoite (top) and cyst (bottom); note identifying morphologic characteristics.

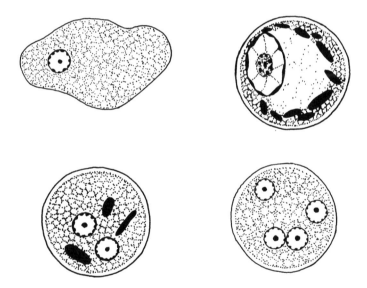

Figure 3 E. histolytica: (A) trophozoite (does not contain ingested red blood cells); (B) precyst (large single nucleus, small chromatoidal bars); (C) Two-nucleated cyst (chromatoidal bars have smooth, rounded ends); and (D) mature cyst containing four nuclei (this particular cyst does not contain chromatoidal bars).

9.4   Clinical disease

The presentations of disease are seen with invasion of the intestinal mucosa and/or dissemination to other organs, the most common being the liver. However, it is estimated that only a small proportion of infected individuals (2 to 8%) will have invasive disease beyond the lumen of the bowel. It has also been documented that organisms may be spontaneously eliminated with no disease symptoms.

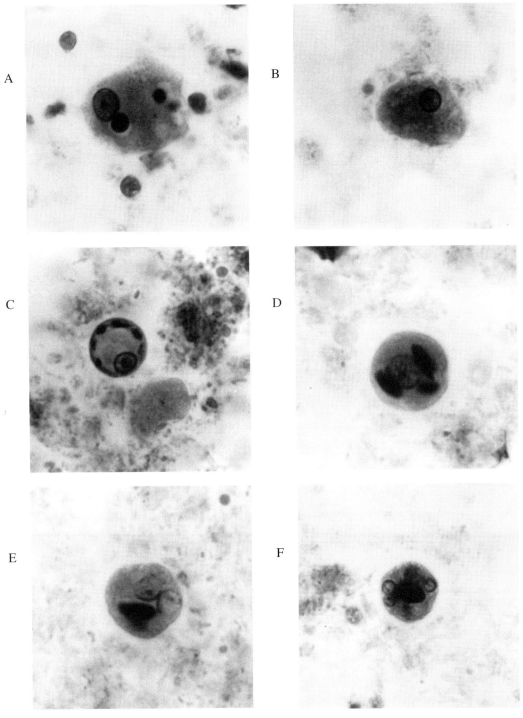

Figure 4 *E. histolytica*: (A) trophozoite containing ingested red blood cells (note evenly arranged chromatin and central, compact karyosome); (B) trophozoite (does not contain ingested red blood cells); (C) precyst containing a single, large nucleus and small chromatoidal bars; (D) precyst containing a single, large nucleus and larger chromatoidal bars; (E) two-nucleated cyst containing chromatoidal bars; and (F) mature cyst containing chromatoidal bars with smooth, rounded ends (only three of the four nuclei are visible).

Table 2 Cysts of Amebae in the Genus *Entamoeba*

Characteristic	E. histolytica	E. hartmanni	E. coli
Pathogenicity	Pathogenic[a]	Nonpathogenic	Nonpathogenic
Size[b] (diameter or length)	10–20 μm; usual range: 12–15 μm	5–10 μm usual range: 6–8 μm	10–35 μm; usual range: 15–25 μm
Shape	Usually spherical	Usually spherical	Usually spherical; may be oval or other shapes; may be distorted or shrunken on permanent stained slide due to inadequate fixation
Nucleus: number and visibility	Mature cyst: 4; immature: 1 or 2 nuclei; nuclear characteristics difficult to see on wet preparation	Mature cyst: 4; immature: 1 or 2 nuclei; two nucleated cysts <u>very common</u>	Mature cyst: 8; occasionally 16 or more nuclei may be seen; immature cysts with 2 or more nuclei are occasionally seen
Peripheral chromatin (stained)	Peripheral chromatin present; fine, uniform granules, evenly distributed; nuclear characteristics may not be as clearly visible as in trophozoite	Fine granules evenly distributed on the membrane; nuclear characteristics may be difficult to see, especially with numerous chromatoidal bars	Coarsely granular; may be clumped and unevenly arranged on membrane; nuclear characteristics not as clearly defined as in trophozoite; may resemble *E. histolytica*
Karyosome (stained)	Small, compact, usually centrally located but occasionally may be eccentric	Small, compact, usually centrally located	Large, may or may not be compact and/or eccentric; occasionally may be centrally located
Cytoplasm, chromatoidal bodies (stained)	May be present; bodies usually elongate, with blunt, rounded, smooth edges; may be round or oval	Usually present; bodies usually elongate with blunt, rounded, smooth edges; may be round or oval	May be present (less frequently than *E. histolytica*); splinter shaped with rough, pointed ends
Glycogen (stained with iodine)	May be diffuse or absent in mature cyst; clumped chromatin mass may be present in early cysts (stains reddish brown with iodine)	May or may not be present as in *E. histolytica*	May be diffuse or absent in mature cyst; clumped mass occasionally seen in mature cysts (stains reddish brown with iodine)

[a] The genus/species name *Entamoeba histolytica* actually includes two different species in the genus *Entamoeba*: *E. histolytica* (pathogenic) and *E. dispar* (nonpathogenic). Unless trophozoites of *E. histolytica* contain ingested red blood cells (RBCs), there is no way to morphologically distinguish *E. histolytica* from *E. dispar*. Most laboratories will continue to report "*Entamoeba histolytica*" when, in fact, the majority of these organisms may be *E. dispar*. (See text for additional information.)

[b] Wet preparation measurements (permanent stains; organisms usually measure 1–2 μm less).

9.4.1   Asymptomatic infection

Individuals harboring *E. histolytica* may have either a negative or weak antibody titer, stools negative for occult blood, and may be passing cysts that can be detected if the routine ova and parasite examination is performed. Although trophozoites may also be found, they will not contain any phagocytized RBCs. Isoenzyme analysis of organisms isolated from asymptomatic individuals generally indicate the isolates belong to non-pathogenic zymodemes.[17] Generally, asymptomatic patients never become symptomatic and may excrete cysts for a short period of time. This same pattern is found for patients with either nonpathogenic or pathogenic strains.[38]

9.4.2   Intestinal disease

Although the exact mode of mucosal penetration is not known, microscopy studies suggest amebae have enzymes which lyse host tissue, possibly from lysosomes on the surface of the amebae or from ruptured organisms. Amebic ulcers most often develop in the cecum, appendix, or adjacent portion of the ascending colon; however, they can also be found in the sigmoidorectal area. From these primary sites other lesions may occur. Ulcers are usually raised with a small opening on the mucosal surface and a larger area of destruction below the surface — "flask shaped." The mucosal lining may appear normal between ulcers.

Although the incubation period may vary from a few days to a much longer time, in an endemic area it is impossible to determine exactly when the exposure took place. Normally, the time frame will range from 1 to 4 months.

Symptoms may range from the individual who is totally asymptomatic to one in whom multiple symptoms are present and which may mimic ulcerative colitis. Patients with colicky abdominal pain, frequent bowel movements, and tenesmus may present with a gradual onset of disease. With the onset of dysentery, bowel movements characterized by blood-tinged mucus are frequent (up to 10 a day). Although dysentery may last for months, it usually varies from severe to mild over that time and may lead to weight loss and prostration. In severe cases, symptoms may begin very suddenly and include profuse diarrhea (over 10 stools per day), fever, dehydration, and electrolyte imbalances. If the clinical picture is acute, the illness may mimic appendicitis, cholecystitis, intestinal obstruction, or diverticulitis.

9.4.3   Hepatic disease

Blood flow draining the intestine tends to return to the liver, most commonly the upper right lobe (Figure 5). The organisms present in the submucosa can therefore be carried via the bloodstream to the liver. Onset of symptoms may be gradual or sudden; upper right abdominal pain with fever from 38 to 39°C is the most consistent finding. Weakness, weight loss, cough, and sweating are less commonly seen. There tends to be hepatomegaly with tenderness; however, liver function tests may be normal or slightly abnormal with jaundice being very rare. There may be changes at the base of the right lung due to the elevated diaphragm. The abscess can be visualized radiologically, ultrasonically, or by radionuclear scan, and the majority of patients have a single abscess in the right lobe of the liver.[39] The most common complication is rupture of the abscess into the pleural space.[40,41] An abscess can also extend into the peritoneum and through the skin. Hematogenous spread to the brain, as well as to lung, pericardium, and other sites is possible.[42]

E. histolytica cysts and trophozoites are found in the stools of only a few patients with liver abscess. Usually 60% of these patients have no intestinal symptoms, nor any previous

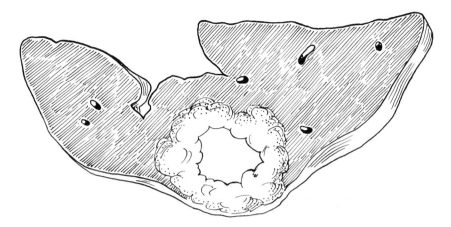

Figure 5 Liver abscess caused by *E. histolytica*. Amebae would be found at the advancing margin of the lesion and the last portion of the aspirated material might reveal the organisms. Illustration by Sharon Belkin. (From Garcia, L.S. and D.A. Bruckner, *Diagnostic Medical Parasitology,* 3rd ed. American Society for Microbiology, ASM Press, Washington, D.C., 1997. With permission.)

Table 3   *Entamoeba histolytica*: Recommended Diagnostic Procedures

Organism	Recommended specimen	Diagnostic procedure
Entamoeba histolytica	Stool	Complete ova and parasite exam
		Immunodiagnostic tests
	Sigmoidoscopy material	Permanent stains
	Hepatic abscess aspirate	Digestion/wet preparations
		Permanent stains
	Biopsy	Routine histology: PAS, H&E
	Serum	Serology

history of dysentery. Stained smears prepared from material obtained at sigmoidoscopy may also be negative.

9.5   Diagnosis

The laboratory diagnosis of amebiasis, particularly intestinal amebiasis, depends on a number of procedures, any one of which can prevent organism recovery if not performed properly (Table 3). Organism detection depends on collection of the correct specimens, the number of specimens submitted, processing methods and diagnostic tests used, and examination by personnel who are well trained in protozoa identification. This diagnosis can be one of the more difficult to achieve. Lack of appropriate training and diagnostic testing may lead to missed infections. In some cases, false-positives may be due to identification of human white blood cells as amebae.[43]

The standard ova and parasite examination is the recommended procedure for recovery and identification of *E. histolytica* in stool specimens. However, eliminating ova and parasite examinations for patients hospitalized for more than three days is becoming more widely accepted.[44] In these cases, an onset of diarrhea is more often linked to the use of antibiotics and subsequent changes in the intestinal flora rather than parasites.

Microscopic examination of a direct saline wet mount may reveal motile trophozoites, which may contain RBCs. However, the number of times these trophozoites with RBCs are present is very limited and they are seen only in cases of true amebic dysentery. In many patients who do not present with acute dysentery, trophozoites may be present but they will not contain RBCs. An asymptomatic individual may have few trophozoites and possibly only cysts in the stool. Although the concentration technique is helpful in demonstrating cysts, *the most important technique for the recovery and identification of protozoan organisms is the permanent stained smear* (normally stained with trichrome or iron hematoxylin). A minimum of three specimens collected over a time frame of not more than ten days is recommended.

The accurate identification of *E. histolytica*, rather than *E. hartmanni*, *E. coli*, or human cells can be very difficult, particularly for those who have little training or experience. As an example, if the permanent stained smear is quite dark, a delicate *E. histolytica* may appear more like the nonpathogen *E. coli*; on a very thin, pale smear, *E. coli* can appear more like *E. histolytica*. Also, when the organisms are dying or have been poorly fixed, they will appear more highly vacuolated, thus looking like *E. coli* trophozoites rather than *E. histolytica*. If the organisms are not properly measured, then *E. histolytica* can also be confused with the nonpathogenic *E. hartmanni*.

If slides are prepared properly and examined carefully, sigmoidoscopy specimens may be very helpful.[43] At least six areas of the mucosa should be sampled. Smears from these areas should be examined after permanent staining. However, this approach does not take the place of the recommended minimum of three stool specimens submitted for ova and parasite examinations (direct, concentration, and permanent stained smear). Refer to Algorithms 1–4 for detailed information.

9.5.1   Immunodetection

Although reagent development has been underway for some time, earlier attempts at immunodetection of organisms in stool were marginally successful. The level of sensitivity and specificity of these reagents was no greater than routine stool examination. However, more recent work indicates definite improvement in reagent quality.[45,46]

To provide clinically relevant information to physicians for treatment of patients infected with pathogenic strains of *E. histolytica*, methods using monoclonal antibodies, purified antigens, or DNA probes would be helpful. Reagents have been developed to differentiate pathogenic *E. histolytica* from nonpathogenic *E. dispar*.[47-50] Although some of these reagents are now available, routine use in clinical laboratories may not be accepted due to cost, limited numbers of cases, and infrequent identification of organisms in the genus *Entamoeba*. Reliable probes based on the hypothesis of zymodeme stability and two separate species (one pathogenic, one nonpathogenic) offer significant improvements over current serologic or direct detection methods. These probes may also help eliminate false-positive results due to misidentification of human cells or other nonpathogenic protozoa in patient specimens.

The laboratory may now have the ability to routinely indicate to the physician whether the *Entamoeba* spp. organisms seen in the stool specimen are pathogenic or nonpathogenic. Without the use of these types of reagents, the only way to morphologically identify true pathogenic *E. histolytica* would be the rare presence of trophozoites containing ingested RBCs. In the event the laboratory does not use these reagents, the presence of *E. histolytica* should be reported to the physician, accompanied by some additional commentary related to the newer information on pathogenicity. Ultimately, the physician will have to decide on the issue of therapy based on the patient's clinical condition. However, without more accurate information on pathogenicity of organisms seen in clinical specimens, from a public health point of view, it may be appropriate to treat all infected patients. Also, based on each state's requirements, *E. histolytica* is generally reported to the public health facility (County).

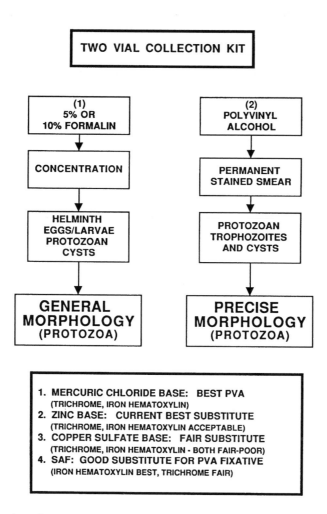

Algorithm 1   Procedure for processing preserved stool for the ova and parasite examination (formalinized material can be used for EIA and FA immunodiagnostic kits; modified acid-fast stains for *Cryptosporidium parvum, Cyclospora cayetanensis,* and *Isospora belli*; and modified trichrome stains for the microsporidia). (Modified from Garcia, L.S. and D.A. Bruckner, *Diagnostic Medical Parasitology,* 3rd ed., American Society for Microbiology, ASM Press, 1997. With permission.)

9.5.2   Antibody detection

Serologic testing for intestinal disease is normally not recommended unless the patient has true dysentery; even in these cases, the titer (indirect hemagglutination as an example) may be low and thus difficult to interpret. Certainly the definitive diagnosis of intestinal amebiasis should not be made without demonstrating the organisms. In cases suspected of extraintestinal disease, serological tests are much more important and helpful. Indirect hemagglutination and indirect fluorescent antibody tests have been reported positive with titers of ≥1:256 and ≥1:200, respectively, in almost 100% of cases of amebic liver abscess.[43,51] Positive serological results, in addition to clinical findings, make the diagnosis highly probable. In the absence of stat serological tests for amebiasis (tests with very rapid turnaround times for results), the decision as to causative agent often must be made on clinical grounds and on results of other diagnostic tests such as scans. Definitive diagnosis of liver abscess can be obtained by identification of organisms from liver aspirate material. However, this procedure is rarely performed and often the specimen obtained is not collected properly. Aspirated material must be aliquoted into several different containers

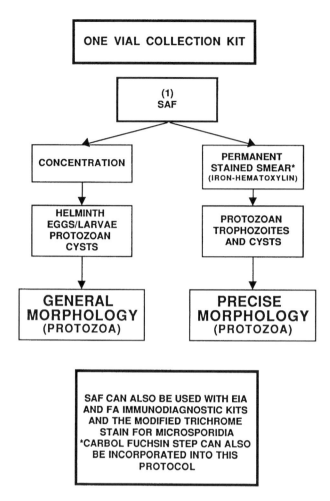

Algorithm 2 Use of SAF-preserved stool for the ova and parasite examination (single vial can be used for EIA and FA immunodiagnostic kits; modified acid-fast stains for *Cryptosporidium parvum*, *Cyclospora cayetanensis*, and *Isospora belli*; and modified trichrome stains for the microsporidia). (Modified from Garcia, L.S. and D.A. Bruckner, *Diagnostic Medical Parasitology*, 3rd ed., American Society for Microbiology, ASM Press, 1997. With permission.)

as it is removed from the abscess; amebae may be found only in the last portion of the aspirated material, theoretically material from the abscess wall, not necrotic debris from the abscess center.[43] Refer to Algorithm 5 for detailed information.

9.5.3 Histologic detection

Histologic diagnosis of amebiasis can be made when the trophozoites within the tissue are identified. Organisms must be differentiated from host cells, particularly histiocytes and ganglion cells. Periodic acid-Schiff (PAS) is often used to help locate the organisms. The organisms will appear bright pink with a green-blue background (depending on the counterstain used). Hematoxylin and eosin (H&E) staining will also allow typical morphology to be seen, thus providing an accurate identification. Due to sectioning, some organisms will exhibit the evenly arranged nuclear chromatin with the central karyosome and some may no longer contain the nucleus.

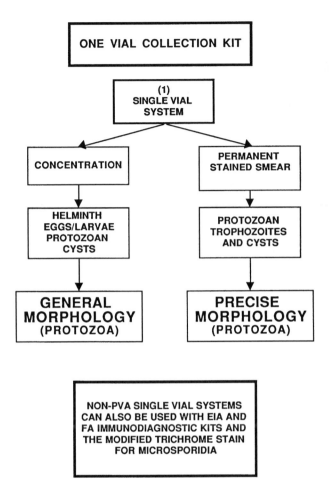

Algorithm 3 Use of preserved stool for the ova and parasite examination (newer fixatives are now available and can be used for the entire stool examination, including EIA and FA immunodiagnostic kits; modified acid-fast stains for *Cryptosporidium parvum, Cyclospora cayetanensis,* and *Isospora belli;* and modified trichrome stains for the microsporidia). (Modified from Garcia, L.S. and D.A. Bruckner, *Diagnostic Medical Parasitology,* 3rd ed., American Society for Microbiology, ASM Press, 1997. With permission.)

9.5.4   Review of laboratory diagnosis

A minimum of three stool specimens should be submitted for the diagnosis of intestinal amebiasis. Any examination for parasites in stool specimens must include the use of a permanent stained smear (even on formed stool); this method is critical for the definitive identification of the intestinal protozoa. Differentiation is particularly important between pathogenic *E. histolytica* and other nonpathogens, and presumptive identification on a wet preparation must always be confirmed using the permanent stained smear.

Six smears should be prepared at sigmoidoscopy; however, this procedure and subsequent examination of the permanent stained smears should not take the place of the routine ova and parasite examinations.

The serology for antibody may or *may not* be positive in intestinal disease, and is much more likely to be positive in extraintestinal disease. Serologic testing is most relevant in patients with extraintestinal disease in which organisms are not routinely seen in the stool.

AMEBIASIS INTESTINE

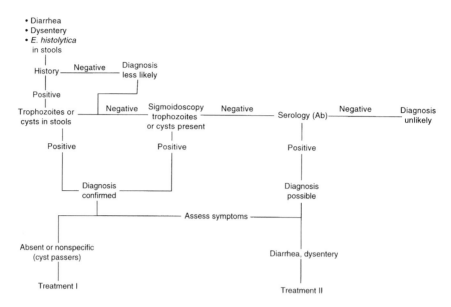

Algorithm 4   Intestinal amebiasis. (From Garcia, L.S. and D.A. Bruckner, *Diagnostic Medical Parasitology,* 3rd ed., American Society for Microbiology, ASM Press, 1997. With permission.)

AMEBIC LIVER ABSCESS

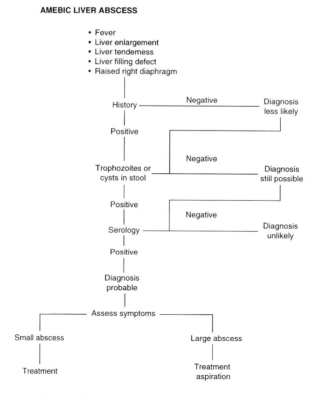

Algorithm 5   Hepatic amebiasis. (From Garcia, L.S. and D.A. Bruckner, *Diagnostic Medical Parasitology,* 3rd ed., American Society for Microbiology, ASM Press, 1997. With permission.)

9.5.5 Differentiation of amebiasis and inflammatory bowel disease

In both the acute and chronic form, amebiasis can mimic idiopathic inflammatory bowel disease (IBD), not only in terms of symptoms, but with radiographic and endoscopic results as well. Differentiation between amebiasis and IBD, including ulcerative colitis (UC) and Crohn's disease (CD), can be very difficult on the basis of clinical grounds, and the correct diagnosis often depends on the recovery and identification of *E. histolytica* organisms from the intestinal tract. Physical examination also offers little specific information. Although proctosigmoidoscopy and colonoscopy are often used in addition to the barium enema, preparation of the patient may prevent the recovery and identification of amebae. The coexistence of IBD and amebiasis must also be considered. The importance of making the appropriate diagnosis should be emphasized; the therapeutic approach to amebiasis and IBD are quite different and an incorrect diagnosis could certainly put the patient at risk for complications.[52]

9.6 Treatment

Over the years there has been much controversy concerning the possibility of pathogenic and nonpathogenic strains of *E. histolytica* and whether or not every patient found to harbor this parasite should be treated. Brumpt is credited with the first suggestion that *E. histolytica* consists of two morphologically identical organisms, one pathogenic and invasive, and the other a harmless commensal.[2] Studies in Durban, South Africa, have provided some information on various zymodemes (strains determined by isoenzyme electrophoresis) of *E. histolytica*.[53] All the strains of *E. histolytica* isolated from cases of proven invasive amebiasis showed the pathogenic zymodeme pattern and all nonpathogenic zymodemes were isolated from individuals without symptoms of amebic disease. Additional studies indicate that 94 to 100% of patients with pathogenic zymodemes were strongly seropositive, compared to 2 to 4% of subjects with nonpathogenic zymodemes.[54] Pathogenic zymodemes are, therefore, thought to be in constant contact with the host's tissues, even in asymptomatic individuals.

Another study suggests that while carriers usually harbor amebae with nonpathogenic isoenzyme patterns, pathogenic patterns also may be found in these individuals.[55] Unfortunately, at the present time, test methodologies which may differentiate between the various zymodemes of *E. histolytica* are not routinely used in diagnostic laboratories. The diagnosis of *E. histolytica* infection is still based on organism morphology. For this reason, in general, patients in the U.S. who harbor this organism may be treated, regardless of the presence or absence of symptoms.[56]

There are two classes of drugs used in the treatment of amebic infections: luminal amebicides such as iodoquinol or diloxanide furoate and tissue amebicides such as metronidazole, chloroquine, or dehydroemetine. Because differences in drug efficacy exist, it is important that the laboratory report for the physician indicate whether cysts, trophozoites, or both are present in the stool specimen.

9.6.1 Asymptomatic patient

Patients found to have *E. histolytica* in the intestinal tract, even if they are asymptomatic, should be treated to eliminate the organisms. Diloxanide furoate, iodoquinol, or paromomycin are available for treatment of patients who have cysts in the lumen of the gut. A recent study involving 14 years' experience in the U.S. using diloxanide furoate for treating asymptomatic cyst passers indicates the drug is safe and effective and may be particularly well tolerated in children.[57] In general, these treatments are ineffective against extraintestinal disease. If the patient is passing both trophozoites and cysts, the recommended treatment is metronidazole plus iodoquinol.

9.6.2　Mild to moderate disease

In these patients metronidazole (Flagyl) should be used when tissue invasion occurs, regardless of the tissue involved. Drugs directed against the lumen organisms should also be used in these instances.

9.6.3　Severe intestinal disease

Metronidazole plus one of the luminal drugs should be used for therapy.

9.6.4　Hepatic disease

Metronidazole plus one of the luminal drugs should be used in these cases. There are also some other combinations which could be used, some of which use emetine where the patient must be monitored very carefully for possible cardiotoxicity. The importance of using both luminal and tissue amebicides is emphasized in a study reviewing the enteric phase of 50 patients with amebic liver abscess. The overall prevalence of asymptomatic colonization was 72% (36/50); however, based on isoenzyme analysis, all of these isolates were pathogenic. Using metronidazole (tissue amebicide), there was 100% clinical response to the hepatic lesions; failure to eliminate the organism from the bowel in 20/36 patients led to second bouts with invasive disease and intestinal colonization. Also, these carriers constitute a public health hazard.[58]

References

1. Lösch, F.A., Massive development of amebas in the large intestine. *Am. J. Trop. Med. Hyg.* 24, 383, 1875.
2. Brumpt, M.E., Etude sommaire de l'*Entamoeba dispa*r n. sp. amibe a kystes quadrinuclues parisite de l'homme. *Bull. Acad. Med. Paris* 94, 943–952, 1925.
3. Imperato, P.J., A historical overview of amebiasis. *Bull. NY Acad. Med.* 57, 175–187, 198.
4. Diamond, L.S., Techniques of axenic cultivation of *Entamoeba histolytica* Schaudinn, 1903 and *E. histolytica*-like amebae. *J. Parasitol.* 54, 1047–56, 1961.
5. Sargeaunt, P.G., The reliability of *Entamoeba histolytica* zymodemes in clinical diagnosis. *Parasitol. Today* 3, 40–43, 1987a.
6. Sargeaunt, P.G., and Jackson, T.F.H.G., Amoebic isoenzymes. *Lancet* 1, 1050, 1985.
7. Sargeaunt, P.G., Jackson, T., and Simjee, A.E., Biochemical homogeneity of *Entamoeba histolytica* isolates, especially those from liver abscess. *Lancet* 1, 1386–1388, 1982a.
8. Sargeaunt, P.G., and Williams J.E., Electrophoretic isoenzyme patterns of the pathogenic and nonpathogenic intestinal amoebae of man. *Trans. R. Soc. Trop. Med. Hyg.* 73, 225–227, 1979.
9. Sargeaunt, P.G., Williams, J.E., and Simjee, A.E., A zymodeme study of *Entamoeba histolytica* in a group of South African school children. *R. Soc. Trop. Med. Hyg.* 76, 401–402, 1982b.
10. Mirelman, D., Ameba-bacterium relationship in amebiasis. *Microbiol. Rev.* 51, 272–84, 1987.
11. Mirelman, D., Effect of culture conditions and bacterial associates on the zymodemes of *Entamoeba histolytica*. *Parasitol. Today* 3, 37–40, 1987.
12. Mirelman, D., Bracha, R., and Chayen, A., *Entamoeba histolytica*: effect of growth conditions and bacterial associates on isoenzyme patterns and virulence. *Exp. Parasitol.* 62, 142–8, 1986.
13. Clark, C.G., and Diamond, L.S., Ribosomal RNA genes of pathogenic and nonpathogenic *Entamoeba histolytica* are distinct. *Mol. Biochem. Parasitol.* 49, 297–302, 1991.
14. McKerrow, J.H., Pathogenesis in amebiasis: Is it genetic or acquired? *Infect. Agents Dis.* 1, 11–14, 1992.

15. Mirelman, D., Pathogenic versus nonpathogenic *Entamoeba histolytica. Infect. Agents Dis.* 1, 15–18, 1992.

16. Orozco, E., Pathogenesis in amebiasis. *Infect. Agents Dis.* 1, 19–21, 1992.

17. Diamond, L.S., and Clark, C.G., A redescription of *Entamoeba histolytica* Schaudinn, 1903 (emended Walker, 1911) separating it from *Entamoeba dispar* Brumpt, 1925. *J. Eur. Microbiol.*, 40, 340–344, 1993.

18. Vargas, M.A., and Orozco, E., *Entamoeba histolytica*: Changes in the zymodeme of cloned non-pathogenic trophozoites cultured under different conditions. *Parasitol. Res.* 19, 353–356, 1993.

19. Orozco, E., Báez-Camargo, M., Gamboa, L., Flores, E., Valdés, J., and Hernández, F., Molecular karyotype of related clones of *Entamoeba histolytica. Mol. Biochem. Parasitol.* 59, 29–40, 1993.

20. Orozco, E., Lazard, D., Sanchez, T., Sanchez, M.A., Hermandez, R., and Silva, E.F., A variable DNA region of *Entamoeba histolytica* is expressed in several transcripts which differ in genetically related clones. *Mol. Gen. Genet.* 241, 271–279, 1993.

21. Petri Jr, W.A., Clark, C.G., and Diamond, L.S., Host-parasite relationships in amebiasis: Conference report. *J. Infect. Dis.* 169, 483–484, 1994.

22. Stanley, S.L., Zhang, T.H., Rubin, D., and Li, E., Role of the *Entamoeba histolytica* cysteine proteinase in amebic liver abscess formation in severe combined immunodeficient mice.*Infect. Immun.* 63, 1587–1590, 1995.

23. Leroy, A., Dubruyne, G., Mareel, M., Nokkaew, C., Bailey, G., and Nelis, H., Contact-dependent transfer of the galactose-specific lectin of *Entamoeba histolytica* to the lateral surface of enterocytes in culture. *Infect. Immun.*, 63, 4253–4260, 1995.

24. Martínez-Cairo, S., Gorab, M., Muñoz, O., and Reyes, M., Coproantibodies in intestinal amebiasis. *Arch. Invest. Med.* 10, 121–126, 1979.

25. Ortiz-Ortiz, L., Amebiasis. In: Kierszenbaum, F. ed. *Parasitic Infections and the Immune System.* San Diego, Academic Press, 1994:145–162.

26. Horstmann, R.D., Target recognition failure by the nonspecific defense system: Surface constituents of pathogens interfere with the alternative pathway of complement activation.*Infect. Immun.* 60, 721–727, 1992.

27. Ravdin, J.I., *Amebiasis: Human Infection by Entamoeba histolytica.* New York, John Wiley & Sons, 1988.

28. Kretschmer, R.R., Immunology of amebiasis. In: Martínez-Palomo, A., ed.*Amebiasis.* Amsterdam, Elsevier, 1986:95–167.

29. Gill, N.J., Ganguly, N.K., Mahajan, R.C., Bhusnurmath, S.R., and Dilawari, J.B., Monocyte functions in human amoebiasis. *Ind. J. Med. Res.* 76, 674–679, 1982.

30. Salata, R.A., Martínez-Palomo, A., Murray, H.W., Canales, L., Treviño, N., Segovia E., Murphy, C.F., and Ravdin, J.I., Patients treated for amebic liver abscess develop cell-mediated immune responses effective *in vitro* against *Entamoeba histolytica. J. Immunol.* 136, 2633–2639, 1986.

31. Walsh, J.A., Prevalence of *Entamoeba histolytica* infection. In: Ravdin, J., ed. *Amebiasis: Human Infection by Entamoeba histolytica.* New York, John Wiley & Sons, 1988:93–105.

32. Kappus, K.D., Lundgren Jr, R.G., Juranek, D.D., Roberts, J.M., and Spencer, H.C., Intestinal parasitism in the United States: Update on a continuing problem. *Am. J. Trop. Med. Hyg.* 50, 705–713, 1994.

33. Beaver, P.C., Jung, R, Sherman, H., Read, T., and Robinson, T., Experimental *Endamoeba histolytica* infections in man. *Am. J. Trop. Med. Hyg.* 500,1000–1009, 1956.

34. Druckman, D.A., and Quinn, T.C., *Entamoeba histolytica* infections in homosexual men, In: Ravdin J., ed. *Amebiasis: Human Infection by Entamoeba histolytica.* New York, John Wiley & Sons, 1988:93–105.

35. Ortega, H.B., Borchardt, K.A., Hamilton, R. et al., Enteric pathogenic protozoa in homosexual men from San Francisco. *Sex. Trans. Dis.* 11, 59, 1983.

36. Markell, E.K., Havens, R.F., Kuritsubo, R.A. et al., Intestinal protozoa in homosexual men of the San Francisco Bay area: Prevalence and correlates of infection. *Am. J. Trop. Med. Hyg.* 33, 239, 1984.

37. Hartskeerl, R.A., Vangool, T., Schuitema, A.R.J., Didier, E.S., and Terpstra, W.F., Genetic and immunological characterization of the microsporidian *Septata intestinalis* Cali, Kotler and Orenstein, 1993: Reclassification to *Encephalitozoon intestinalis. Parasitology* 110, 277–285, 1995.

38. Bruckner, D.A., Amebiasis. *Clin. Microbiol. Rev.* 5, 356–369, 1992.

39. Katzenstein, D., Rickerson, V., and Braude, A., New concepts of amebic liver abscess derived from hepatic imaging, serodiagnosis, and hepatic enzymes in 67 consecutive cases in San Diego. *Medicine* 61, 237–246, 1982.

40. Adams, E.B., and MacLeod, I.N., Invasive amebiasis. I. Amebic dysentery and its complications. *Medicine* 56, 315–323, 1977a.

41. Adams, E.B., and MacLeod, I.N., Invasive amebiasis. II. Amebic liver abscess and its complications. *Medicine* 56, 325–334, 1977b.

42. Ohnishi, K., Murata, M., Kojima, H., Takemura, N., Tsuchida, T., and Tachibana, H., Brain abscess due to infection with *Entamoeba histolytica*. *Am. J. Trop. Med. Hyg.* 51, 180–182, 1994.

43. Garcia, L.S., and Bruckner, D.A., *Diagnostic Medical Parasitology*, 3rd ed., American Society for Microbiology, ASM Press, Washington, D.C., 1997.

44. Garcia, L.S., Bullock-Iacullo, S., Palmer, J., and Shimizu, R.Y., Diagnosis of parasitic infections: Collection, processing and examination of specimens, In: *Manual of Clinical Microbiology*, ed. 6 (Murray, P.R., Baron, E.J., Pfaller, M.A., Tenover, F.C., and Yolken, R.H., Eds.) American Society for Microbiology, Washington, D.C., 1995.

45. Merino, E., Glender, W., del Muro, R., and Ortiz-Ortiz, L., Evaluation of the ELISA test for detection of *Entamoeba histolytica* in feces. *J. Clin. Lab. Anal.* 4, 39–42, 1990.

46. Wonsit, R., Thammapalerd, N., Tharavanij, S., Radomyos, P., and Bunnag, D., Enzyme-linked immunosorbent assay based on monoclonal and polyclonal antibodies for the detection of *Entamoeba histolytica* antigens in faecal specimens. *Trans. R. Soc. Trop. Med. Hyg.* 86, 166–169, 1992.

47. Abd-Alla, M.D., Jackson, T.F.H.G., Gathiram, V., El-Hawey, A.M., and Ravdin, J.J., Differentiation of pathogenic *Entamoeba histolytica* infections from nonpathogenic infections by detection of galactose-inhibitable adherence protein antigen in sera and feces. *J. Clin. Microbiol.* 31, 2845–2850, 1993.

48. Haque, R., Kress, K., Wood, S., Jackson, T.F., Lyerly, D., Wilkins, T., and Petri, W.A.J., Diagnosis of pathogenic *Entamoeba histolytica* infection using a stool ELISA based on monoclonal antibodies to the galactose-specific adhesin. *J. Infect. Dis.* 167, 247–249, 1993.

49. Haque, R., Neville, L.M., Wood, S., and Petri Jr., W.A., Short report: Detection of *Entamoeba histolytica* and *E. dispar* directly in stool. *Am. J. Trop. Med. Hyg.* 50, 595–596, 1994.

50. Katzwinkel-Wladarsch, S., Loscher, T., and Rinder, H., Direct amplification and differentiation of pathogenic and nonpathogenic *Entamoeba histolytica* DNA from stool specimens. *Am. J. Trop. Med. Hyg.* 51, 115–118, 1994.

51. Wilson, M., Schantz, P., and Pieniazek, N., Diagnosis of parasitic infections: Immunologic and molecular methods, In: *Manual of Clinical Microbiology*, ed. 6 (Murray, P.R., Baron, E.J., Pfaller, M.A., Tenover, F.C., and Yolken, R.H., Eds.) American Society for Microbiology, Washington D.C., 1995.

52. Schleupner, C.J., and Barritt III, A.S., Differentiation and occurrence of amebiasis in inflammatory bowel disease, In: Ravdin J., ed. *Amebiasis: Human Infection by Entamoeba histolytica*. New York, John Wiley & Sons, 1988:93–105.

53. Elsdon-Dew, R. The epidemiology of amoebiasis. *Adv. Parasitol.*, 6, 1–62, 1968.

54. Jackson, T. F. H. G., and V. Gathiram, Seroepidemiological study of antibody responses to the zymodemes of *Entamoeba histolytica*. *Lancet* 1, 716–718, 1985.

55. Meza, I., de la Garza, M., Meraz, M.A., Gallegos, B., de la Torre, Tanimoto, M., and Martínez-Paloma, A., Isoenzyme patterns of *Entamoeba histolytica* isolates from asymptomatic carriers: Use of gradient acrylamide gels. *Am. J. Trop. Med. Hyg.* 35, 1134–1139, 1986.

56. Ravdin, J.I., and Jones, T.C., *Entamoeba histolytica* (Amebiasis), In: G.L. Mandell, R. G. Douglas, and J. E. Bennett (Eds.), *Principles and Practice of Infectious Diseases,* John Wiley & Sons, New York, 1985.

57. McAuley, J.B., Herwaldt, B.L., Stokes, S.L., Becher, J.A., Roberts, J.M., Michelson, M.K., and Juranek, D.D., Diloxanide furoate for treating asymptomatic *Entamoeba histolytica* cyst passers: 14 years' experience in the United States. *Clin. Inf. Dis.* 15, 464–468, 1992.

58. Irusen, E.M., Jackson, T.F.H.G., and Simjee, A.E., Asymptomatic intestinal colonization by pathogenic *Entamoeba histolytica* in amebic liver abscess: prevalence, response to therapy, and pathogenic potential. *Clin. Inf. Dis.* 14, 889–893, 1992.

chapter ten

Cryptosporidiosis

Lynne S. Garcia

10.1   Introduction..189
     10.1.1   Historical information 189
     10.1.2   Pathogenicity..190
     10.1.3   Host defense mechanisms 191
10.2   Epidemiology and prevention 191
     10.2.1   Overview 191
     10.2.2   Sources of infection and transmission....................................192
     10.2.3   Distribution and relevance to human health 193
     10.2.4   Infectivity..193
     10.2.5   Prevention..193
10.3   Life cycle and morphology...194
     10.3.1   Taxonomy 194
     10.3.2   Life cycle..195
     10.3.3   Morphology...197
10.4   Clinical disease 197
     10.4.1   Immunocompetent individuals 197
     10.4.2   Immunocompromised individuals..197
10.5   Diagnosis 198
     10.5.1   Clinical laboratory...198
     10.5.2   Histology 201
     10.5.3   Water testing 201
10.6   Treatment...202
References...202

10.1   Introduction

10.1.1   Historical information

Some of the important historical dates related to *Cryptosporidium* are indicated below.[1] The first reported description of *Cryptosporidium* was in 1907 in the gastric crypts of a laboratory mouse.[2] It has also been found in chickens, turkeys, mice, rats, guinea pigs, horses, pigs, calves, sheep, rhesus monkeys, dogs, cats, and humans. [3] In the early 1970s, it was found to be an important cause of diarrhea in calves. Information also supports previous suggestions that cryptosporidiosis is a zoonosis, is not host-specific, and is transmitted via the fecal-oral route. This infection is now well recognized as causing disease in humans and was first reported in 1976. In 1981, the first case of cryptosporidiosis in a patient with the acquired immune deficiency syndrome (AIDS) was diagnosed, and this organism has become one of the more important opportunistic agents seen in patients with AIDS. The first child care center outbreak was reported in 1983. Unfortunately, to date, no totally effective therapy for cryptosporidiosis has been identified, in spite of extensive drug trials. Consequently, diagnosing this infection in the immunocompromised host, especially those with AIDS, usually carries a poor prognosis. Documented respiratory tract and biliary tree infections confirm that the developmental stages of this organism are not always confined to the gastrointestinal tract.

Prior to 1980 less than 30 publications were available, and now more than 1,500 published papers appear in the literature related to cryptosporidiosis, many of which include information on nosocomial transmission, daycare center outbreaks, and a number of waterborne outbreaks. During the past few years, there have been definite improvements in diagnostic procedures, particularly those using newer monoclonal-based reagents.[4]

10.1.2 Pathogenicity

The pathogenesis of cryptosporidial diarrhea, even in patients with AIDS, is not fully understood. However, patients with no intestinal symptoms and who are passing formed stool containing few oocysts contrast sharply with those who are symptomatic with watery diarrhea and are passing large number of oocysts. These findings imply a relationship between intestinal dysfunction and injury and the number of organisms infecting the intestinal mucosa. In a study by Goodgame et al., they reviewed the intensity of infection in a group of AIDS patients by counting the total number of fecal oocysts excreted in 24 h.[5] They also determined the percent of duodenal epithelium covered by organisms. Intestinal function was assessed by vitamin B-12 absorption and the serum D-xylose test. Assessment of intestinal injury was based on the morphology of the duodenal mucosa, differential urinary excretion of lactulose and mannitol, and fecal alpha(1)-antitrypsin clearance. They found that vitamin B-12 and D-xylose absorption were negatively correlated with the intensity of infection and villus atrophy occurred only in patients with oocyst excretion of >10(8) oocysts/24 h. Both intestinal function and injury improved in patients whose oocyst counts were reduced using paromomycin therapy. Based on this particular study, the authors concluded that cryptosporidiosis in AIDS patients causes malabsorption and intestinal injury in proportion of the number of organisms infecting the intestine.[5]

In another study, human colon adenocarcinoma cells (Caco-2 cell monolayers) were used to detect enterotoxic effect of fecal specimens from 11 patients with enteric cryptosporidiosis.[6] Using osmotic gap determinations, Caco-2 monolayers were grown on filters and mounted in Ussing chambers. Electrical parameters were measured before and after the addition of fecal supernatant fluid. In 9/11 patients, a significant increase in short-circuit current was seen. This enterotoxic effect was time- and dose-dependent, saturable, and Cl$^-$- and Ca^{2+}-dependent. The fecal osmotic gap was consistent with secretory diarrhea in the 9/11 patients. Based on this report of the establishment of a cell line model for studying the pathophysiology of enteric cryptosporidiosis, enterotoxic activity was observed in most patients with enteric cryptosporidiosis and was strictly associated with secretory diarrhea.[6]

In a study using the piglet model, villus architecture changes corresponded to the extent of infection, and increased numbers of lamina propria inflammatory cells were evident at 36 h postinoculation. They also concluded that passive solute and macromolecular permeability in infected tissues is not significantly increased during parasite-host cell interactions 12–48 h postinoculation. Electrogenic glucose stimulated Na$^+$ absorption (function of the villus absorptive cells) is impaired, but electrogenic Cl$^-$ secretion (function of crypt epithelial cells) remains the same. These findings parallel structural observations that include loss of the Na$^+$/glucose-transporting villus epithelium without loss of crypt epithelium.[7]

10.1.3   Host defense mechanisms

In humans, age and immune status at the time of primary exposure to *C. parvum* do not appear to be primary factors influencing susceptibility to infection. Symptomatic intestinal and respiratory cryptosporidiosis has been seen in both immunocompetent and immunodeficient patients of all ages. However, once the primary infection has been established, the immune status of the host plays a very important role in determining the length and severity of the illness. People who are immunocompetent usually develop a short-term, self-limited diarrhea lasting approximately 2 weeks.

C. parvum preparations were studied for their ability to induce specific proliferation of cultures of human peripheral blood mononuclear cells (PBMC) from both immunocompetent and HIV-positive individuals, some of whom had transient cryptosporidiosis. PBMC from immunocompromised patients did not proliferate in response to *C. parvum*-specific antigens. However, the supernatants of PBMC obtained from immunocompetent donors contained interleukin-10 and interferon (IFN)-gamma after PBMC were exposed to *C. parvum* preparations. High IFN-gamma values were found in patients who had recovered from symptomatic cryptosporidiosis, suggesting that IFN plays a role in resolving this infection.[8]

In contrast, those who are immunocompromised initially develop the same type of illness; however, it becomes more severe with time and results in a prolonged, life-threatening, cholera-like illness. These severe infections have been seen in patients undergoing immunosuppressive chemotherapy with drugs that affect both T- and B-lymphocyte function, in patients with hypogammaglobulinemia, and in those with AIDS. From many observations on these types of patients, the difference in outcome can probably be explained by the development of an immune response in the immunocompetent host sufficient to eradicate the parasite from the infected individual. This explanation is also supported by the fact that individuals whose immunosuppressive therapy has been discontinued will rapidly clear the body of *C. parvum* once their immune function is restored. Studies also suggest that the overall immune response to cryptosporidiosis is probably an antibody-dependent, cell-mediated, cytotoxic effect of unknown mechanism.

10.2   Epidemiology and prevention

10.2.1   Overview

Cryptosporidiosis is now recognized as a leading cause of protozoal diarrhea and has been reported worldwide. Patients range from newborn infants to the elderly, however, symptoms tend to be more severe in infants and young children, probably due to the potential for fecal-oral contamination and insufficient protection immunity.[9]

Cryptosporidium is transmitted by oocysts that are usually fully sporulated and infective at the time they are passed in stool. Oocysts are resistant to some of the disinfectants which are routinely used in medical care facilities. They are susceptible to ammonia, 10% formalin in saline, freeze-drying, and exposure to temperatures below freezing or above

65°C for 30 min.[10] Commercial bleach in a 50% solution is also effective; however, lower concentrations, even up to 2 h exposure time, are ineffective.[11] Although some specialized stool specimen collection kits contain a vial of potassium dichromate specifically for *Cryptosporidium,* the oocysts remain viable in this solution for a period of at least 12 months (W. L. Current, personal communication).

10.2.2   Sources of infection and transmission

Studies have shown that calves, and perhaps other animals, serve as potential sources of human infections. Contact with these animals may be an unrecognized cause of gastro-enteritis in humans, both in rural and urban settings.

Direct person-to-person transmission is also likely and may occur through direct or indirect contact with stool material. Direct oral-anal contact (anilingus) is a common practice among homosexual men which leads to both fecal exposure and oral contact with a variety of intestinal pathogens. Although anilingus has often been listed as a key risk factor in potential exposure, transmission can also occur during oral-genital sex after anal intercourse has occurred. It has also been shown that active heterosexuals can acquire infection with *Cryptosporidium* through sexual activities that provide an opportunity for fecal-oral contamination. The key factor is not necessarily homosexuality, but the frequency of sexual activity and potential for fecal-oral contact.

Indirect transmission may occur through exposure to positive specimens in a laboratory setting or from contaminated surfaces or food or water. Overall, increased rates of infection are linked to contaminated water, poor sanitation, crowding, and the potential for human and domestic animal contact.

In January and February of 1987, cryptosporidiosis was associated with an estimated 13,000 cases of gastroenteritis in Caroll County, GA.[12] *Cryptosporidium* oocysts were identified in the stools of 39% of the persons examined during the outbreak; a randomized telephone survey indicated probable attack rates of 54% within the city of Carollton and 40% overall for the county. The only significant risk factor associated with illness was exposure to the public water supply which was filtered and chlorinated. It was interesting to note that according to records kept during the outbreak, the treatment facility was operating within Environmental Protection Agency (EPA) guidelines. However, this outbreak was thought to be related to the removal of mechanical agitators in the water treatment plant resulting in decreased efficiency of the flocculation step and incomplete particulate removal.

Other waterborne outbreaks within the U.S. include: Milwaukee, WI; (2) Braun Station (near San Antonio) TX (first well-water outbreak — contaminated with sewage); Jackson County, OR; (4) New Mexico (untreated surface water); and (5) Los Angeles (first swimming pool outbreak).[13-16] With the exception of the New Mexico outbreak, all were associated with treated water that met both EPA coliform and turbidity standards.

This increase in the number of reported waterborne disease outbreaks associated with *Cryptosporidium* can be attributed to improved techniques for oocyst recovery and identification. The use of high-volume filters and immunofluorescent detection methods has resulted in the demonstration of oocysts in surface and drinking waters and in sewage effluents from many geographic regions.[2,17,18] The importance of agricultural waste water and runoff, particularly from lambs and calves, is also now recognized as a potential source of infective *Cryptosporidium* oocysts.

Regardless of whether the patient has diarrhea or is passing formed stool, the oocysts are considered infective as soon as they are passed in stool and can remain viable and infective outside the body for 2–6 months.

10.2.3   Distribution and relevance to human health

Prevalence rates reported from various surveys indicate a rate of 1 to 2% (Europe), 0.6 to 4.3% (North America), and higher rates of 3 to 20% from other areas of the world (Asia, Australia, Africa, and Central and South America). It has been suggested that the infection rate for individuals with diarrheal illness is 2.2% for persons living in industrialized countries and 8.5% for those residing in developing countries. Based on available data, predictions indicate that there are 250 to 500 million *Cryptosporidium* infections annually in persons living in Asia, Africa, and Latin America. Generally, young children tend to have higher infection rates and all patients appear to have symptoms. Available serologic data support the prevalence rates with figures from Europe and North America normally between 25 and 35% and rates from South America indicating rates up to 64%.[19]

The epidemiologic considerations for cryptosporidiosis emphasize transmission by environmentally resistant oocysts, numerous potential reservoir hosts for zoonotic transmission, documentation of person-to-person transmission in daycare centers, nosocomial transmission within the healthcare setting, occurrence of asymptomatic infections (infective, carrier state), widespread environmental distribution resulting in the probability of waterborne transmission, and the link between cryptosporidiosis and severe, life-threatening disease in individuals with impaired immune function. Prevalence data from the Centers for Disease Control and Prevention (CDC) for patients with AIDS are thought to be an underestimate of actual cases (2 to 5%), particularly when other figures indicate percentages of 15% (National Institutes of Health in Bethesda, MD) and 11% (Great Britain).[20]

10.2.4   Infectivity

It has been well documented that small numbers of *C. parvum* oocysts can contaminate drinking water, even if it has been treated. Ingestion of oocysts can cause diarrhea in both immunocompetent and immunosuppressed individuals. In a recent study by DuPont and colleagues,[21] 29 healthy volunteers without evidence of previous infection with *C. parvum* were given a single dose of 30 to 1 million oocysts obtained from an infected calf. The volunteers were monitored for clinical illness and oocyst excretion for a total of eight weeks. Household contacts were also monitored for infection. Subjects (14/16, 88%) receiving a dose of ≥300 oocysts became infected. After a dose of 30 oocysts, 1/5 (20%) became infected and 7/7 subjects became infected at a dose of 1000 or more oocysts. The median infective dose was 132 oocysts. Of the 18 people who excreted oocysts after the challenge dose, 11/18 had symptoms and 7 (39%) had clinical disease consisting of diarrhea plus one other symptom. All of the volunteers recovered and there were no secondary cases of diarrhea among household contacts. This study emphasizes the point that in healthy adults with no serologic evidence of past infection with *C. parvum*, a low dose of oocysts is sufficient to initiate infection.[21]

10.2.5   Prevention

Because effective treatment is not available for cryptosporidiosis, prevention of infection is the most realistic method of infection control.[22] Some general guidelines are available and should become a routine part of any educational effort directed toward disease prevention. One issue that is relatively minor, but worth mentioning, is pet ownership. Although the risk related to cryptosporidiosis is small, HIV-positive individuals should avoid contact with animal feces. If contact is required (cat litter box, etc.), then gloves should be worn. Also, the risk from pets is greatest when the animal is less than 6 months of age or has diarrhea. It is also important that people who work in urban and rural farms, and animal sanctuaries where the public can come in contact with farm livestock and other animals, should be notified and reminded to take appropriate precautionary measures to prevent transmission of infections.[23] Although animal-to-human transmission is well recognized, most recommendations concerning cryptosporidiosis are directly related to water consumption and include information regarding HIV status, water source, and water treatment (both municipal and individual).

HIV-infected individuals should avoid drinking water directly from environmental sources such as lakes or rivers, including accidental ingestion associated with recreational water activities such as swimming or water skiing. Swimming pools are also a potential source of infection; chlorine is not effective in killing the oocysts and asymptomatic individuals can continue to shed infective organisms for several weeks after symptoms resolve.

The risks associated with municipal drinking water are difficult to assess, in spite of the number of documented waterborne outbreaks. There is insufficient data to recommend that immunocompromised individuals boil or refrain from drinking tap water. However, if individuals want to take independent action to reduce any potential risk, all drinking water can be boiled for 1 min.

Other options would include the use of appropriate filters or high quality bottled water. There are many different types of filters commercially available; it is important to select one that can remove particles that are 0.1–1 μm in size. Acceptable filters include those that work by reverse osmosis, those that have "absolute" 1-μm filters, and those that meet the National Sanitation Foundation (NSF) standard no. 53 for "cyst removal." The "nominal" 1-μm filter rating is not acceptable; filters in this category may not be capable of removing >99% of the oocysts. Filter systems that only use ultraviolet light, activated carbon, or pentiodide-impregnated resins are not effective against *Cryptosporidium* oocysts. It is also important to remember that filter descriptions indicating removal of *Giardia* cysts may not be effective for oocyst removal.[22]

Not all brands of bottled water can be substituted for tap water as a preventive measure against cryptosporidiosis. There are a number of parameters that need to be examined: water source, microbial quality, and possible treatment prior to the bottling process. Water that originates from underground sources not subject to possible contamination from periodic surface water and shown to be free from coliform bacteria are generally considered to be free of oocysts. However, it may be very difficult to determine this information from labels that appear on the bottles. If the water has been filtered or treated prior to bottling, the same guidelines apply that were discussed for tap water.

10.3 Life cycle and morphology

10.3.1 Taxonomy

Protozoan parasites of the genus *Cryptosporidium* are closely related to the other coccidia infecting humans, *Isospora belli*, *Sarcocystis* spp., and *Toxoplasma gondii*. These organisms are obligate intracellular protozoan parasites assigned to the phylum Apicomplexa, class Sporozoasida, subclass Coccidiasina, order Eucoccidiorida, suborder Eimeriorina (true coccidia), and family Cryptosporidiidae. Most species designations of *Cryptosporidium* in the literature were done so with the assumption that these coccidia were very host specific. However, cross-transmission studies have demonstrated little or no host specificity for more than 20 species of *Cryptosporidium* isolated from mammals. Based on oocyst morphology, *C. parvum* has been designated the species that causes disease in humans.

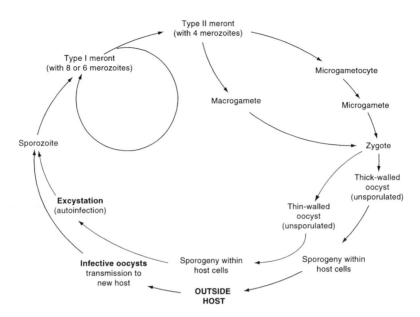

Figure 1 Life cycle of *Cryptosporidium parvum*. (Adapted from Current, W.L. and P.L. Long. 1983. Development of human and calf Cryptosporidium in chicken embryos. *J. Infect. Dis.* 148:1108–1113; from Garcia, L.S. and D.A. Bruckner, *Diagnostic Medical Parasitology*, 3rd ed. American Society for Microbiology, ASM Press, Washington, D.C., 1997. With permission.)

Using random amplified polymorphic DNA (RAPD) analysis, genetic variation in 25 *Cryptosporidium* isolates from humans and other animals were analyzed to determine groupings. Two *C. serpentis* isolates from snakes formed a distinct group of their own. *C. parvum* isolates were divided into two main groups: one containing mostly human isolates and the other containing mostly domestic animals plus two human isolates. Based on the sensitivity of RAPD technology, isolates can now be analyzed genetically, directly from fecal specimens without further biological amplification.[24]

10.3.2   Life cycle

Cryptosporidium differs from other coccidia infecting warm-blooded vertebrates in that its developmental stages do not occur deep within host cells, but are confined to an intracellular, extracytoplasmic location. Each stage is within a parasitophorous vacuole of host cell origin; however, the vacuole containing the organism is located at the microvillous surface of the host cell. Details of the life cycle can be seen in Figure 1.[2]

The presence of a thin-walled autoinfective oocyst may explain why a small inoculum can lead to an overwhelming infection in a susceptible host and why immunosuppressed patients may have persistent, life-threatening infections in the absence of documentation of repeated exposure to oocysts (Figure 1). The stages found on the microvillous surface measure ~1 μm and the oocysts recovered in stool specimens measure 4–6 μm (Figure 2).

Each intracellular stage of *C. parvum* resides within a parasitophorous vacuole within the microvillous region of the host cell. Oocysts undergo sporogony while they are in the host cells and are immediately infective when passed in the stool. This is in contrast to the oocysts of *I. belli* which do not sporulate until they are passed from the host and are exposed to oxygen and temperatures below 37°C. Approximately 20% of the oocysts of *C. parvum* do not form the thick, two-layered, environmentally resistant oocyst wall. The

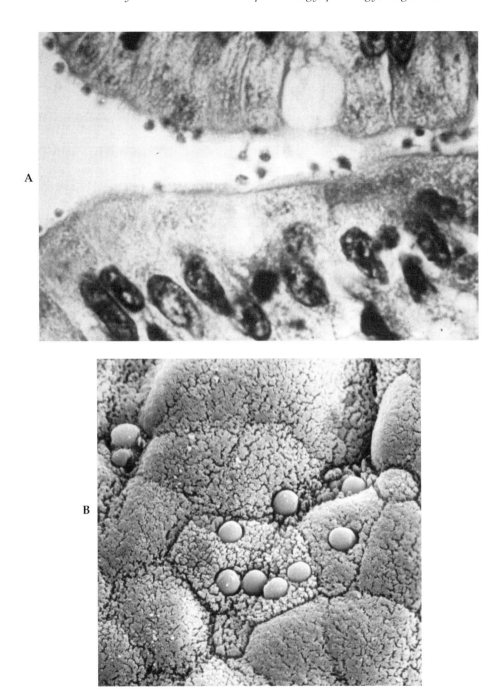

Figure 2 *Cryptosporidium parvum.* (A) Organisms on the brush border of the mucosal surface. (Photo courtesy of Wilfred M. Weinstein.) (B) Organisms on the mucosal surface, human tissue (scanning electron micrograph × 4000). (Photo courtesy of Marietta Voge.) (From Garcia, L.S. and D.A. Bruckner, *Diagnostic Medical Parasitology,* 3rd ed. American Society for Microbiology, ASM Press, Washington, D.C., 1997. With permission.)

four sporozoites within this autoinfective stage are surrounded by a single unit membrane. After being released from a host cell, this membrane ruptures and the invasive sporozoites penetrate the microvillous region of other cells within the intestine and reinitiate the life cycle. As mentioned earlier, the presence of these thin-walled oocysts that can recycle are thought to be responsible for the development of severe, life-threatening disease in immunocompromised patients, even those who are no longer exposed to the environmentally resistant oocysts.

10.3.3 Morphology

Oocysts recovered in clinical specimens are difficult to see without special stains, such as the modified acid fast, Kinyoun's method, Giemsa preparations, or the newer direct fluorescent antibody (DFA) method. Using modified acid-fast stains, the four sporozoites may be seen within the oocyst wall in some of the organisms, although in freshly passed specimens they are not always visible. Occasionally, the oocysts can be seen lightly stained in a routine fecal smear stained with trichrome stain.

10.4 Clinical disease

10.4.1 Immunocompetent individuals

Clinical symptoms include nausea, low grade fever, abdominal cramps, anorexia, and 5 to 10 watery, frothy bowel movements a day, which may be followed by constipation. Some patients may present with diarrhea as described above and others may have relatively few symptoms, particularly later in the course of the infection. In patients with the typical watery diarrhea, the stool specimen contains very little fecal material and is mainly water and mucous flecks. Often the organisms are entrapped in the mucus and diagnostic procedures are performed accordingly. Generally a patient with a normal immune system will have a self-limited infection; however, those patients who are compromised may have a chronic infection with a wide range of symptoms (asymptomatic to severe).

Occasionally, these patients may require fluid replacement and the diarrhea may persist for more than two weeks. This is particularly true in infants where excessive fluid loss may last over three weeks. Failure-to-thrive has also been attributed to chronic cryptosporidiosis in infants. Since diarrheal illness is a major cause of morbidity and mortality in young children living in developing countries, it is likely that cryptosporidiosis plays a major role in the overall health status of these children. It has also been suggested that *Cryptosporidium* may be implicated in respiratory disease that often accompanies diarrheal illness in malnourished children.[25]

10.4.2 Immunocompromised individuals

The duration and severity of diarrheal illness will depend on the immune status of the patient. In most severely immunocompromised patients, they cannot self-cure, the illness becomes progressively worse with time, and the sequelae may be a major factor leading to death. Length and severity of illness may also depend on the ability to reverse the immunosuppression. In these patients *C. parvum* infections are not always confined to the gastrointestinal tract; additional symptoms have been associated with extraintestinal infections including respiratory problems, cholecystitis, hepatitis, and pancreatitis that have also been demonstrated in simian AIDS.[26] In a small series of patients, data indicate that those with CD4$^+$ counts of 180 cells/mm^3 or greater cleared the infection with *C. parvum* over a period of seven days to one month. This data is important in predicting the natural progression of the infection and in designing therapeutic trials. Frequent diagnosis of *C. parvum* infection in patients with neoplasia and diarrhea who are undergoing chemotherapy suggests that in this patient group it is appropriate to routinely submit fecal specimens for examination for oocysts and the cost of laboratory testing is justified.[27]

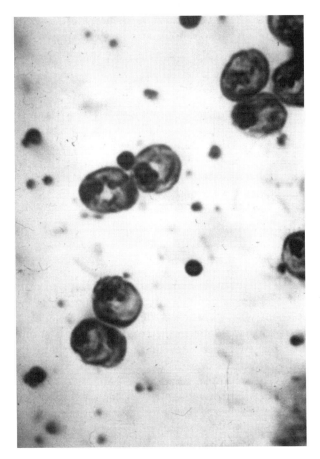

Figure 3 *Cryptosporidium* oocysts from stool; stained with modified acid-fast stain.

10.5   Diagnosis

10.5.1   Clinical laboratory

Previously most human cases have been diagnosed after examination of small or large bowel biopsy material, often using both light and electron microscopy (Figure 2). However, because biopsy specimens might miss the infected area of the mucosa, cases are now routinely diagnosed by recovering oocysts from fecal material using concentration and staining methods. Fresh fecal specimens can be concentrated using Sheather's sugar solution and coverslip preparations examined using both phase-contrast and bright-field microscopy. The oocysts will float and one must focus directly under the glass coverslip. Most laboratories no longer use this approach and have switched to modified acid-fast stains performed on concentrated stool sediment or the newer monoclonal-based reagents using the enzyme immunoassay (EIA) or fluorescent (FA) formats.

Although examination of flotation material using phase-contrast microscopy is an excellent procedure for the recovery and identification of *Cryptosporidium* oocysts, most laboratories have neither access to such equipment nor experience using phase-contrast microscopy. Also, since the organism is considered to be infectious to laboratory personnel, fixed specimens can be processed using several acid-fast stains, many of which are very satisfactory in demonstrating the organisms in stool material (Figures 3 and 4).[28] The more formed and normal the specimen, the better the chance for artifact material which can be confused with *Cryptosporidium*. It is important to remember that the number of oocysts is

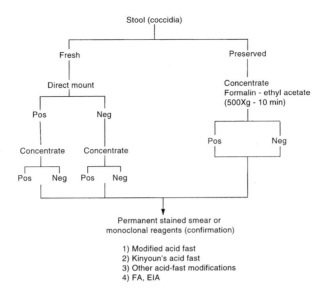

Figure 4 Diagnostic work flow diagram leading from submission of stool specimen to final permanent stained smear (examination for coccidia: permanent stained smear, particularly for *Cryptosporidium parvum*). (Adapted from Garcia, L.S. and D.A. Bruckner, *Diagnostic Medical Parasitology*, 3rd ed. American Society for Microbiology, ASM Press, Washington, D.C.,1997. With permission.)

directly correlated with the consistency of the stool; the more diarrheic the stool, the more oocysts are present.

For the diagnosis of cryptosporidiosis, stool and other body fluid specimens should be submitted as fresh material or in 5% or 10% formalin, sodium acetate-acetic acid-formalin (SAF), or one of the newer single vial stool collection systems (PVA prepared with zinc sulfate-based Schaudinn's fixative). Fixed specimens are recommended because of potential biohazard considerations. In some research laboratories potassium dichromate solution (2 to 3% [wt/vol] in water) is used routinely as a storage medium to preserve oocyst viability; it is not a fixative and not recommended for the routine clinical laboratory. Either fresh or preserved specimens can be examined using the routine stool formalin-ethyl acetate concentration and one of the modified acid-fast stains or the newer monoclonal-based kit reagents. Both FA and enzyme-linked immunosorbent assay (ELISA) methods are currently available. It is recommended that the stool specimen be centrifuged at $500 \times g$ for 10 min prior to performance of any of the stains or monoclonal reagents; centrifugation at this speed and time ensures maximum recovery of the oocysts. Centrifugation at lower speeds and times (often mentioned in some procedures) may not guarantee recovery of the oocysts. Multiple stool specimens may have to be examined in order to diagnose the infection; this is particularly true when dealing with formed stool specimens.[28]

Various screening approaches have been used and the approach varies from testing all specimens submitted for a routine stool examination to testing limited risk groups or testing only on request. There are numerous pros and cons to each approach. Each laboratory will have to select its own approach based on: patient base, client preferences, single vs. batch testing, opportunity for in-service education for clients, availability of personnel, level of personnel training and expertise, clinical relevance, and cost. Prevalence data tend to be low unless specific risk groups are screened. A comprehensive approach would be to screen all symptomatic patients; however, even this approach often results in the identification of very few patients and is certainly not that cost effective. A selective approach might be more reasonable, all compromised patients or compromised patients with diarrhea. However, this assumes the laboratory will always have access to this type of patient information, an assumption that is not realistic. Many laboratories have elected to provide in-service education to their physician clients and will perform these procedures only on request.

Although there is evidence that regional and seasonal variability may occur with cryptosporidiosis, these possibilities will probably have little impact on the laboratory's overall approach to diagnostic testing.

Respiratory cryptosporidiosis has been reported in AIDS patients.[29] Sputum specimens from immunodeficient patients with undiagnosed respiratory illness should be submitted in 10% formalin and examined for *Cryptosporidium* oocysts using the same techniques used for stool samples. Infection of the gallbladder and biliary tree should result in oocysts being passed in the stool.

Preliminary results from serologic methods for the diagnosis of cryptosporidiosis look promising; however, additional patients must be studied before the actual diagnostic potential of these methods can be evaluated.[30] Serologic tests should be very useful in estimating the prevalence of the infection in different parts of the world.

The use of monoclonal antibodies has proven to be very helpful in providing more sensitive methods of detecting organisms in stool specimens.[4] A DFA procedure has been developed with excellent specificity and sensitivity and results in a significantly increased detection rate over conventional staining methods.[31] EIA procedures also provide excellent specificity and sensitivity for those laboratories using this approach.[32] Some of these reagents, particularly the combination DFA product used to identify both *Giardia lamblia* cysts and *C. parvum* oocysts, are being widely used in water testing and outbreak situations.

A flow cytometric method for the quantitation of *Cryptosporidium* oocysts in stool specimens has been developed as an alternative method. Studies indicate results are approximately 10 times more sensitive than conventional immunofluorescent assays.[33] Unfortunately, this approach may be somewhat impractical for most clinical laboratories.

C. parvum coproantigens (CCAg) have been identified in stool eluates of both calves and humans infected with these organisms. Antibodies raised to one of these antigens recognized 18- and 20-kDa CCAg in all positive but no negative samples. These antibodies were used to react with *C. parvum* sporozoites in an immunofluorescence assay. These CCAg remained stable in commonly used stool preservatives and may be useful in designing additional diagnostic tests for the diagnosis of cryptosporidiosis.[34]

Cryptosporidium spp. Key points — laboratory diagnosis.

1. If the specimen represents the typically watery diarrhea, there should be numerous organisms that may be caught up in mucus.
2. The more normal the stool (semi-formed, formed), the fewer the organisms and the more artifact material will be present.
3. Several concentrates and at least five or six acid-fast smears should be examined before a patient is called negative, especially if the patient has been on experimental medications.
4. The most common permanent stains (trichrome, iron hematoxylin) usually do not adequately stain *Cryptosporidium* spp.
5. Although the oocysts can be stained with auramine rhodamine stains, identification should be confirmed using acid-fast stains or the monoclonal reagents (most sensitive). This is particularly true if the stool contains other cells or a lot of artifact material (more normal stool consistency).

6. Sputum specimens should be submitted in 5% or 10% formalin and processed the same way as a stool sample.
7. It is important to remember that in severely immunocompromised patients (≥100 CD4+ cells), microsporidia may also be present in approximately 30% of those patients who have cryptosporidiosis. The diagnostic procedures for the identification of *C. parvum* will not be appropriate for the identification of microsporidial spores. Modified trichrome stains and optical brightening agents (Calcofluor white) can be used for that purpose.[35]

10.5.2   Histology

Developmental stages in the life cycle of *Cryptosporidium* can be found at all levels of the intestinal tract, with the jejunum the most heavily infected site. Routine hematoxylin and eosin (H&E) staining is sufficient to demonstrate these parasites. Using regular light microscopy, the organisms are visible as small (~1–3 μm) round structures aligned along the brush border. They are intracellular, but extracytoplasmic, and are found in parasito-phorous vacuoles. Developmental stages are more difficult to identify without using transmission electron microscopy. It is also important to remember that in the severely compromised patient, *Cryptosporidium* has been found in other body sites, primarily the lung, as a disseminated infection. Within tissue, confusion with *Cyclospora cayetanensis* is unlikely as the oocysts of this coccidian are approximately 8–10 μm and the developmental stages occur within a vacuole at the luminal end of the enterocyte, rather than at the brush border. Developmental stages of *I. belli* also occur within the enterocyte, so should not be confused with *Cryptosporidium*.[36]

Newer methods have also been used to detect *Cryptosporidium* DNA in fixed, paraffin-embedded tissue using the polymerase chain reaction (PCR).[37] This approach could provide a sensitive and specific method for detection of parasite material in paraffin-embedded tissues and could be very valuable in retrospective studies of archival material.

10.5.3   Water testing

Since the late 1980s, most of the water utilities have either set up in-house water quality testing laboratories or contracted with commercial water laboratories for the recovery and identification of *Cryptosporidium* and *Giardia*. In a recent study, two methods were evaluated for the recovery of *Cryptosporidium* and *Giardia*. The American Society for Testing and Materials involves sampling a minimum of 100 l of water through a polypropylene yard cartridge filter, extracting the particulates, flotation concentration of the extracted particulates using a Percoll-sucrose gradient, using the commercially available *Cryptosporidium/Giardia* combination FA reagent, and reviewing the slides for the presence of either *Cryptosporidium* oocysts and/or *Giardia* cysts. This method tends to be labor intensive, complex, lengthy, and depends on the skill and experience of the personnel and quality control measures in use within the laboratory. Recovery rates tend to be low with this approach. The second method uses sampling by membrane filtration, Percoll-Percoll step gradient, and immunofluorescent staining. This method was characterized by higher recovery rates in all three types of waters tested: raw surface water, partially treated water from a flocculation basin, and filtered water. Using seeded specimens, much higher recovery rates were obtained when the flotation step was eliminated from the protocol. Oocyst and cyst recovery rates decreased with both methods as the turbidity of the water increased. Using smaller tubes for flotation, the membrane filter method was less time consuming and cheaper. However, the lack of a confirmatory step might be a problem, particularly if cross-reacting algae are present in water samples.[38] A number of other test options, including PCR, are currently being used.[39] Unfortunately, these procedures emphasize organism detection; the issue of organism viability has not yet been resolved.

10.6   Treatment

Cryptosporidiosis tends to be self-limiting in those patients who have an intact immune system. In those patients who are receiving immunosuppressives, one method of therapy would be to discontinue such a regimen. Other approaches with specific therapeutic drugs such as spiramycin have been tried, but to date the results are still somewhat controversial. Tissue culture systems using cell lines such as human ileocecal adenocarcinoma (HCT-8) cells and animal models that support the entire life cycle have been developed which may provide excellent opportunities for *in vitro* drug studies.[40] Unfortunately, even the studies reported for oral treatment with spiramycin, a macrolide antibiotic related to erythromycin, have been inconclusive.[5,41] Studies indicate a statistically significant reduction in median oocyst excretion after 2 weeks of therapy with paromomycin. Long-term effectiveness of this agent needs to be examined in future studies.[42] Data indicate that severely immunocompromised AIDS patients with refractory cryptosporidiosis may show a variable response to letrazuril with a high rate of relapse and rash as a major side effect.[43] In a group of 129 AIDS patients with refractory diarrhea, response rates based on CD4[+] counts, diarrhea duration, body weight, HIV risk factor, and presence or absence of pathogens showed no benefit of octreotide.[44]

Recent studies using halofuginone in immunosuppressed rats with *C. parvum* indicated the drug's activity was dose-related and both prophylaxis and treatment reduced the rate and severity of infection in the small intestine and cecum. Treatment may reduce the severity of acute cryptosporidiosis, but is less effective for chronic cryptosporidiosis involving the colon and extraintestinal tissues.[45]

Ongoing studies with immunologic intervention hold promise, but are not currently being widely used. A study in mice using two human serum immunoglobulin (HSIG) products indicated HSIG may be beneficial when given prophylactically, but cannot eradicate cryptosporidia from mucosal surfaces in an established infection.[46]

In both animal and clinical studies of *Cryptosporidium* infection, counting the oocysts in fecal specimens is often critical to data interpretation. Results indicate several counting methods are acceptable, and comparisons between different experiments are now possible and scientifically valid.[47]

References

1. Berkelman, R.L., Emerging infectious diseases in the United States, 1993. *J. Inf. Dis.* 70, 272–277, 1994.
2. Current, W. L., Garcia, L.S., Cryptosporidiosis. *Clin. Microbiol. Rev.* 3, 325–358, 1991.
3. Webster, J.P., Macdonald, D.W., Cryptosporidiosis reservoir in wild brown rats (*Rattus norvegicus*) in the UK. *Epidemiology Infect.* 115, 207–209, 1995.
4. Zimmerman, S.K., Needham, C.A., Comparison of conventional stool concentration and preserved-smear methods with Merifluor *Cryptosporidium/Giardia* direct immunofluorescence assay and ProSpect T *Giardia* EZ microplate assay for detection of *Giardia lamblia*. *J. Clin. Microbiol.* 33, 1942–1943, 1995.
5. Goodgame, R.W., Kimball, K., Ou, C.N., White, A.C., Genta, R.M., Lifschitz, C.H., Chappell, C.L., Intestinal function and injury in acquired immunodeficiency syndrome — Related cryptosporidiosis. *Gastroenterology* 108, 1075–1082, 1995.
6. Guarino, A., Canani, R.B., Casola, A., Pozio, E., Russo, R., Bruzzese, E., Fontana, M., Rubino A., Human intestinal cryptosporidiosis: Secretory diarrhea and enterotoxic activity in Caco-2 cells. *J. Infect. Dis.* 171, 976–983, 1995.

7. Moore, R., Tzipori, S., Griffiths, J.K., Johnson, K., Demontigny, L., Lomakina, I., Temporal changes in permeability and structure of piglet ileum after site-specific infectioin by *Cryptosporidium parvum*. *Gastroenterology* 108, 1030–1039, 1995.

8. Gomez Morales, M.A., Ausiello, C.M., Urbani, F., Pozio, E., Crude extract and recombinant protein of *Cryptosporidium parvum* oocysts induce proliferation of human peripheral blood mononuclear cells in vitro. *J. Infect. Dis.* 172, 211–216, 1995.

9. Fang, G.D., Lima, A.A.M., Martins, C.V., Nataro, J.P., Guerrant, R.L., Etiology and epidemiology of persistent diarrhea in northeastern Brazil: A hospital-based, prospective, case-control study. *J. Pediatr. Gastroenterol. Nutr.* 21, 137–144, 1995.

10. Campbell, I., Tzipori, S., Hutchison G., Angus, K.W., Effect of disinfectants on survival of *Cryptosporidium* oocysts. *Vet. Rec.* 111, 414–415, 1982.

11. Fayer, R., Effect of sodium hypochlorite exposure on infectivity of *Cryptosporidium parvum* oocysts for neonatal BALB/c mice. *Appl. Environ. Microbiol.* 61, 844–846, 1995.

12. Hayes, E. B., Matte, T.D., O'Brien, T.R., McKinley, T.W., Logsdon, G.S., Rose, J.B., Ungar, B.L.P., Word, D.M., Pinsky, P.F., Cummings, M.S., Wilson, M.A., Long, E.G., Hurwitgs, E.S., Juranek, D.D., Large community outbreak of cryptosporidiosis due to contamination of a filtered public water supply. *N. Engl. J. Med.* 320, 1372–1376, 1989.

13. Mackenzie, W.R., Hoxie, N.J., Proctor, M.E., A massive outbreak in Milwaukee of *Cryptosporidium* infection transmitted through the public water supply. *N. Engl. J. Med.* 331, 161–167, 1994.

14. Mackenzie, W.R., Schell, W.L., Blair, K.A., Addiss, D.G., Peterson, D.E., Hoxie, N.J., Kazmierczak, J.J., Davis, J.P., Massive outbreak of waterborne cryptosporidium infection in Milwaukee, Wisconsin: Recurrence of illness and risk of secondary transmission. *Clin. Inf. Dis.* 21, 57–62, 1995.

15. Skeels, M.R., Sokolow, R., Hubbard, C.V., Andrus, J.K., Baisch, J., *Cryptosporidium* infection in Oregon public health clinic patients, 1985–1988: The value of statewide laboratory surveillance. *Am. J. Public Health* 80, 305–308, 1990.

16. Sorvillo, F.J., Fujioka, K., Nahlen, B. et al., Swimming-associated cryptosporidiosis. *Am. J. Public Health* 82, 742–744, 1992.

17. Bell, A., Guasparini, R., Meeds, D., et al., A swimming pool-associated outbreak of cryptosporidiosis in British Columbia. *Can. J. Public Health* 84, 334–337, 1993.

18. Atherton, F., Newman, C.P., Casemore, D.P., An outbreak of waterborne cryptosporidiosis associated with a public water supply in the UK. *Epidemiol. Infect.* 115, 123-131, 1995.

19. Ungar, B. L. P., Burris, J.A., Quinn, C.A., Finkelman, F.D., Seroepidemiology of *Cryptosporidium* infection in two Latin American populations. *J. Infect. Dis.* 157, 551–556, 1990.

20. Public Health Laboratory Service Study Group. Cryptosporidiosis in England and Wales: prevalence and clinical and epidemiological features. *Br. Med. J.* 300, 774–777, 1990.

21. DuPont, H.L., Chappell, C.L., Sterling, C.R., Okhuysen, P.C., Rose, J.B., Jakubowski, W., The infectivity of *Cryptosporidium parvum* in healthy volunteers. *N. Engl. J. Med.* 332, 855–859, 1995.

22. Juranek, D.D., Cryptosporidiosis: Sources of infection and guidelines for prevention. *Clin. Inf. Dis.* 21, S57-S61, 1995.

23. Dawson, A., Griffin, R., Fleetwood, A., Barrett, N.J., Farm visits and zoonoses. *Commun. Dis. Rep CDR Rev.* May 26, 5(6), R81-6, 1995.

24. Morgan, U.M., Constantine, C.C., O'Donoghue, P., Meloni, B.P., O'Brian, P.A., Thompson, R.C., Molecular characterization of *Cryptosporidium* isolates from humans and other animals using random amplified polymorphic DNA analysis. *Am. J. Trop. Med. Hyg.* 52, 559–564, 1995.

25. Egger, M., Mausezahl, D., Odermatt, P., Marti, H.P., Tanner, M., Symptoms and transmission of intestinal cryptosporidiosis. *Arch. Dis. Child.* 65, 445–447, 1990.

26. Baskerville, A., Ramsay, A.D., Millwardsadler, G.H., Cook, R.W., Cranage, M.P., Greenaway, P.J., Chronic pancreatitis and biliary fibrosis associated with cryptosporidiosis in simian AIDS. *J. Comparative Pathol.* 105, 415–421, 1991.

27. Tanyuksei, M., Gun, H., Doganci, L., Prevalence of *Cryptosporidium* sp in patients with neoplasia and diarrhea. *Scand. J. Inf. Dis.* 27, 69–70, 1995.

28. Garcia, L.S., Bruckner, D.A., *Diagnostic Medical Parasitology*, 3rd. ed. American Society for Microbiology, ASM Press, Washington, D.C., 1997.

29. Moore, J.A., Frenkel, J.K., Respiratory and enteric cryptosporidiosis in humans. *Arch. Pathol. Lab. Med.* 115, 1160–1162, 1991.

30. Laxer, M. A., Alcantara, A.K., Javato-Laxer, M., Menorca, D.M., Fernando, M.T., Ranoa, C.P., Immune response to cryptosporidiosis in Philippine children. *Am. J. Trop. Med. Hyg.* 42, 131–139, 1990.

31. Alles, A.J., Waldron, M.A., Sierra, L.S., Mattia, A.R., Prospective comparison of direct immunofluorescence and conventional staining methods for detection of *Giardia* and *Cryptosporidium* spp. in human fecal specimens. *J. Clin. Microbiol.* 33, 1632–1634, 1995.

32. Rosenblatt, J.E., Sloan, L.M., Evaluation of an enzyme-linked immunosorbent assay for detection of *Cryptosporidium* spp. in stool specimens. *J. Clin. Microbiol.* 31, 1468–1471, 1993.

33. Arrowood, M.J., Hurd, M.R., Mead, J.R., A new method for evaluating experimental cryptosporidial parasite loads using immunofluorescent flow cytometry. *J. Parasitol.* 81, 404–409, 1995.

34. Elshewy, K., Kilani, R.T., Hegazi, M.M., Makhlouf, L.M., Wenman, W.M., Identification of low-molecular-mass coproantigens of *Cryptosporidium parvum. J. Infect. Dis.* 169, 460–463, 1994.

35. Garcia, L.S., Shimizu, R.Y., Bruckner, D.A., Detection of microsporidial spores in fecal specimens from patients diagnosed with cryptosporidiosis. *J. Clin. Microbiol.* 32, 1739–1741, 1994.

36. Orihel, T.C., Ash, L.R., *Parasites in Human Tissues*, ASCP, Chicago, IL, 1995.

37. Laxer, M.A., D'Nicuola, M.E., Patel, R.J., Detection of *Cryptosporidium parvum* DNA in fixed, paraffin-embedded tissue by the polymerase chain reaction. *Am. J. Trop. Med. Hyg.* 47, 450–455, 1992.

38. Nieminski, E.C., Schaefer, F.W., Ongerth, J.E., Comparison of two methods for detection of *Giardia* cysts and *Cryptosporidium* oocysts in water. *Appl. Environ. Microbiol.* 61, 1714–1719, 1995.

39. Johnson, D.W., Pieniazek, N.J., Griffin, D.W., Misener, L., Rose, J.B., Development of a PCR protocol for sensitive detection of *Cryptosporidium* oocysts in water samples. *Appl. Environ. Microbiol.* 61, 3849–3855, 1995.

40. Woods, K.M., Nesterenko, M.V., Upton, S.J., Development of a microtitre ELISA to quantify development of *Cryptosporidium parvum in vitro, FEMS Microbiol. Lett.* 128, 89–93, 1995.

41. Flanigan, T.P., Soave, R., Cryptosporidiosis. In Sun, T. (Ed.) *Progress in Clinical Parasitology, Vol III.* Springer-Verlag, New York, p. 1–20, 1993.

42. White, A.C., Chappell, C.L., Hayat, C.S., Kimball, K.T., Flanigan, T.P., Goodgame, R.W., Paromomycin for cryptosporidiosis in AIDS: A prospective, double-blind trial. *J. Infect. Dis.* 170, 419–424, 1994.

43. Loeb, M., Walach, C., Phillips, J., Fong, I., Salit, I., Rachlis, A., Walmsley, S. Treatment with letrazuril of refractory cryptosporidial diarrhea complicating AIDS. *J. AIDS, Human Retrovirol.* 10, 48–53, 1995.

44. Simon, D.M., Cello, J.P., Valenzuela, J., Levy, R., Dickerson, G., Goodgame, R., Brown, M., Lyche, K., Fessel, W.J., Grendell, J., Wilcox, C.M., Afdhal, N., Fogel, R., Reevesdarby, V., Stern, J., Smith, O., Graziano, F., Pleakow, D., Flanigan, T., Schubert, T., Loveless, M., Eron, L., Basuk, P., Bonacini, M., Orenstein, J., Multicenter trial of octreotide in patients with refractory acquired immunodeficiency syndrome-associated diarrhea. *Gastroenterology* 108, 1753–1760, 1995.

45. Rehg, J.E., The activity of halofuginone in immunosuppressed rats infected with *Cryptosporidium parvum, J. Antimicrob. Chemother.* 35, 391–397, 1995.

46. Kuhls, T.L., Orlicek, S.L., Mosier, D.A., Crawford, D.L., Abrams, V.L., Greenfield, R.A., Enteral human serum immunoglobulin treatment of cryptosporidiosis in mice with severe combined immunodeficiency. *Infect. Immun.* 63, 139–95, 1995.

47. Kao, T.C., Ungar, B.L.P., Comparison of sequential, random, and hemacytometer methods for counting *Cryptosporidium* oocysts. *J. Parasitol.* 80:816–819, 1994.

chapter eleven

Trichomoniasis

Kenneth A. Borchardt

11.1   Introduction...205
11.2   Epidemiology..205
11.3   Clinical disease 207
11.4   Diagnosis 209
11.5   Treatment..210
References..212

11.1   Introduction

The genus *Trichomonas* has more than a 100 species. All of these flagellated protozoa are parasitic except for a few free-living forms. Generally they are less than 25 μm in length and reproduce asexually.

Trichomonas gallinae (Figure 1) occurs in pigeons, doves, and chickens. It produces an infection in the mouth, esophagus, and crop, with potential dissemination to internal organs. Mortality in infected pigeons and doves can be 90%.

Trichomonas foetus (Figure 2) is an important pathogen of cattle worldwide. The bull is either asymptomatic or acutely infected after dissemination of the trichomonads to the distal penis and prepuce. In the cow *T. foetus* infects the vagina, cervix, and uterus. It can result in infertility and abortion, but the infection is subsequently self-limiting. *T. foetus* infection is untreatable in the bull and makes the animal unsuitable for breeding.

Three species of trichomonads have been identified in humans and exist only in the trophozoite stage. *Trichomonas tenax*, a commensal, inhabits the oral cavity. *Pentatrichomonas hominis* colonizes the large intestine and has questionable pathogenicity. *Trichomonas vaginalis* (Figure 3) produces genitourinaty tract infections in both males and females.

In 1836 Donné identified the flagellated protozoan *T. vaginalis* microscopically from a patient's vaginal discharge after mixing the clinical specimen with saline.[1] His laboratory discovery established the saline wet mount as a diagnostic method for identifying the pathogen from human infections.

11.2   Epidemiology

The World Health Organization estimates that 180 million cases of trichomoniasis occur annually worldwide.[2] Trichomoniasis is considered by others to be the most disseminated nonviral infection of all sexually transmitted diseases (STD).[3] The accuracy of any estimate is questionable because the infection is not a reportable STD in the U.S. and other countries

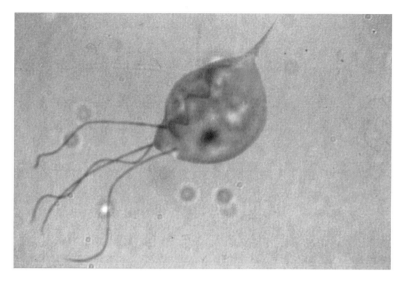

Figure 1   *Trichomonas gallinae.* (Photo courtesy of John Semnan, M.S.)

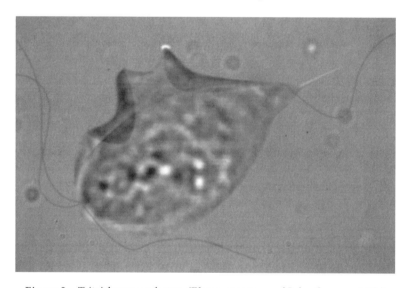

Figure 2   *Tritrichomonas foetus.* (Photo courtesy of John Seman, M.S.)

of the world.[4] Other factors influence the reports of infection because of questionable accuracy of diagnosis. *T. vaginalis* infections frequently are subclinical in either sex and misdiagnosed. Laboratory tests employed for identifying *T. vaginalis* vary in their sensitivity which effects an accurate identification.

Population groups differ in their incidence of reported trichomoniasis. High risk populations are found in the lower socioeconomic populations, those with multiple sex partners, prostitutes, illiterates, and individuals with poor genital hygiene. Depending on the patient groups studied, third world countries have reported rates of trichomoniasis that vary from 19 to 47.1%.[4,5]

For many years trichomoniasis was perceived as an insignificant or self-limiting infection. Contemporary clinical studies have described the cervical inflammation of this STD and its resistance to treatment.[6,7] Viral research has demonstrated that *T. vaginalis* is capable of phagocytizing viral particles while maintaining its viability. The role of *T. vaginalis* in transmission of viral infections such as herpes simplex has been postulated. Trichomonads

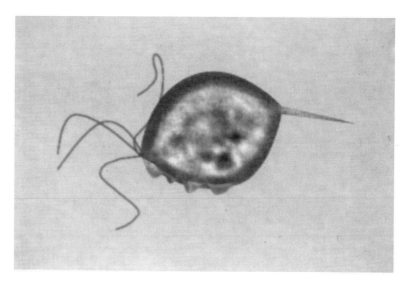

Figure 3   *Trichomonas vaginalis.* (Photo courtesy of John Seman, M.S.)

are phagocytic and can maintain the viability of the virus.[8] Because trichomoniasis produces an inflammatory reaction in the host, the infection increases the host's predisposition to a retrovirus infection such as the human immunodeficiency virus (HIV).[9]

11.3   Clinical disease

Clinically, the disease can be a diagnostic problem in either male or female patients. Trichomoniasis is asymptomatic in approximately 50% of infected females, while the majority of males present a self-limiting or subclinical infection.[10] Both sexes remain reservoirs for trichomoniasis because of the failure of the host's humoral and cell-mediated immune responses.

The ameboid movement of trichomonads and their adherence to urethral or vaginal epithelium tissue results in mechanical damage to the tissue. A toxic secretion may be released by the organisms.[11]

Provenzano and Alderete[12] demonstrated the degradation of human IgG, IgM, and IgA by cysteine proteinases produced by *T. vaginalis.* These proteinases were recoverable in the vaginal washings from infected patients which possibly predisposed the vagina to other STDs.

It is estimated that one of five sexually active women will be infected with *T. vaginalis* in their lifetime.[13] The incubation period before clinical symptoms occur in women varies from a few days to four weeks.[14] In the female infection, trichomonads invade the vagina, endocervix, and the urethra resulting in vaginitis, pruritis, dysuria, and dyspareunia.[15] Vaginal discharge varies in quantity and appearance. Frequently it appears greenish-gray in color, bubbly, and malodorous. Other symptoms include backache and pelvic pressure. A STD study on 63,365 Indian women included the diagnosis for trichomoniasis. Those diagnosed as positive were evaluated for statistically significant symptoms. The most frequently noted were vaginitis, cervical erosion of an unhealthy cervix, and cervicitis.[16]

In pregnancy an infected patient may experience either premature rupture of her membranes resulting in death of the fetus or a neonate with an abnormal birth weight.[17] An infected mother can transmit the infection to her newborn female by direct vulvovaginal contamination during a vaginal delivery. Infection can occur after an infant's ingestion of trichomonads. Because of the neutral pH of the digestive tract, the trichomonads pass through the digestive tract while maintaining their viability. Subsequently, feces containing

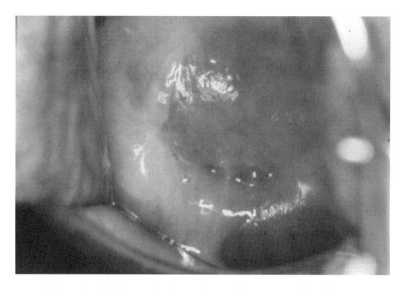

Figure 4 Trichomoniasis patient with a cervical discharge.

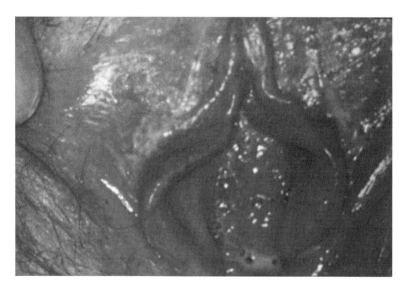

Figure 5 Trichomoniasis patient with a profuse discharge and vulvar hyperemia.

trichomonads contaminate either the vagina or urethra. The newborn is susceptible because of an appropriate vaginal environment, which possesses an akaline pH and high glycogen content.[18]

Both premenarchal girls and postmenopausal women offer an unfavorable environment for growth of *T. vaginalis*. The deficiency of vaginal estrogen results in a more akaline pH with decreased glycogen.[19]

Trichomoniasis has been reported in lesbians although STDs are less frequently diagnosed than in hetersosexual women. This infection has been reported as being transmissible between lesbian partners.[20]

The infected untreated female experiences periods of remission and exacerbation of symptoms approximating the period of menstruation or during prenancy. This may be the result of the organism's invasion of the endocervix producing a cervicitis.

T. vaginalis infections in the male are characterized as non-gonoccocal urethritis, prostatitis, epididymitis, balanoposthitis, urethral stricture, and infertility.[21] Trichomonads in

Table 1 Evaluation of Diagnostic Tests for *T. vaginalis*

Test	Sensitivity
Papanicolaou stain	Cytological smears frequently inaccurate
ELISA	Not as sensitive as culture
Latex agglutination	95.5% sensitivity
DNA probe	90% sensitivity
DFA staining	Sensitivity better than saline wet mount
Saline wet mount	Sensitivity variable from 40–75%
Culture-Hollander's	Sensitivity better than 80%
Culture-Trichosel	Sensitivity better than 80%
Culture-modified Diamonds	Sensitivity 20 CFU/0.5 ml[a]
Culture-InPouch TV	Sensitivity 2 CFU/0.5 ml

[a] Compared to agar dilution.

the male have been isolated from urine, semen, urethral discharge, and prostatic fluid. Urogenital trichomoniasis has been classified as an asymptomatic carrier state, acute symptomatic, or as a symptomatic disease. The asymptomatic carrier state is determined by recovering *T. vaginalis* from a patient who has had sexual contact with an infected person. An acute symptomatic infection is characterized by either a burning sensation during urination, purulent urethral discharge, or other genitourinary complications. Symptomatic males present symptoms similar to nongonococcal urethritis. The incubation period for urethritis varies to 10 days.[21]

T. vaginalis has been observed within the prostate gland by employing an immunoperoxide procedure.[22] Both acute and chronic inflammatory changes were observed. Trichomonads were identified in the prostatic urethra, glandular lamina, submucosa, and stroma.

Semen does not have an inhibitory effect on the survival of *T. vaginalis*. Spermatozoa in an infected patient are not adversely affected by trichomonads either in their motility or density for at least 24 h. Thus, semen can serve as an effective transport for transmitting the infection.[23]

11.4 Diagnosis

Laboratory methods that have been employed for demonstrating *T. vaginalis* infections include: staining, enzyme-linked immunosorbent assay (ELISA), direct fluorescent antibody (DFA) staining, latex agglutination, DNA probe, saline wet mount, and culture (Table 1).[24]

The sensitivity and specificity of the Papanicolaou stain as a diagnostic test for *T. vaginalis* is frequently inaccurate and requires routine culturing for quality control for both laboratory personnel and clinicians.[25]

ELISA methods have only detected antibodies of the IgG and IgA class in vaginal washes from patients with acute trichomoniasis. Serum samples from both infected patients and experimental animals have been false-negative for IgE antibody.[26]

Currently a dual latex agglutination test is available in the U.S.[27] In one study 352 patients were evaluated comparing the latex agglutination test to wet mount microscopy. The latex agglutination test identified 42 infected patients (95.5% sensitivity) compared to 31 (73.8% sensitivity) with the wet mount, but 40 of these 42 positive patients had a clinical diagnosis of trichomoniasis.

The Affirm VPIII is a DNA probe test for identification of *Candida albicans*, *Gardnerella vaginalis*, and *T. vaginalis*.[28] In one study the DNA probe evaluated 852 samples which were sampled both by the wet mount and Diamond's medium. The Affirm test demonstrated a relative sensitivity of 90% and a specificity of 99.9% when compared to Diamond's 5–7 day culture.

DFA staining has a better sensitivity than the wet mount (80-90%) but is not comparable to the most sensitive culture methods.[29] This procedure requres fluorescent microscopy, which limits the test's availability.

The variability in the sensitivity of the saline wet mount method is due to several factors that are not easily controlled: (1) the source of the specimen; (2) the patient with a polymicrobic STD infection, which can limit visualization of the trichomonads; (3) the clinical stage of infection; (4) transport time; (5) method of specimen preparation; (6) time allocated for microscopic examination; and (7) the experience of the microscopist in recognizing *T. vaginalis*. Only 60–70% of infections will be positive with the wet mount procedure.[30] A sensitivity of 40% has been reported for wet mount compared to agar dilution.[25]

In vitro culture is considered the gold standard for diagnosis of trichomoniasis.[23] Hollander's, Trichosel, modified Diamond's, and the InPouch TV test have been used for culture. In evaluating a culture method, various parameters must be considered in addition to the sensitivity and specificity of the medium: storage temperature, shelf-life of the medium, technology time required in performing the test, and the volume of medium examined.

The InPouch TV test has demonstrated a greater sensitivity then either the saline wet mount, Hollander's, Trichosel, or modified Diamond's media.[31-33] The shelf-life of the InPouch test when stored at room temperature is 15 months, while the others have a shelf-life of 3–6 months when stored at 4°C.

The InPouch test serves first as a specimen transport vessel and growth chamber during incubation, then as a viewing chamber during microscopy. It consists of a clear, gas-impermeable, plastic pouch that is double-chambered. The medium has both polymicrobic antibacterial and antifungal activities. Once it is inoculated, it requires no opening for viewing. After incubation at 37°C. positive growth occurs within 24–48 h, infrequently at 5 days.[28]

Hollander's, Trichosel, and modified Diamond's are tubed media that require an aliquot being transferred to a glass slide before microscopic examination. This quantitates the amount of medium that can be placed under the coverslip. The InPouch method is superior because: (1) it eliminates the glass slide and coverslip, (2) a larger volume of medium is viewed per field, (3) the medium restricts the growth of yeast and bacteria, and (4) the characteristic motility of the trichomonads is easier to observe.[32]

11.5   Treatment

Of the 5-nitroimidazole derivatives, tinidazole, ornidazole secnidazole, and ninorazole, metronidazole is almost the exclusive treatment for trichomoniasis.[34] The first evaluation of its efficacy against *T. vaginalis* began in France in 1958.[35] Metronidazole is the only nitroimidazole available for treatment in the U.S. The treatment regimen is described in Table 2. It is important that the sexual partner be treated for trichomoniasis to prevent reinfection. The wet mount test is not recommended to determine infection in the sexual partner. It has demonstrated significant insensitivity when compared to culture in male patients who had sexual contact with infected females.[36]

Metronidazole therapy of 250 mg t.i.d. for 7 days has been effective in 90–99% of incarcerated women,[37] but studies in outpatient clinics vary in treatment success between 81–99%.[38] Treatment failures have been attributed to failure of patient compliance in taking the drug as prescribed, inadequate drug absorption from the intestine, an inability of the drug to reach therapeutic concentrations in the vagina, or degradation of metronidazole

Table 2 Treatment for Trichomoniasis

Recommended regimen	Oral metronidazole 2 g in a single dose
Alternative regimen	Oral metronidazole in 250 mg t.i.d. for 7 days
Management of sex partner	Oral metronidazole 2 g
Treatment in pregnancy	Contraindicated in first trimester and avoided subsequently. Clotrimazole 100 mg intravaginally for 1 week. Lactation treat with 2 g metronidazole orally, stop breast-feeding for 24 h
Treatment of children	Newborn: for infection beyond 4th week of life metronidazole 10–30 mg/kg daily for 5–6 days; Older (consider sexual abuse): oral metronidazole 15 mg/kg daily in 3 doses for 7 days
Treatment failure	Retreat patient and partner. CDC recommends 2 g oral metronidazole for 3 days

From McGregor, J. Trichomoniasis: a common challenge in STD treatment. *STD Bull.* Jan., 8 (6): 1-11. 1989. With permission.

by bacterial flora in the vagina.[34,36] A study evaluated 11 patients who were repeated treatment failures to oral metronidazole.[41] Oral dosages of metronidazole were first prescribed at 200 mg, 3 times per day, for 7 days, then at an increased dosage of 200 mg, 3 times per day for 2 days, and 800 mg from days 3–7. Measurements for metronidazole and its metabolite were obtained from patients after both treatments by employing a specific, highly sensitive pressure chromatographic method. The results indicated that with lower dosages, the levels of metronidazole and its metabolite in plasma and vaginal content were normal (mean of 8.3 mg/l). A proportionately higher level was obtained with an increased dosage. These results from both treatment regimens indicated that neither malabsorption from the gut nor abnormal levels in the vagina were directly related to treatment failures. These data disproved the concept that metronidazole was unable to reach the site of infection in therapeutic levels. An additional important therapeutic conclusion was defined in treatment of resistant cases of trichomoniasis. Intravenous therapy was applicable only when a patient was incapable of taking the drug orally. This study substantiated the resistance of *T. vaginalis* to metronidazole.

Various *in vitro* methods have been employed to identify metronidazole resistant strains of *T. vaginalis*. Meingassner and Thurner used both stoppered tubes and multi-well plates to test the resistance of a trichomonad isolated from a patient with recurrent trichomoniasis.[42] The isolate only demonstrated resistance under aerobic conditions, indicating that assay conditions were important in identifying resistant organisms. This was confirmed in an *in vitro* study using Trichosel broth in tubes, with disks containing 5, 15, and 30 µg of metronidazole, and incubated under aerobic and anaerobic conditions.[43] Only 2 of 12 clinical isolates were resistant to metronidazole, but anaerobic incubation significantly decreased the minimum inhibitory concentration (MIC) for a resistant isolate against metronidazole. Another study employed a broth dilution procedure using modified Diamond's medium without antibiotics and under aerobic incubation.[44] Patients were treated with either single 1- or 2-g doses of metronidazole. The results indicated that the MICs for resistant organisms were significantly greater than the MICs from patients that were cured. In comparing the MICs from those patients responding to treatment with either 1 or 2 g of metronidazole, it was evident that the MICs for trichomonads isolated from those receiving 2 g were higher than those patients treated with 1 g.

A study of 53 isolates of metronidazole-resistant *T. vaginalis* were tested for both aerobic and anaerobic metronidazole susceptibility employing a modification of Meingasser's method.[45] The results indicated a better correlation of clinical resistance to metronidazole aerobically (79%) than anaerobically (53%). Although the aerobic minimum lethal concentrations MLCs were more sensitive to clinical resistance, the values obtained were biologically unfeasible.

A recent method for determining resistance of trichomonads to metronidazole utilized the InPouch TV test. This test enabled the determination of both a MIC and MLC. *T. vaginalis* patients responding to metronidazole treatment demonstrated MLCs between 0.4 to 3.1 µl/mL. The MLCs from those tested from initial treatment failures were between 6.2–50 µg/mL.[46]

References

1. Donne, M.A., Animalcules observes dans les matieres purulents et le produit des secretiones des organes genitaux de l'homme et de le femme. *Compt. Rendus Acad. Sci. (Paris)* 3, 385–6, 1836.
2. Brown, M.T., Trichomoniasis. *Practitioner* 209, 639–43, 1972.
3. Krieger, J.N., Urologic aspects of trichomoniasis. *Invest. Urol.* 18, 411–17, 1981.
4. Borchardt, KA., Hernandez, V., Miller, S., et al., A clinical evaluation of trichomoniasis in San Jose, Costa Rica using the InPouch TV test. *Genitourin. Med.* 68, 328–30, 1992.
5. Wawer, M.J., McNairn, D., Wabwire-Mergen, F., et al., Self-administered vaginal swabs for population-based assessment of *Trichomonas vaginalis* prevalence. *Lancet* 345, 131, 1995.
6. O'Farrell N.O., Risk factors for susceptibility to heterosexual human immunodeficiency virus infection in women. *J. Inf. Dis.* 173, 1520–1, 1996.
7. Hamed, K.A., Studemeister, A.E., Successful response of metronidazole-resistant trichomonas vaginitis to tinidazole. *Sex. Trans. Dis.* November-December, 339–40, 1992.
8. Wasserheit, J.N., Homes, K.K., Reproductive tract infections: Challenges for international health policy, programs, and research. In: *Reproductive Tract Infections: Global Impact and Priorities for Women's Reproductive Health.* Edited by Germain, A., Holmes, K.K., Piot, P., Wasserheit, J.N., New York, Plenum Press, 7–33, 1992.
9. Pindak, F.F., dePindak, M.M., Hyde, B.M., Gardner, W.A., Acquisition and retention of viruses by *Trichomonas vaginalis*. *Genitourin. Med.* 65, 366–71, 1989.
10. Laga, M., Manoka, A., Kivuvu, M., Malele, B., et al., Nonulcerative sexually transmitted diseases as risk factors for HIV-1 tramsission in women: results from a cohort study. *AIDS* 7(1), 95–102, 1993.
11. Nielsen, M.H., Nielsen, R., Electron microscopy of *Trichomonas vaginalis* Donne: interaction with vaginal epithelium trichomoniasis. *Acta Pathol. Microbiol. Immunol. Scand.* [B] 83, 305–20, 1975.
12. Provenzano, D., Alderete, J.F., Analysis of human immunoglobulin-degrading cysteine proteinases of *Trichomonas vaginalis*. *Infect. Immun.* 63, 3388–95, 1995.
13. Bickly, L.S., Krish, K.K., Punsalagk, A., et al., Comparison of direct fluorescent antibody, acridine orange, wet mount, and culture for detection of *Trichomonas vaginalis* in women attending a sexually transmitted disease clinic. *Sex. Trans. Dis.* 16, 127–31, 1989.
14. Rein, M.F., Muller, M., *Trichomonas vaginalis*. In: *Sexually Transmitted Diseases.* Holmes, K.K., Mardh, P.A., Sparling, P.F., Weisner, P.J. Eds. New York, McGraw Hill, 325–36, 1984.
15. Catteral, R.D., Trichomonal infection of the genital tract. *Med. Clin. N. Am.* 56, 1203, 1972.
16. Sardana, S., Sodhani, P., Agarwal, S., et al., Epidemiologic analysis of *Trichomonas vaginalis* infection in inflammatory smears. *Acta Cytolog.* 38, 693–7, 1994.
17. Cotch, M.F., Pastorak, M., Effects of *T. vaginalis* (TV) carriage on pregnancy outcome. 4th International Society of Sexually Transmitted Disease, Abstr. C-104, 1991.
18. Al-Salihi, F.L., Curran, J.P., Wange, J.S., Neonatal *Trichomonas vaginalis*: Report of three cases and review of the literature. *Pediatrics* 53, 196–200, 1874.
19. Postelethwaite, R.J., *Trichomonas vaginalis* and *Escherichia coli* urinary tract infection in a newborn infant. *Clin. Pediatr.* 14, 866–7, 1975.
20. Sivakumar, K., De Silva, A.H., Roy, R.B., *Trichomonas vaginalis* in a lesbian. (Letter). *Genitourin. Med.* 65, 399–400, 1989.

21. Krieger, J.N., Trichomoniasis in men: old issues and new data. *Sex. Trans. Dis.* March–April, 83–96, 1995.

22. Gardner, W.A., Jr., Culberson, D.E., Bennett, B.D., *Trichomonas vaginalis* in the prostate gland. *Arch. Pathol. Lab. Med.* 110, 430–32, 1986.

23. Daly, J.J., Sherman, J.K., Green, L., Hostetler, T.L., Survival of *Trichomonas vaginalis* in human semen. *Genintourin. Med.* 65, 106–8, 1989.

24. Borchardt, K.A., Trichomoniasis: Its clinical significance and diagnostic challenges. *Am. Clin. Lab.* Sept, 20–1, 1994.

25. Lossick, J.G., Kent, H.L., Trichomoniasis: trends in diagnosis and management. *Am. J. Obstet. Gynecol.* 165, 1219–22, 1991.

26. Quik-Tri/Can™, A dual latex test for differential detection of *Trichomonas vaginalis* and/or Candida antigens in vaginal swab specimens. Integrated Diangostics, Inc. Baltimore, MD, 12120, 7.

27. Affirm VPIII, Microbial identification test. Becton Dickinson and Company, 7 Loveton Circle, Spanks, MD, PP-120, 12.

28. Alderete, J.F. Enzyme linked immunosorbent assay for detecting antibody to *Trichomonas vaginalis*: Use of whole cells and aqueous extract as antigens. *Br. J. Vener. Dis.* 60, 164–70, 1984.

29. Phillip, A., Carter-Scott, P., Rogers, C., An agar culture technique to quantitate *Trichomonas vaginalis* from women. *J. Inf. Dis.* 155(2), 304–8, 1987.

30. Rein M.F., *Trichomonas vaginalis*. In: Mandel, G.L., Douglas, R.G., Jr., Bennett, J.E. Eds. *Principles and Practices of Infectious Diseases.* 3rd ed. New York, Churchill Livingstone, 2115–8, 1990.

31. Borchardt, K.A. Smith, R.F., An evaluation of an InPouch™ TV culture method for diagnosing *Trichomonas vaginalis* infection. *Genitourin. Med.* 67, 49–52, 1991.

32. Borchardt, K.A., Zhang, M.Z., Shing, H., A comparison on the sensitivity of the InPouch, Diamonds, and Trichosel media for detection of *Trichomonas vaginalis*. American Society For Microbiology, New Orleans, LA, Abstr. #721, May 19–23, 1996.

33. Borchardt, K.A., Al-Haraci, S., Maida, N., Prevalence of *Trichomonas vaginalis* in a male sexually transmitted disease clinic by interview, wet mount microscopy, and InPouch TV culture. *Genitourin. Med.* 71, 405–6, 1995.

34. Muller, M., Meingassner, J.G., Miller, W.A., Ledger, W.J., Three metronidazole-resistant strains of *Trichomonas vaginalis* from the United States. *Am. J. Obstet. Gynecol.* 138, 808–12, 1980.

35. Roe, F.J., Metronidazole: Review of uses and toxicity. *J. Antimicrob. Chemother.* 3, 205–12, 1977.

36. Hager, W.D., Brown, S.T., Kraus, S.J., et al., Metronidazole for vaginal trichomoniasis. Seven-day vs. single-dose regimens. *JAMA* 244, 1219–20, 1980.

37. Pereyra, A.J., Lansing, J.D., Urogenital trichomoniasis: Treatment with metronidazole in 2,002 incarcerated women. *Obstet. Gynecol.* 24, 499–508, 1964.

38. Underhill, R.A., Peck, J.H., Causes of therapeutic failure after treatment of trichomonal vaginitis. *Br. J. Clin. Pract.* 28, 134–6.

39. Kane, P.O., McFadzean, J.A., Squires, S., Absorption and excretion of metronidazole. Part II. Studies on primary failures. *Br. J. Vener. Dis.* 37, 276–7, 1961.

40. Nicol, C.S., Evans, A.J., McFadzean, J.A., Squires, S., Inactivation of metronidazole. *Lancet* 6, 441, 1966.

41. Robertson, D.H., Heyworth, R., Harrison, C., Lumsden, W.H., Treatment failure in *Trichomonas vaginalis* infections in females. I. Concentrations of metronidazole in plasma and vaginal content during normal and high dosage. *J. Antimicrob. Chemother.* 21, 373–8, 1988.

42. Meingassner, J.G., Thurner, J., Strain of *Trichomonas vaginalis* resistant to metronidazole and other 5-nitroimidazoles. *Antimicrob. Agents Chemother.* 15, 254–7, 1978.

43. Smith, R.F., Di Domenico, A., Measuring the *in vitro* susceptibility of *Trichomonas vaginalis* to metronidazole. *Sex. Trans. Dis.* July–Sept., 120–24, 1980.

44. Ralph, E.D., Darvish, R., Austin, T.W., Susceptibility of *Trichomonas vaginalis* to metronidazole treatment. *Sex. Trans. Dis.* 10(3), 119–22, 1983.

45. Lossick, J.G., Miller, M., Gorreil, T.E., *In vitro* drug susceptibility and doses of metronidazole required for cure in cases of refractory vaginal trichomoniasis. *J. Inf. Dis.* 153(2), 948–55, 1986.

46. Borchardt, K.A., Li, Z., Zhang, M.Z., Shing, H., An *in vitro* susceptibility test for trichomoniasis using the InPouch™ TV. test. *Genintourin. Med.* 72, 132–5, 1996.

Viral

---

chapter twelve

Herpesviruses

Dawn M. Sokol and Robert F. Garry

12.1   Introduction..218
12.2   Structure and replication of herpesviruses...218
    12.2.1   Structure..218
    12.2.2   Replication...222
        12.2.2.1   Attachment..222
        12.2.2.2   Penetration..222
        12.2.2.3   Uncoating 222
        12.2.2.4   Gene expression..222
        12.2.2.5   Viral DNA synthesis 223
        12.2.2.6   Assembly, maturation, and egress 223
12.3   Cellular effects of herpesviruses..224
    12.3.1   Herpesvirus-induced cytopathogenesis 224
    12.3.2   Establishment and maintenance of herpesvirus latency 224
    12.3.3   Cell transformation by herpesviruses...225
12.4   HSVs..226
    12.4.1   Epidemiology of HSVs..226
    12.4.2   Clinical manifestations of gentital infection by HSVs..............226
    12.4.3   Diagnosis of HSV infections...229
    12.4.4   Treatment of HSV infections 230
12.5   Herpesvirus infections with concurrent HIV disease............................231
    12.5.1   HIV and HSVs...231
    12.5.2   HIV and CMV..233
        12.5.2.1   Epidemiology of CMV 233
        12.5.2.2   Clinical manifestations of CMV infection.................233
        12.5.2.3   Diagnosis of CMV infection 234
        12.5.2.4   Treatment of CMV infection in HIV-infected patients..............235
    12.5.3   HIV and EBV 236
        12.5.3.1   Epidemeology of EBV 236
        12.5.3.2   Clinical manifestations of EBV in HIV-infected patients 236
    12.5.4   HIV and varicella-zoster virus...237
    12.5.5   HIV and HHV-6 and HHV-7..238
    12.5.6   HIV and HHV-8 238
12.6   Conclusions 240
References..243

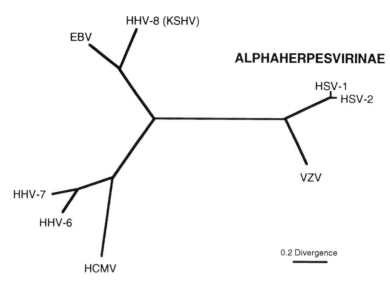

Figure 1 Phylogenetic analysis of the human herpesviruses. (Adapted from Moore et al. *J. Virol.* 70, 549, 1996. With permission.)

12.1 Introduction

Herpesviruses are large, enveloped, morphologically complex DNA viruses. Members of the herpesvirus family are widely distributed in nature, and isolates have been found in mammals, birds, fish, reptiles, and amphibians as well as certain invertebrate species. This diverse family of viruses includes herpes simplex virus type 2 (HSV-2), the prototypic sexually transmitted virus. The herpesvirus family also contains at least seven other human viruses which are, with the possible exception of human herpes virus type 7 (HHV-7), important human pathogens (Figure 1; Table 1). A defining characteristic of herpesviruses is their capacity to remain latent in their natural host.

  The herpesviruses are divided into three subfamilies. The alphaherpesvirinae, which include HSV-1 and -2, have relatively short replication cycles, spread rapidly with high cytopathogenicity in cell culture, and have the ability to establish latency in sensory ganglia. Betaherpesvirinae, including cytomegalovirus (CMV), have long replication cycles and spread slowly in culture. Although cytopathic effects in the form of enlarged cells are often observed, persistently infected cultures are established by betaherpesvirinae more easily than in the case of alphaherpesviruses. The gammaherpesvirinae, including Epstein-Barr virus (EBV), are all capable of replication in lymphoid cells, and may establish either latent, transforming, or cytolytic infections in lymphoid cells and other cell types.

12.2 Structure and replication of herpesviruses

12.2.1 Structure

Herpesvirus virions contain an icosadeltahedral capsid (approximately 100 nm in diameter) comprised of 162 capsomers (150 hexameric and 12 pentameric hollow capsomers; T = 16); (Figure 2).[1] The viral capsid is composed of viral protein 5 (VP5), VP19C, VP23, VP24, and VP26 among other proteins.[2] The capsid contains the DNA genome within a

Table 1 Herpesviruses of Humans

Designation	Common name	Subfamily	Diseases	Transmission	Treatment
Human herpesvirus-1	Herpes simplex type 1 virus	α	Gingivostomatitis; encephalitis; keratoconjunctivitis; genital lesions (rare)	Contact; sexual	Acyclovir
Human herpesvirus-2	Herpes simplex type 2 virus	α	Genital lesions; neonatal herpes meningitis; keratoconjunctivitis	Sexual	Acyclovir
Human herpesvirus-3	Varicella-zoster virus	α	Chickenpox, zoster	Contact	Acyclovir
Human herpesvirus-4	Epstein-Barr virus	γ	Infectious mononucleosis; Burkitt's and other lymphomas; nasopharyngeal carcinoma; AIDS-associated oral hairy leukoplakia	Contact; blood; allograft	Acyclovir Interferon-α[a]
Human herpesvirus-5	Cytomegalovirus virus	β	Mononucleosis; cytomegalic inclusion disease	Contact; sexual; blood; allograft	Gancyclovir; foscarnet
Human herpesvirus-6	Human B-lymphotropic virus	β	Exanthum subitum (roseola infantum; sixth disease)	Contact; allograft	Gancyclovir[b] Foscarnet[b]
Human herpesvirus-7	None	β	Unknown	Unknown	Unknown
Human herpesvirus-8	Kaposi's sarcoma-associated herpesvirus	α	Kaposi's sarcoma	Unknown	Unknown

[a] Antiviral efficacy unknown.
[b] Clinical efficacy unknown.

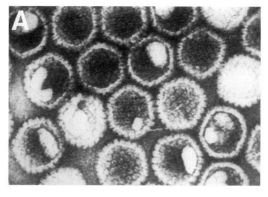

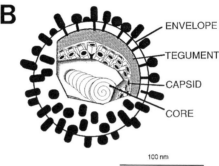

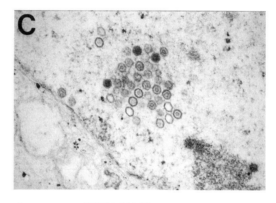

Figure 2   Morphology and structure of HSV. (A) Electron microscopic image of purified HSV type 2. (Centers for Disease Control and Prevention.) (B) Ultrastructural analysis of HSV type 2 in the brain of a patient with encephalitis. (Courtesy of Dr. Russell Van Dyke, Tulane Medical School.) (C) Structure of HSV.

toroidal structure. A fibrous "tegument" surrounds the capsid. The tegument contains a number of important proteins including the α-*trans*-inducing factor (αTIF) and the virion host shut off (VHS) protein (see below). The tegument is surrounded by a lipid-containing envelope from which protrude numerous spikes. The envelope spikes are composed of at least 11 glycosylated proteins including gB, gC, gG, gI, gK, gL, and gM and a few intrinsic membrane proteins.[2] Herpesvirus virions contain more than 30 virus-specified proteins and essentially no detectable host proteins or other components except for the envelope lipids.

The bulk of the nucleic acid packaged by herpesviruses is linear, double-stranded DNA, although a limited number of ribonucleotides may also be associated.[3] In the virion the ends of this genomic DNA appear to be held together by a large virion-associated

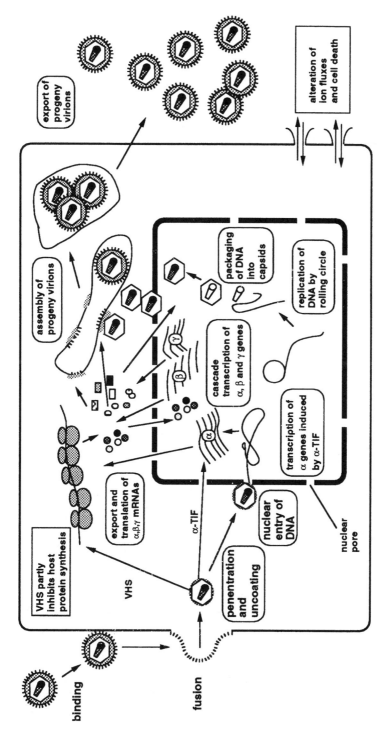

Figure 3 Replication cycle of herpesviruses. See text for details.

protein (VP1-2). The organization of the DNA is complex, consisting of various permutations of two covalently linked components designated L (long) and S (short). The unique gene sequences of L and S are flanked by inverted repeats. L and S can be arranged in four possible linear isomers each of which appear to be equally infectious.

12.2.2 Replication

Replication of herpesviruses follows steps which are similar for most other obligate intracellular parasites (Figure 3).

12.2.2.1 Attachment

The initial step in the replication cycle of all viruses is attachment to a cellular receptor. Heparin sulfate has been implicated as a cellular receptor for both HSV-1 and –2.[4] Heparin sulfate is widely distributed on mammalian cells which may explain why these viruses can attach to and penetrate many types of cultured mammalian cells. Heparin partially inhibits HSV-1 and -2 attachment and enzymatic removal of heparin sulfate substantially reduces attachment. However, because inhibition is only partial it is likely that other receptors can also be utilized by HSV. The fact that HSVs are capable of infecting both epithelial cells and cells of the nervous system further suggests that these viruses may be capable of utilizing multiple receptors. The question of which viral envelope protein(s) is involved in attachment to the cellular receptors is also complex. Mutation of each of the 10 glycoprotein genes individually fails to totally abrogate infection in a variety of cell types. This provides further evidence for multiple pathways involving multiple cellular receptors and viral proteins for attachment of herpesviruses to their host cell.

12.2.2.2 Penetration

Herpesvirus penetration into the host cell is rapid and appears to involve direct fusion of the virion envelope with the plasma membrane. There is little evidence for penetration via endocytosis and entry by this route may result in a nonproductive infection. Glycoproteins gB, gD, gL, and gH have each been implicated in penetration of various cell types. As with attachment, multiple pathways for viral fusion with various types of host cells may be utilized by different herpesviruses.

12.2.2.3 Uncoating

After penetration, herpesvirus virions are transported via the cytoskeleton to the vicinity of the nucleus. Empty capsids are often found by electron microscopic analysis in the vicinity of nuclear pores suggesting that DNA enters the nucleus through these structures.

12.2.2.4 Gene expression

Herpesvirus genes are expressed during productive infection by a cascade mechanism (Figure 4). The α genes, which map near the termini or within the inverted repeats of the L and S components of the viral DNA, are the first to be expressed. The virion-associated protein designated αTIF (VP16) acts in trans to induce synthesis of the α gene products, formerly referred to as immediate early proteins. In HSV-infected cultured cells the synthesis of the 5 proteins specified by the α genes designated intracellular protein 0 (ICP0), ICP4, ICP22, ICP27, and ICP47, peaks at 2–4 h postinfection, but continues throughout infection at reduced rates. Each of these proteins appears to have a regulatory function(s) that is required for the synthesis of subsequent proteins in the cascade.

The genes for the subsequent two classes of herpesvirus proteins, designated β and γ, are generally located in the unique sequences of the L and S components. Expression of the β genes begins early after infection and peaks at 5 to 7 h postinfection. This class of herpesvirus genes can be divided into two subclasses. The β_1 gene products ICP6, part of the viral ribonucleotide reductase, and ICP 8, a DNA binding protein, are synthesized

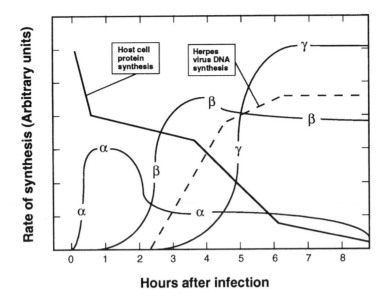

Figure 4 Cascade regulation of herpesvirus gene expression. Temporal sequence of expression of the three classes of herpesvirus genes. Relative expression of the α, β, and γ gene products is not to scale.

very early after infection, but are classified as β genes because their synthesis requires expression of α4. Most of the β_2 gene products, such as the viral thymidine kinase (TK) and DNA polymerase, are involved in synthesis of viral DNA.

The γ gene products are generally expressed late in infection. However, γ_1 gene products (also referred to as βγ), such as gB and gD are synthesized relatively early, prior to the onset of the bulk of viral DNA synthesis. In contrast, the γ_2 gene products, such as gC, are expressed later, and are not expressed in the presence of DNA synthesis inhibitors.

12.2.2.5 Viral DNA synthesis

Herpesvirus DNA synthesis takes place in the nucleus. A large number of virally encoded enzymes participate in herpesvirus DNA synthesis. These proteins include a DNA polymerase (a product of at least seven genes), single- and double-stranded DNA-binding proteins, and primases and helicases. Herpesviruses also encode a number of proteins that are involved in nucleic acid metabolism, such as the TK, ribonucleotide reductase, deoxyuridine triphosphatase, and certain nucleases. Some of these virally encoded enzymes, such as TK, have been targeted for antiviral drug therapies.

In HSV-infected cells viral DNA synthesis begins at about 3 h postinfection, however, most viral DNA is made later in infection. After entering the nucleus through the nuclear pore, the viral DNA circularizes. The best available evidence suggests that the viral DNA is synthesized by a rolling circle mechanism that yields concatomeric DNA. For HSVs and perhaps other herpesviruses, there appears to be three origins of replication, two within the repeated region of the S component and one in the middle of the L component. During the processing steps of herpesvirus DNA synthesis the sequences contained in the inverted repeats of the concatomeric DNA are amplified.

12.2.2.6 Assembly, maturation, and egress

The capsids of herpesviruses are assembled in the nucleus.[5] The monomeric subunits are assembled into preformed capsid structures in the nucleus of the infected cell. It has been suggested that the catomeric DNA is cleaved into the genome-length monomeric subunits during the assembly process. In principle this could occur by a mechanism analogous to that used by certain T-even bacteriophages in which a "head-full" of DNA is inserted into each virion. It has been suggested that the DNA-containing viral capsids acquire an envelope by "budding" through the inner lamnellar nuclear membranes. The virion may be "de-enveloped" at the outer lamnella, then re-enveloped by the endoplasmic reticulum where virions acquire the tegument. Subsequently viruses may be released by vesicles into the extracellular environment or, perhaps, enveloped at the plasma membrane. Whatever their source, modified membrane that is retained by progeny viruses contains viral glycoproteins on the outer surface and tegument proteins on the inner surface. On the other hand, the viral membrane appears to be devoid of cellular proteins.

12.3 Cellular effects of herpesviruses

Infection of herpesviruses can result in several outcomes including cytolysis or death, latency, or transformation. Studies of these phenomena have involved both the use of animal models and cultured cells. It is plausible that certain mechanisms underlying the events that occur in cultured cells and experimental animal systems are related to events that occur in persons infected with herpesviruses. For example, it is a reasonable presumption that cytopathic mechanisms employed by HSVs in cells cultured *in vitro* could also contribute to the formation of epithelial or nervous cell lesions *in vivo*.

12.3.1 Herpesvirus-induced cytopathogenesis

Productive infection of cultured cells by HSVs inevitably results in cell death, a phenomenon used in diagnosis of these infections. Herpesviruses may induce multiple alterations to host cell metabolism and structure that culminate in cytolysis of the infected cell. For example, the nucleolus of the HSV-infected cell often becomes enlarged and displaced within the nucleus. Host cell chromatin also becomes displaced, and late in infection the nucleus itself may become distorted and lobated. Cellular membranes are also extensively modified throughout the course of HSV-1 and -2 infection either by insertion of viral glycoproteins or other membrane proteins or by association with tegument proteins on the inner surface. Certain HSV mutants (syn+) induce cell-cell fusion resulting in polykaryon formation. It is likely even in wild type HSV (syn-) that membrane modifications actively contribute to the demise of the host cell. Ultimately the accumulation of damage to the cells induced by HSV-1 and 2 causes the infected cells to detach from the surface of the culture vesicle, round up, and aggregate. Other herpesviruses such as CMV, EBV, and HHV-6 can also induce lytic infections.

Herpesviruses, like most other cytolytic viruses, actively terminate host macromolecular synthesis early after infection. This shutoff may permit the virus to compete for components of the synthesizing machinery of the cell and/or for amino acids, nucleotides, and other building blocks required from progeny virus production. As in other cytolytic viruses the ability to terminate host macromolecular synthesis is tightly linked to the cytopathic potential of the viruses. The shutoff of cell macromolecular synthesis by herpesvirus is complex and involves several viral products. It is known that HSV encodes a virion-associated protein designated VHS which contributes to the shutoff of host macromolecular synthesis. Thus, partial shutoff can occur even in the absence of *de novo* herpesvirus gene expression. A second phase of shutoff occurs later in infection and is associated with expression of β (or γ_1) gene products.

12.3.2 Establishment and maintenance of herpesvirus latency

The ability to remain latent in the host organism is a defining characteristic of herpesviruses. Although the molecular mechanisms that permit the herpesviruses to enter a latent state are poorly understood, studies of herpesviruses in both animal models and in cultured cell systems have begun to elucidate the requirements for establishment and maintenance of the latent state of HSVs. As will be discussed in more detail below, after a period of replication in mucosal tissues HSV-1 and -2 can gain entry into nerves of mucosal tissues. After a brief period, which may include a few rounds of replication, HSVs can establish a latent state in which few, if any, viral genes are expressed. Subsequently, the virus can become reactivated and infectious virus is carried back to peripheral tissues by axonal transport. The factors that contribute to reactivation *in vivo* are not well understood, but in many cases they seem to correlate with the physical or emotional stress or hormonal imbalance of the host.

Mice, rabbits, and guinea pigs have each been established as experimental models of herpesvirus latency. The best available animal model appears to be the female Hartley guinea pig. When infected by vaginal inoculation of high doses of HSV-2 the guinea pig readily demonstrates establishment of viral latency and frequently shows viral reactivation. Explantation of neurons from experimental animals infected with HSV-2 generally results in reactivation and replication of latent virus. Models which have used various combinations of cytokines or growth factors such as interferon or nerve growth factor (NGF) have shown promise for either establishing or maintaining HSV-2-infected cultured neurons in a latent state, but the reliability of these systems requires improvement.

Of all the HSV genes, only the so-called latency associated transcript (LAT) has been detected in latently infected neurons.[6] Although this transcript is conserved in various strains of HSVs, defining the function of the transcript has remained an elusive task. The LAT is approximately 2 kb and represents transcription from an intron. Despite it's derivation from an intron, LAT may be spliced. LAT is derived in part from the antisense strand of the α0 gene, and potentially could function as a transcriptional or translational inhibitor of this gene. However, experiments using mutants in LAT do not sustain this hypothesis. Indeed, both latency and reactivation can occur in the absence of LAT expression.

The conclusion from most experimental studies of latency is that few, if any, HSV gene products are required for maintaining the latent state. This has focused attention of the infected neuron itself as the regulator of herpesvirus latency. During latency the potent herpesvirus promoters that are active in other cell types are inactive. Perhaps, the cellular transcription factors that are required along with the virion-associated αTIF for activation of the α genes are not active in sensory ganglia. The possibility of active suppression of transcription in these cell types should also be considered.

In contrast to HSV, a number of gene products of EBV are expressed during the latent state established in lymphoblastoid cells.[7,8] Although virion structural gene products are generally not expressed, the list of products expressed in some latently infected cells includes Epstein-Barr nuclear antigens (EBNAs), latency membrane proteins (LMPs), and Epstein-Barr encoded small nonpolyadenylated RNAs (EBERs). Different subsets of these products can be expressed depending on the cell type or lineage. It is possible that in the case of EBV some of these viral gene products have evolved to actively maintain the virus in a latent state.

12.3.3   Cell transformation by herpesviruses

Several herpesviruses have been implicated in the induction of human cancers. The prototype among these is EBV which is associated with Burkitt's lymphoma, nasopharyngeal carcinoma, and other human malignancies. EBV can readily transform human lymphocytes *in vitro*. Lymphocytes transformed by EBV resemble normal B-lymphocytes stimulated to grow by antigens, mitogens, or cytokines. The distinguishing characteristic of the lymphocytes transformed by EBV is immortalization and a relative degree of independence

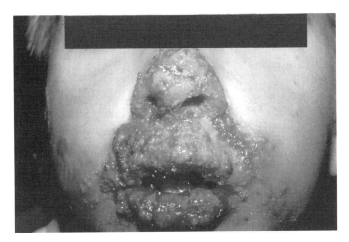

Figure 5 Herpes simplex type 1 perioral lesions with impetiginization. (Courtesy of Dr. Cathy Newman, University of Texas at Galveston.)

from exogenous growth factors. In general, EBV structural proteins are not expressed in transformed cells. In contrast, the EBV proteins that are expressed in latently infected lymphocytes are also expressed in transformed lymphocyte. Some of the products expressed during EBV latency have been shown to also have roles in transformation. For example, LMP1 has been shown to upregulate the expression of various adhesion proteins, to increase expression of *bcl-2* (an inhibitor of apoptosis), and to increase the intracellular concentration of calcium. These changes, as well as numerous others induced by LMP1, occur in a cell line or lineage dependent manner, but each could contribute to the transformed state. Most current models of cellular transformation by EBV suggest that LMPs, EBNAs, or EBERs affect the expression of various cellular oncogenes that sustained the transformed phenotype.

12.4   HSVs

12.4.1   Epidemiology of HSVs

The HSV has a worldwide distribution. The number of new cases of genital HSV infections which occur each year in the U.S. has been estimated to range from 300,000 to 500,000 individuals.[9] Seroprevalence data of HSV infections among individuals in the U.S. estimates 40–60 million cases of genital infections with HSV-2.[9] Genital herpesvirus infections have been found in highest prevalence in 19–39 year olds, and are often found in association with other sexually transmitted diseases. Risk factors for the acquisition of a genital HSV infection include female gender, age, black race, divorced individuals, urban residence, and a greater number of sex partners.

Transmission occurs by contact with secretions from an infected person with either overt infection or asymptomatic excretion of virus. Genital infections are primarily due to HSV-2 strains, though a small proportion of cases are attributable to HSV-1. The majority of HSV-1 lesions are perioral (Figure 5). Recurrent genital lesions are more common with HSV-2 than with HSV-1.

12.4.2   Clinical manifestations of genital infection by HSVs

Primary HSV infection has a wide range of disease manifestations which can vary from mild to life threatening.[10] Primary genital HSV infection occurs following an incubation period of 2-7 days and the average duration to complete healing of lesions is 3 weeks.

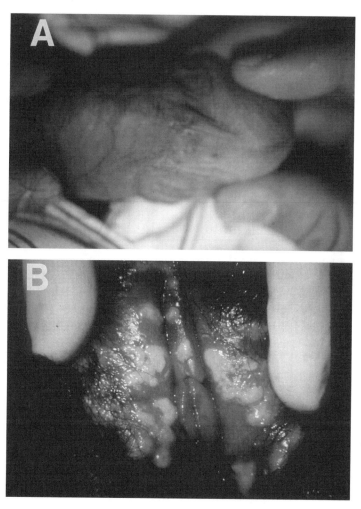

Figure 6   Primary HSV type 2 genital lesions: (A) Male and (B) female. (Courtesy of Dr. Steve Tyring, University of Texas at Galveston.)

Disease manifestations may vary among men and women, but systemic complaints of fever, chills, headache, malaise, dysuria, anorexia, and tender inguinal adenopathy are seen in up to 70% of cases. Local symptoms include a burning sensation or mild paresthesias which precedes the eruption of vesicles. Small clusters of vesicles on an erythematous base develop and ulcerate after 3–5 days. The lesions in men initially appear as a cluster of vesicles located primarily on the prepuce, glans, or shaft of the penis which crust before re-epithelialization (Figure 6A). Painful lesions in women can appear on the vulva, perineum, buttocks, cervix, and less frequently the vagina in association with a light vaginal discharge (Figure 6B). In female subjects, the lesions are quick to ulcerate and become covered by a whitish-gray exudate. The majority of women (80%) are likely to experience dysuria, discharge from the vagina, and have prolonged painful adenopathy during a primary genital herpesvirus infection. In contrast, less than 45% of men experience dysuria or a clear urethral discharge and the tender inguinal adenopathy is of shorter duration than in women. The severity of symptoms peaks during the second week of illness with the painful adenopathy usually the last symptom to resolve. Shedding of virus from genital lesions persists for about 10–12 days after the onset of the rash. Women are more likely than men to have HSV isolated from the urethra and the majority also shed the virus from the cervix.

Complications of primary genital HSV infection are related to either local extension or spread to extragenital sites, particularly the central nervous system. Women develop complications of HSV infection more frequently than men. For example, aseptic meningitis occurs in greater than 30% of women but less than 15% of men during primary genital HSV infection. Clinical features include a stiff neck, headache, photophobia, and a lymphocytic pleocytosis in the cerebral spinal fluid. Long-term neurologic sequelae is rare after HSV meningitis, but short-term residual neurologic symptoms can include urinary retention, neuralgia, dysesthesias, paresthesias, and difficulties with concentration which often resolves gradually over a period of 3-6 months. Less frequently, autonomic nervous system dysfunction involving a neurogenic bladder, poor rectal sphincter tone, constipation, and impotence in males is seen as a complication of primary genital HSV infection. The autonomic involvement is transient and symptoms gradually resolve over a period of weeks.

Extragenital lesions involving the adjacent skin of the thighs, perineum, and buttocks have been reported in 10–20% of cases. Other sites of extragenital spread occur with greater frequency in women and include the lip, breast, finger, and eye. In addition, a genital herpes infection can lead to pharyngitis in a sexual partner of couples following orogenital contact. Symptoms include sore throat, fever, malaise, and myalgia if the illness involves a primary HSV infection and may include genital lesions as well. The pharyngeal lesions are initially vesicular in appearance and then ulcerate before healing over a period of 2–4 weeks.

Recurrent genital HSV infection occurs in 75% of cases following infection with HSV-2 but in only 50% of cases involving HSV-1 infection (Figure 7). Numerous factors can precipitate an episode of recurrent HSV infection including a systemic infection, development of a malignancy, menstruation, and local trauma to the skin such as a sunburn. A prodrome of burning, itching, or tingling is often reported by the individual prior to eruption of lesions and systemic symptoms are usually lacking. Recurrent genital HSV infections are generally less severe than the primary infection. There is a tendency in the recurrent episodes for fewer vesicles to develop, for the vesicles to be more localized, and for the healing period to be shorter, usually 7–10 days. Recurrence rates are greater in males than females with estimates of 2.7 per 100 patient days versus 1.9 per 100 patient days, respectively.[10] Females are more likely to experience painful lesions associated with dysuria than males during recurrent episodes. Shedding of virus from the genital lesions during recurrent infection occurs for 2–5 days and in lower quantity than during primary disease. Women are less likely to shed virus from the cervix during recurrent genital infection compared to the primary episode.

An indirect but serious consequence of a genital HSV infection is the transmission of virus from mother to infant during the passage through the infected genital tract. The risk of neonatal infection is significantly greater in mothers with a primary infection during pregnancy compared to women who experience reactivation of infection. Other factors which influence the transmission of HSV infection to the newborn include rupture of membranes of greater than six hours and use of fetal scalp electrodes which can provide a site of entry for the virus. Disease manifestations in the newborn may be limited to the mucous membranes of the skin, eyes, and mouth or present as a disseminated infection or encephalitis. Immunocompromised adult patients are at increased risk to develop severe disseminated HSV-1 or -2 infections. In HIV-infected patients cutaneous dissemination of HSV-1 or -2 lesions can occur by autoinoculation to multiple sites and can progress to involve the respiratory tract, esophagus, or gastrointestinal tract (see below). Reactivation of HSV can be a frequent occurrence in HIV-infected patients.

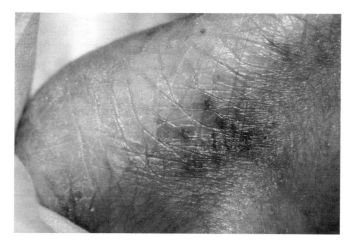

Figure 7 Reactivation of HSV type 1 on S1 dermatome. (Courtesy of Dr. Mark Beilke, Tulane Medical School.)

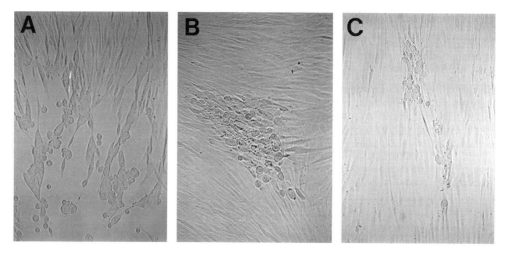

Figure 8 Cytopathology of herpes viruses during replication in cultured human foreskin fibroblasts. (A) HSV type 2; (B) CMV; and (C) varicella-zoster virus. (Dr. Dawn Sokol, Tulane Medical School.)

12.4.3   Diagnosis of HSV infections

The diagnosis of HSV infection can be confirmed by a variety of laboratory methods. As with other herpesviruses, isolation of HSV remains the standard technique employed by large viral diagnostic laboratories (Figure 8). Numerous cell lines can support the propagation of HSV with the characteristic cytopathic effect demonstrated in 24–48 h after inoculation. Proper collection and handling of the specimen is essential to maximize the identification of HSV. A newly formed vesicular lesion should be scraped, the specimen placed in viral transport media, and then delivered to the laboratory promptly for inoculation. If a delay in the delivery of the specimen to the laboratory is unavoidable, then the specimen should be placed on ice. Other specimens which may yield HSV depending on the clinical manifestations of disease include cerebrospinal fluid, urethral swabs, vaginal or cervical specimens, throat, and conjunctivae.

A second approach to the diagnosis of genital HSV infection is the cytology examination of cells collected from lesions of the skin, cervix, or conjunctivae. Although the sensitivity and specificity of this method is less than culture, cytology examination is more readily available in laboratories without viral diagnostic facilities. Cellular specimens obtained from scraping the base of the lesion are stained according to the methods of Papanicolaou, Giemsa, or Wright and examined for the presence of multinucleated giant cells. The presence of multinucleated giant cells is indicative of an HSV or varicella infection. The use of newer staining methods which employ immunohistochemical or immunofluorescent tagged monoclonal antibodies have improved the specificity and the sensitivity of cytology examination. The quality of the specimen, the staining method used, and the experience of the cytologist can all influence the sensitivity of this method.

Another method utilized for the diagnosis of HSV infection is the detection of HSV DNA by the polymerase chain reaction (PCR). Specimens from skin, genital swabs, and cerebrospinal fluid have all been analyzed by PCR for the presence of HSV DNA. While detection of HSV DNA in cerebrospinal fluid has proven useful in the diagnosis of encephalitis, its usefulness in the rapid detection of HSV genital infections is less clear. The routine clinical use of PCR for the diagnosis of HSV infection will require standardization of the testing method in order to maximize the sensitivity and specificity.

Serologic diagnosis of HSV infection is of limited value due to the inability of the current commercially available serologic assays to distinguish between antibodies to HSV-1 and HSV-2. A variety of methods have been used to measure HSV antibodies including complement fixation, neutralization, passive hemagglutination, indirect immunofluorescence and enzyme-linked immunosorbent assays. Occasionally serology can be useful to diagnose a primary HSV infection by demonstration of a fourfold rise in antibody titer in acute and convalescent sera. Serology is unable to predict a recurrent infection due to a lack of correlation between a rising antibody titer and the presence of genital lesions.

12.4.4   Treatment of HSV infections

Acyclovir, a nucleoside analog, inhibits HSV DNA polymerase through the intracellular production of acyclovir triphosphate from the monophosphate form by TK. Acyclovir is available as a topical ointment, intravenous solution, and as several oral formulations for the treatment of primary genital herpes infection. Acyclovir given orally at a dose of 200 mg 5 times a day for 10 days can reduce the duration of the acute genital infection. The duration of pain, new lesion formation, and time to lesion healing is reduced in some patient groups. Individuals who present early in the course of the infection or those with severe disease are more likely to benefit from acyclovir therapy. In patients with severe disease manifested by marked systemic symptoms, central nervous system involvement, urinary retention, or an inability to take oral medication, intravenous acyclovir may be indicated. Intravenous acyclovir is given at a dose of 5–10 mg/kg every 8 h depending on the age of the patient and the severity of the infection. Treatment can continue for a period of 7–14 days depending on the clinical resolution. In disseminated infection or encephalitis in the newborn the duration of treatment may extend for a period of 21 days.

Recurrent genital HSV infections can be reduced in frequency with acyclovir prophylaxis and severity in individuals who experience more than six episodes per year. In patients with severe complications such as recurrent aseptic meningitis suppressive therapy is beneficial. Oral suppressive therapy with acyclovir has been safe and effective when continued for periods of up to three years. The need for ongoing suppressive therapy should be accessed yearly to determine if the pattern of recurrences has decreased and therefore the use of acyclovir is no longer necessary. A variety of suppressive regimens have been evaluated and in the normal host either 200 mg given 3 times a day or 400 mg given twice a day appear effective. Side effects are infrequent with the long-term use of oral acyclovir at these doses and include nausea, diarrhea, and headache in less than 5% of patients. Adjustment in the dose is indicated in the patient with renal impairment.

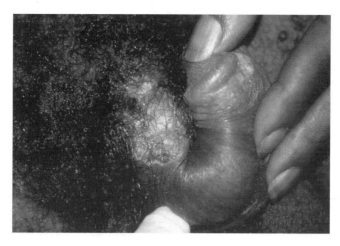

Figure 9 Genital HSV type 2 lesions in an AIDS patient. (Courtesy of Dr. Cathy Newman, University of Texas at Galveston.)

Acyclovir-resistant mutants of HSV have been observed, particularly in the immunosuppressed patient. The appearance of these drug-resistant variants provides incentive for development of additional, more effective agents to control HSV infection.

Experimental vaccines against HSV have shown promise in animal models, but human trials have been less rewarding. Recently, genetically engineered HSV vaccines have been developed which include subunit vaccines and a live attenuated recombinant HSV product. Animal data and preliminary human trials with these engineered products have shown some promise for the eventual development of a HSV vaccine.

12.5 Herpesvirus infections with concurrent HIV disease

HIV, the retrovirus that induces the acquired immune deficiency syndrome (AIDS), has profound effects on the immune system. The hallmark of HIV infection is a progressive depletion of CD4+ T lymphocytes. The loss of these critical immune regulatory cells perturbs virtually all aspects of the immune system, including both humoral and cellular immunity. AIDS patients have increased susceptibility to opportunistic pathogens and an increased risk for developing otherwise rare cancers such as Kaposi's sarcoma (KS). It is not surprising that the course of various herpesvirus infections is altered dramatically as a consequence of concurrent HIV infection or AIDS. In addition, there are several plausible interactions that may occur at the molecular level between various herpesviruses and HIV that can influence replication of either virus or possibly change the outcome of virus:cell or virus:host interactions.

12.5.1 HIV and HSVs

Genital HSV infection in the HIV-infected patient is similar in presentation as in the non-HIV-infected host except recurrences tend to be more frequent and prolonged (Figure 9). In addition, chronic nonhealing ulcers may form and become granulated and bloody. HSV may involve a chronic proctitis in HIV-infected homosexual males practicing receptive anorectal sexual intercourse. Clinical features include fever, severe rectal pain, constipation, urinary retention, and tenesmus. External cutaneous lesions may be absent and the diagnosis is made by examination and cultures obtained on sigmoidoscopy. HSV genital infections in HIV-infected individuals may also be complicated by giant nonhealing perianal and anal lesions which become confluent grayish-white ulcerative lesions prone to

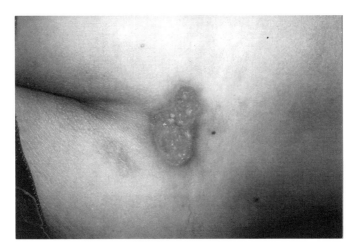

Figure 10   Perianal HSV type 2 lesions in an AIDS patient. (Courtesy of Dr. Cathy Newman, University of Texas at Galveston.)

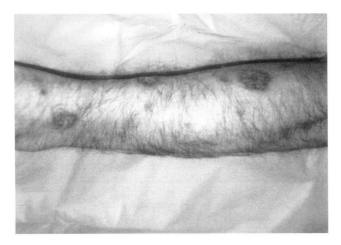

Figure 11   HSV type 1 cutaneous lesions in an AIDS patient. (Courtesy of Dr. Cathy Newman, University of Texas at Galveston.)

secondary bacterial infections (Figure 10). Other sites of HSV infection in patients with AIDS include colon, esophagus, oropharynx, and the central nervous system. HSV-1 cutaneous lesions in AIDS patients may also occur in a variety of locations in addition to periorally. As with genital HSV-2 lesions in this population, HSV-1 cutaneous lesions may persist and be difficult to heal (Figure 11).

Genital lesions due to HSV infection may be typical or atypical in appearance and therefore the diagnosis should be confirmed by culture. Another advantage of tissue culture diagnosis is that testing for acyclovir resistance can be readily performed if the virus is propagated in culture. Other diagnostic methods such as staining of skin or mucous membrane lesions may not be able to differentiate varicella-zoster virus from HSV if a nonspecific staining method is utilized.

Acyclovir is often the initial therapy for genital HSV infection given in a dosage regimen similar to the non-HIV-infected host. Recurrent genital HSV infection can be decreased in severity and frequency with regimens of 200 mg by mouth 5 times a day or 400 mg 3 times a day over a period of 1 year. However, with prolonged use in an immunocompromised host, acyclovir-resistant mutants lacking TK may be associated with progressive HSV disease. Foscarnet has proven to be effective in controlling acyclovir-resistant HSV infections in an HIV-infected population. The majority of patients responded with complete healing of lesions when given foscarnet at a dose of 120 to 180 mg/kg/day in three divided doses.

12.5.2   HIV and CMV

12.5.2.1   Epidemiology of CMV

CMV has a worldwide distribution with an antibody prevalence ranging from 40–100%, depending on the socioeconomic status of the population. In the U.S., there is a wide range in the seroprevalence in different regions of the country with some large urban areas exceeding 80% of the population positive for CMV antibody. A variety of modes of transmission have been defined and include blood transfusions, organ and tissue transplant, breast milk, sexual contact, and congenital or perinatal routes of infection.

The role sexual contact plays in the transmission of CMV is difficult to define because contact with oral secretions also plays a role in the transmission of the virus. However, both cervical and semen specimens have been identified as sites of viral shedding. Shedding of virus from the cervix has been correlated with the number of sex partners and a younger age at the time of first intercourse. Additional evidence for the sexual transmission of CMV can be found in an abrupt increase rate of infection in a seronegative population during the second and third decades of life as individuals reach their reproductive years. Among homosexual men the rate of CMV infection is nearly 100% and has been correlated with passive anal sex and a greater number of sex partners, again suggesting the transmission of CMV during sexual contact.

12.5.2.2   Clinical manifestations of CMV infection

The majority of children and adults experience a subclinical infection with CMV marked only by seroconversion of CMV antibody. In those who develop clinical symptoms, a CMV-associated mononucleosis is the most frequent manifestation. Fever is the most prominent feature of the illness with enlarged lymph nodes, mild hepatitis, and hepatosplenomegaly less frequently reported. The fever can last for greater than two weeks and a lymphocytosis marked by atypical lymphocytes is often found. In the majority of patients the illness is self-limited and symptoms resolve over a period of two to four weeks. Occasionally a complication of CMV infection develops in an otherwise healthy individual. Guillain-Barré syndrome, myocarditis, thrombocytopenia, and hemolytic anemia and meningoencephalitis have been described in patients with a recent CMV infection. Disease manifestations of CMV infection in immunocompromised patients are often more severe, particularly when a primary infection develops in the face of severe, immunosuppression. In transplant recipients CMV can cause a life-threatening interstitial pneumonitis or a fulminant hepatitis depending on the type of organ transplanted and the degree of immunosuppression.

In AIDS patients, retinitis is the most common manifestation of CMV infection (Figure 12). Infection of the retina in HIV-infected and other immunocompromised patients poses a serious threat to sight. Up to 25% of HIV-infected patients will develop CMV retinitis, and the majority of CMV-infected AIDS patients will develop bilateral disease in the absence of specific antiviral therapy. CMV can be found in all retinal layers and is commonly absent from the underlying choroidal tissue. While the pathogenesis of CMV in the retina is still poorly understood, nerve infarcts, hemorrhages, and opacifications are known to occur. Hemorrhages and retinal detachment are the most common complications of CMV retinitis that result in blindness. CMV infection can also occur in many other different organ systems in AIDS patients, including the skin (Figure 13). As in other immunosuppressed patients, CMV interstitial pneumonitis can be a significant problem

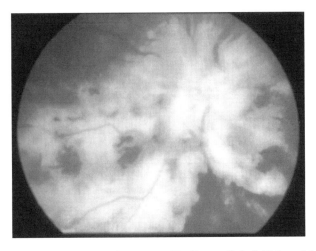

Figure 12 CMV retinitis in an AIDS patient. (Dr. Dawn Sokol, Tulane Medical School.)

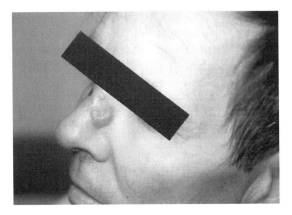

Figure 13 CMV facial lesion in an AIDS patient. (Courtesy of Dr. Vibhagool, University of Texas at Galveston.)

in AIDS patients, but the exact impact of the infection is difficult to determine because CMV is often found in association with other pathogens such as pneumocystis. Likewise, CMV infection involving the central nervous system has been described in HIV-infected patients including encephalitis, radiculopathy, and myelopathy. The gastrointestinal tract is also a frequent site of CMV infection in AIDS patients, where clinical syndromes of gastritis and enterocolitis may result.

12.5.2.3 Diagnosis of CMV infection

The diagnosis of a primary CMV infection can be difficult because of the high frequency of asymptomatic shedding of CMV seen during reactivation of latent virus. In addition, the production of CMV IgM antibody occurs in some episodes of reactivation. Therefore, careful interpretation of laboratory tests and correlation with the clinical illness is needed to accurately diagnose a symptomatic CMV infection. Virus can be isolated and cultured from many sites including urine, saliva, peripheral blood leukocytes, breast milk, semen, and cervical secretions, as well as biopsy material of infected liver or lung. Typical cytopathic effect can be seen in the first week, but more typically isolation in cell culture requires two to four weeks (Figure 8B). Definitive identification can be confirmed by immunofluorescent (IF) or immunoperoxidase (IP)-labeled CMV-specific antibody.

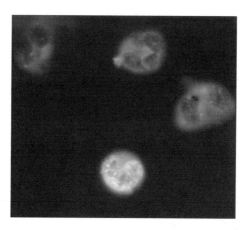

Figure 14   CMV immunofluorescence. CMV detected in PMNs by direct immunofluorescence using antibodies to pp65.

Early diagnosis of CMV infection is desirable if antiviral therapy if to have its greatest benefit. More recently developed techniques have attempted to achieve this goal. A rapid form of culture technique employs a shell vial assay in which the virus is propagated on cell monolayer attatched to a round coverslip in a 1-dram vial. After 16–36 h of incubation, the coverslip is removed and stained with either an IF- or IP-labeled monoclonal antibody against the immediate early antigen (Figure 14). Antigen detection methods have also been developed to enhance the detection of CMV in histologic samples and antigenemia in circulating neutrophils. A commercially available CMV antigenemia assay has been evaluated in transplant and HIV-infected hosts and is a rapid and sensitive method for the detection of CMV. In addition, diagnosis of CMV infection through the use of PCR techniques is a promising approach.[11] Positive results for viremia detected by PCR or the CMV antigenemia assay may be seen transiently in an immunosuppressed host and do not always correlate with overt disease.

12.5.2.4   Treatment of CMV infection in HIV-infected patients

CMV retinitis is progressive unless treated. Although a number of antiviral genes have been utilized in the past, derivatives of acyclovir, specifically the 9-(1,3-dihydroxy-2-propomethyl)guanine congener (ganciclovir), and phosphonoformic acid (foscarnet) have been demonstrated to have the most significant clinical benefit for CMV infections.[12-14] Treatment with ganciclovir is begun at a dose of 5 mg/kg given twice daily for a period of 14–21 days followed by a maintenance dose of 5 mg/kg given as a single dose 5–7 days per week which is required to prevent or delay relapses. During ganciclovir therapy, myelosuppression, particularly neutropenia, is a common dose-limiting toxicity which can lead to premature treatment discontinuation. Foscarnet can be used as an alternative therapy for CMV retinitis given at a dose of 60 mg/kg three times a day for a period of 14–21 days.[12] Foscarnet maintenance therapy is continued at a dose of 90–120 mg/kg/day indefinitely and requires careful monitoring of renal function and serum electrolytes to reduce toxicity.

Although conflicting results have been obtained preliminary studies have also shown that ganciclovir may have prophylactic value, particularly in patients with AIDS and those otherwise immunosuppressed. However, toxicities can result from long-term use, or mutations in the DNA polymerase(s) or impaired phosphorylation can render CMV-resistant ganciclovir. Under these conditions resistance to foscarnet does not occur due to separate mechanisms of action. Other CMV targets, such as the viral proteases, are important in future efforts at anti-CMV drug development.

12.5.3   HIV and EBV

12.5.3.1   Epidemiology of EBV

In most human populations infection by EBV almost always occurs in the first three years of life and is asymptomatic. Most if not all persons subclinically infected by EBV establish a carrier state in which circulating B cells contain latent EBV. In this carrier state replication of EBV and EBV-infected cells appears to be under control by the immune system. When infection is delayed until the second decade of life or later as occurs in some Western populations, EBV can induce infectious mononucleosis (IM) in as many as 50% of infected individuals. IM is commonly known as the "kissing disease" because EBV can easily be detected in throat washings and salivary and parotid glands and is assumed to be transmitted by direct infection of the oral cavity. It appears that EBV replication in the oral epithelium or in infiltrating B lymphocytes can result in seeding of the B cells in the circulation and lymphoid organs. As discussed above, EBV establishes persistent, latent, and productive (lytic) infections in B cells. In IM patients EBV maintains a chronic state of infection in spite of vigorous immune responses. The atypical mononuclear cells in the blood that are the key diagnostic feature of IM are T lymphocytes presumed to be involved in the cellular response to chronic EBV infection. The strong immune responses, both humoral and cellular, to EBV could account for many, if not all, of the pathognomonic features of IM. In particular, abnormal expression of cytokines, perhaps interferons or tumor necrosis factor (TNF), may induce the persistent fevers and chronic fatigue of IM. Eventually, most IM patients also establish a carrier state in which replication of EBV and EBV-infected cells is under control of the immune system.

12.5.3.2   Clinical manifestations of EBV in HIV-infected patients

The first evidence that the immune system plays a critical role in control of the EBV during the carrier state came in studies of renal allograft recipients given immunosuppressive doses of either azothioprene/prednisolone or cyclosporin A in which a subset of patients developed a mononucleosis-like syndrome. Increased shedding of EBV in immunosuppressed renal allograft recipients is accompanied by increases in circulating antibodies and cytotoxic T lymphocytes with specificity for EBV. Patients with other immune dysregulatory diseases, such as autoimmune diseases, can also experience reactivation of EBV and an IM-like disease. A severe IM-like syndrome is linked to a rare X-linked immunodeficiency which causes EBV infection to be fatal in about 75% of afflicted boys. Those individuals that survive the X-linked syndrome are at greatly increased risk of developing lymphoproliferative diseases and lymphomas.

HIV-infected patients also may experience reactivation of their latent EBV infections. A significant percentage of HIV-infected patients develop oral hairy leukoplakia (OHL); (Figure 15). This is a wart-like lesion typically on the lateral borders of the tongue. *In situ* hybridization and immunohistochemical studies have convincingly demonstrated that OHL represents a focal activation of EBV in the oral epithelium. Although viral DNA and antigens are not present in the basal and parabasal layers of the tissue, viral DNA and proteins are abundantly present in the upper epithelial strata. Latency-associated transcripts such as LMP1 are also not present in large amounts in the OHL lesions. However, a gene product of EBV named BHRF1, a protein required neither for latency or transformation, is expressed abundantly in OHL lesions. BHRF1 is a distant structural analog of the apoptosis inhibiting/cell survival protein Bcl-2. Expression of this EBV protein could account for the abnormal proliferation/differentiation of the OHL lesion. Clinically, OHL lesions respond to acyclovir or its derivative desciclovir.

Given its preeminent role as a human tumor virus, it is not surprising that EBV has been associated with several malignancies in AIDS patients. Burkitt's lymphoma (BL) is one of the best studied human tumors induced by EBV and occurs both endemically in

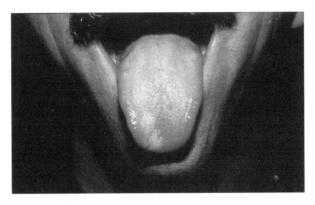

Figure 15   Oral hairy leukoplakia caused by Epstein-Barr virus. (Courtesy of Dr. Angela Yen, University of Texas at Galveston.)

Africa and sporadically in other parts of the world. Endemic BL is the most prevalent childhood cancer of equatorial Africa, an area with epidemic malaria. The tumors of endemic BL present usually at extranodal sites and are found frequently in the jaw in association with molar eruption. All the tumor cells of endemic BL display reciprocal translocations between the locus for the *c-myc* cellular oncogene (chromosome 8), and either the immunoglobulin heavy chain locus (chromosome 14; 80% of cases) or one of two light chain loci (chromosome 2 or 22; variant translocations). In other parts of the world, sporadic childhood lymphomas with the identical karyotypic markers have also been shown to be due to EBV infection. In contrast to the Africa BL, the presentation of the tumor rarely involves the jaw, but is usually present in the abdomen. Sporadic BL can also involve the bone marrow in which case it presents as an acute lymphoblastic leukemia.

The pandemic of HIV infections has now produced a third form of BL. Up to 10% of HIV-infected persons in Western societies develop B-cell malignancies. A high portion of these contain the characteristic BL t(8:14), t(8:2), or t(8;22) translocations and present clinically and histopathologically as sporadic cases of BL. The combination of the HIV-induced immunosuppression which permits reactivation of latent EBV, coupled with deficient immune surveillance against tumor cells are two factors contributing to the development of BL in AIDS patients. Given that EBV is associated with a number of human cancers besides BL, including rare T-cell lymphomas/leukemias, the role of this agent in various AIDS-associated malignancies should remain an active area of investigation.

12.5.4   HIV and varicella-zoster virus

Varicella-zoster virus (VZV) is the etiologic agent of chickenpox, primarily an illness of childhood manifested by a generalized vesicular rash, moderate fever, and systemic symptoms. Complications are rare in children and include arthritis, hepatitis, pneumonitis, encephalitis, and glomerulonephritis. In immunocompromised hosts, a progressive varicella infection can develop marked by prolonged fever and continued eruption of vesicles into the second week of the illness. Complications are more common in this group of individuals and pneumonia is the most frequently seen feature leading to significant morbidity and mortality.

As with other herpesviruses infection typically results in a life-long association with the host. In most persons this association is uneventful, but in a small percentage of persons VZV can be reactivated as the painful cutaneous lesions of herpes zoster or shingles. The dermatomal distribution of the zoster lesions typically follow precisely the unilateral distribution of one to three adjacent sensory nerves. As with HSV-1 and -2 diseases herpes zoster can be recurrent.

Immunocompromised patients, such as those infected with HIV, often experience reactivation of VZV. In addition to typical zoster, unusual chronic verrucous lesions have been described in AIDS patients. These lesions are characterized by epithelial hyperplasia and extensive hyperkeratosis. VZV is readily detected in the lesions by culture or PCR. VZV can also disseminate in HIV to multiple dermatomes and organs with similar pathology as occurs in progressive varicella.

Acyclovir is the drug of choice for treatment of VZV infection, because it elicits fewer side effects than vidarabine and interferon-alpha, two other drugs that inhibit VZV. High dose acyclovir at a dose of 500 mg/m^2 given intravenously every 8 h for 7–10 days is the recommended dose for chickenpox or zoster in an immunocompromised host. HIV-infected patients who have recurrent episodes of zoster requiring repeated treatment with acyclovir are prone to the development of resistance. Under these circumstances, 120 mg/kg/day of foscarnet given in 3 doses divided for 14–26 days has been effective in treating acyclovir-resistant zoster.

12.5.5   HIV and HHV-6 and HHV-7

The two subtypes of HHV-6, HHV-6A and HHV-6B, and HHV-7 represent recently identified members of the herpesvirinae that infect humans.[15-17] The biological and sequence properties of these viruses suggest that they are closely related members of the betaherpesvirinae subfamily. HHV-6B has been established as the etiological agent of exantum subitum (roseola infantum, sixth disease), a common childhood rash. This infection is usually mild and uneventful, but can cause cases of extremely high fever or more rarely hepatosplenomegaly, aseptic meningitis, hepatitis, thrombocytopenia, and other potentially fatal conditions. HHV-6B has also been established as a cause of bone marrow suppression in bone marrow transplant recipients and reactivation of this virus can contribute to rejection of either kidney or liver transplants. Neither HHV-6A or HHV-7 have been clearly linked to any disease.

Both HHV-6 subtypes and HHV-7 are capable of infecting cultured CD4+ T-lymphoblastoid cells, the same cell type which is the primary target for HIV. HHV-6A and -6B and HHV-7 are also capable of inducing an acute cytopathic effect in CD4+ T-lymphoblastoid cells that resembles the "balloon degeneration" induced by HIV. *Trans*-activating transcription factors encoded in these human herpesviruses can activate transcription mediated by the HIV long terminal repeat (LTR). These observations have suggested that HHV-6 and/or HHV-7 might represent cofactors for HIV disease progression. However, epidemiological evidence has generally not supported this conclusion. Persons that progressed rapidly to AIDS did not seem to express higher levels of HHV-6 or -7 than persons with a more extended disease course. Reactivation HHV-6 has been noted in AIDS patients where it has been associated with cases of pneumonitis.

Because HHV-6B can induce bone marrow suppression in iatrogenically immunosuppressed patients, the possibility that this might also occur in HIV disease should be investigated. Controlled clinical trials are also needed to determine if antiviral drugs, such as ganciclovir or foscarnet, that inhibit HHV-6 and HHV-7 replication in culture and have clinical benefit in other herpesvirus infections have utility in treatment. Because HHV-6 and -7 and HIV have a common target cell, the CD4+ T lymphocyte, HHV-6 or -7 might also be considered as a vector for targeted delivery of molecular therapeutics, such as ribozymes or antisense constructs, that could specifically inhibit HIV.

12.5.6   HIV and HHV-8

KS is the most frequently observed malignancy in persons with HIV infection (Figures 16 and 17). KS also occurs in non-HIV-infected persons, most often in elderly men of

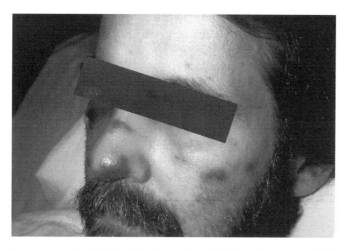

Figure 16 Kaposi's sarcoma in AIDS patients — facial lesions (courtesy of Dr. Cathy Newman, University of Texas at Galveston).

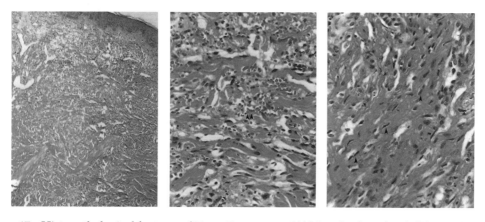

Figure 17 Histopathological features of Kaposi's sarcoma. (A) Macule phase (×80); (B) macule phase demonstrating early formation of spindle cells (arrowheads); (×400); and (C) macule phase demonstrating slit-like primative blood vessels (arrowheads); (×400). (Courtesy of Dr. Aizen Marrogi, Tulane Medical School.)

Mediterranean, Middle Eastern, or Eastern European descent. Endemic KS occurs in Africa where it tends to a less aggressive clinical course. Cases of KS have also been diagnosed in non-HIV-infected homosexual men and in xenograft recipients. Several epidemiological studies have suggested the possibility that KS is caused by an infectious agent.[18] Evidence supporting a possible sexual transmission is the observation that KS is as much as 20 times more prevalent in HIV-infected homosexual men than in HIV-infected persons in other risk groups.

Chang, Moore, and co-workers used representational difference analysis (RDA), a PCR-based technique that can amplify DNA sequences uniquely present in one but not another DNA sample, to identify a previously unknown herpesvirus in association with KS.[19] KS lesions of AIDS patients were found by RDA to contain DNA sequences closely related to genes for the capsid and tegument proteins of the gammaherpesvirinae. These sequences were usually not found in uninvolved tissues of KS patients or in tissues from uninfected patients. Subsequent studies have confirmed these results and found that similar herpesvirus sequences are also present in lesions of patients with classic KS.[20] Sequences of the KS herpesvirus were found in 95% of nearly 200 samples of KS tissues by PCR. The sequences were also found in 52% of PBMC from AIDS patients with AIDS KS, but in only 11-13% of AIDS patients without KS. This later observation may indicate that infection with this herpesvirus precedes the onset of KS. Sequences of the KS-associated herpesvirus have also been found in body cavity lymphomas of HIV-infected patients, suggesting that this virus may also have a role in these AIDS-associated cancers.

Recently, an additional 20 kbp of the sequence of the KS-associated herpesvirus has been obtained allowing a more precise phylogenetic placement within the gammaherpesvirinae (Figure 1).[21] The newly identified human herpesvirus should tentatively be designated HHV-8. At present it is not known whether the agent is actually localized within the spindle-shaped KS tumor cells or whether it is present in adjacent cells within the tumor. Further studies are required to conclusively define its role in KS and to elucidate the mechanism by which it induces tumorigenesis. Successful growth of HHV-8 in cultured cells should further this investigative process.

12.6   Conclusions

HSV-2 continues to represent one of the most important sexually transmitted human viral pathogens. Research toward improved anti-herpesvirus drugs against HSV-2 should continue with high priority. It should also be recognized that the need for improved antiherpetic drugs in the context of HIV infection will continue to increase in dramatic fashion. The HIV pandemic is expanding at a steady rate in developed countries, not only among the initial risk groups of homosexuals and intravenous drug abusers, but increasing by heterosexual transmission. In nonindustrial nations the spread of HIV is progressing at an even more alarmingly rapid rate. Research toward a better understanding of herpesvirus-induced cancers, with and without concurrent HIV infection, should also continue with urgency. The possibility that a newly discovered sexually transmitted human herpesvirus HHV-8 has a role in an important cancer should advance and further intensify research efforts on herpesvirus-induced malignancies. The recent discoveries of HHV-6 through 8 suggests that other, as yet unrecognized, human herpesviruses may exist with roles in cancers or other important diseases. Advances in highly sensitive molecular and immunological techniques should hasten the discovery of new disease agents. Finally, in recognizing the limitations of effectiveness and cost of most antiviral drugs, the search for effective vaccination strategies against HSV and other members of the herpesvirus family should also be considered extremely worthwhile.

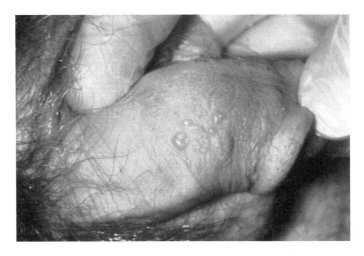

Cluster of early primary herpetic veicles. (Photo courtesy of A.W. Hoke, M.D.)

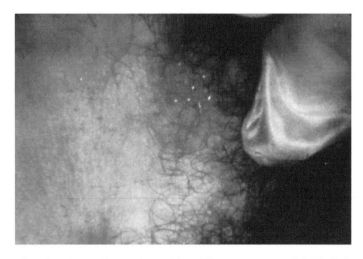

Cluster of early primary herpetic vesicles. (Photo courtesy of A.W. Hoke, M.D.)

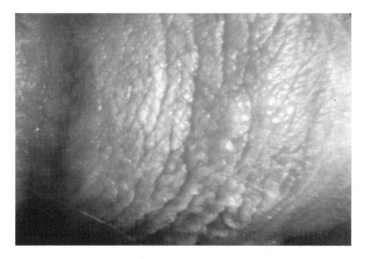

Primary herpes. (Photo courtesy of A.W. Hoke, M.D.)

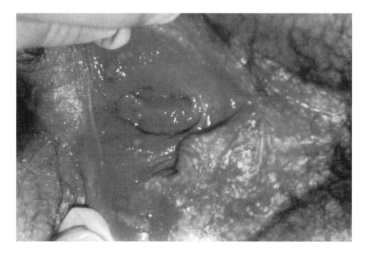

"Kissing" herpetic vesicles. (Photo courtesy of A.W. Hoke, M.D.)

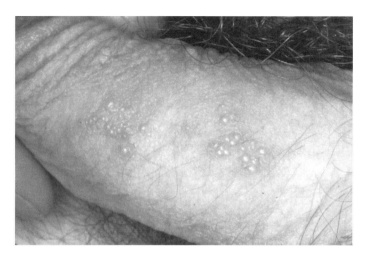

Multiple herpetic vesicles. (Photo courtesy of R. Odom, M.D.)

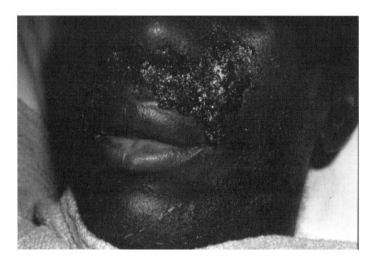

Herpes in an AIDS patient. (Photo courtesy of A.W. Hoke, M.D.)

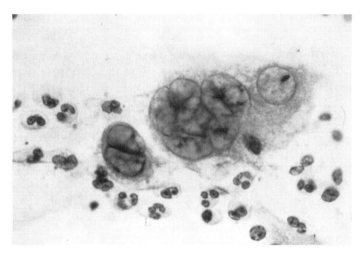

A Tzank stain of herpes. (Photo courtesy of K. Hadley, M.D.)

References

1. Roizman, B., Carmicheal, L., Deinhardt, F., de The, G., Nahmias, A., Plowright, W., Rapp, F., Sheldrick, P., Takahashi, M., and Wolfe, K. Herpesviridae: definition, provisional nomenclature and taxonomy. *Intervirology* 16, 201, 1981.
2. Spear, P., and Roizman, B. Proteins specified by herpes simplex virus. V. purification and structural proteins of the herpesvirion. *J. Virol.* 9, 431, 1972.
3. Roizman, B. The organization of herpes simplex virus genomes. *Ann. Rev. Genet.* 13, 25, 1979.
4. Shieh, M., WuDunn, D., Montgomery, R., Esko, J., and Spear, P. Cell surface receptors for herpes simplex virus are heparin sulfate proteoglycans. *J. Cell Biol.* 116, 1273, 1992.
5. Morgan, C., Rose, H., Holden, M., and Jones, E. Electron microscopic observations on the development of herpes simplex virus. *J. Exp. Med.* 110, 643, 1959.
6. Stevens, J., Haarr, L., Porter, D., Cook, M., and Wagner, E. Prominence of the herpes simplex virus latency-associated transcript in trigeminal ganglia from seropositive humans. *J. Infect. Dis.* 158, 117, 1988.
7. Milman, G., and Wang, E. Epstein-Barr virus nuclear antigen forms a complex that binds with high concentration dependence to a single DNA-binding site. *J. Virol.* 61, 465, 1987.
8. Wang, F., Tsang, S., Kurilla, M., Cohen, J., and Keiff, E. Epstein-Barr virus nuclear antigen 2 transactivates the latent membrane protein (LMPI). *J. Virol.* 64, 3407, 1990.
9. Johnson, R. E., Nahmias, A. J., Magder, L. S., Lee, F. K., Brooks, C. A., and Snowden, C. B. A seroepidemiologic servey of the prevalence of herpes simplex virus type 2 infection in the United States. *N. Engl. J. Med.* 321, 7, 1989.
10. Corey, L. M., Adams, H. G., Brown, Z. A., and Holmes, K. K. Gential herpes simplex virus infections: Clinical manifestations, course, and complications. *Ann. Int. Med.* 98, 958, 1983.
11. Spector, S., Merrill, R., Wolf, D., and Danker, W. Detection of human cytomegalovirus in plasma of AIDS patients during acute viceral diseaes by DNA amplification. *J. Clin. Microbiol.* 30, 2359, 1992.
12. Sokol, D. M. Foscarnet. *Semin. Pediatr. Infect. Dis.* 7, 1, 1996.
13. Mills, J., Jacobson, M. J., O'Donnell, J. J., Cederberg, D., and Holland, G. N. Treatment of cytomegalovirus retinitis in patients with AIDS. *Rev. Infect. Dis.* 10, S522, 1988.
14. Spector, S., Weingeist, T., Pollard, R., et al. A randomized, controlled study of intravenous ganciclovir therapy for cytomegalovirus peripheral retinitis in patients with AIDS. *J. Infect. Dis.* 168, 557, 1993.
15. Lopez, C., Pellett, P., Stewart, J., Goldsmith, C., Sanderlin, K., Black, J., Warfield, D., and Feorino, P. Characterization of human herpesvirus-6. *J. Infect. Dis.* 157, 127, 1988.
16. Frenkel, N., Schirmer, E., Wyatt, L., Katsafanas, G., Roffman, E., Danovitch, R., and June, C. Isolation of a new herpesvirus from human CD4+ T cells. *Proc. Natl. Acad. Sci. U.S.A.* 87, 748, 1990.
17. Salahuddin, S., Ablashi, D., Markham, P., et al. Isolation of a new virus, HBLV, in patients with lymphoproliferative disorders. *Science* 234, 596, 1986.
18. Beral, V., Peterman, A., Berkelman, R., and Jaffe, H. Kaposi's sarcomas among persons with AIDS: a sexually transmitted infection. *Lancet* 335, 123, 1990.
19. Chang, Y., Cesarman, E., Pessin, M., Lee, F., Culpepper, J., Knowles, D., and Moore, P. Identification of herpesvirus-like DNA sequences in AIDS-associated Kaposi's sarcoma. *Science* 266, 1865, 1994.
20. Chang, Y., and Moore, P. Detection of herpesvirus-like DNA sequences in Kaposi's sarcoma in patients with and those without HIV infection. *N. Eng. J. Med.* 332, 1181, 1995.
21. Moore, P., Gao, S. -J., Dominguez, G., Cesarman, E., Lungu, O., Knowles, D., Pellett, P., McGeogh, D., and Chang, Y. Primary characterization of a herpesvirus agent associated with Kaposi's sarcoma. *J. Virol.* 70, 549, 1996.

chapter thirteen

Infection with the human immunodeficiency virus and the acquired immunodeficiency syndrome

Julio S.G. Montaner, Michael V. O'Shaughnessy and Martin T. Schechter

13.1   Introduction..246
13.2   Pathophysiology..246
13.3   Transmission 246
13.4   Epidemiology...246
13.5   Definition and classification...246
13.6   Medical history and review of systems 251
13.7   Physical examination..251
13.8   General approach to the symptomatic patient.......................................252
13.9   Laboratory markers of disease progression..253
13.10 Baseline laboratory investigations..255
13.11 Follow-up assessment 255
13.12 Prophylactic treatments and vaccinations 256
13.13 Antiretroviral therapy 256
13.14 The goal of antiretroviral therapy 257
13.15 When to start antiretroviral therapy..257
13.16 Relative potency of current antiretroviral therapy regimens 258
       13.16.1 Initiating antiretroviral therapy..258
       13.16.2 When to change therapy...258
       13.16.3 Modifying therapy due to drug intolerance 259
       13.16.4 Modifying therapy due to treatment failure 260
13.17 Specific antiretroviral agents..260
       13.17.1 Cerebrospinal fluid (CSF) penetration of antiretrovirals............263
       13.17.2 Newer antiretrovirals 263
References..266

13.1 Introduction

Infection with the human immunodeficiency virus (HIV) leads to the development of the acquired immunodeficiency syndrome, or AIDS. This is characterized by severe cellular immunodeficiency which is responsible for the development of a variety of opportunistic infections and cancers. AIDS was first identified and defined in 1981 by the U.S. Center for Disease Control (CDC), but studies suggest the virus has been present in Africa since the late 1950s and that it first appeared in North America in the mid-1970s. HIV was isolated in 1984, and a second related virus, HIV-2, has since been described. The latter appears to be less pathogenic than HIV-1 and is largely prevalent in western Africa. The HIV antibody tests currently in use detect both HIV-1 and HIV-2 antibodies.

13.2 Pathophysiology

HIV is a retrovirus pathogenic in humans. Other retroviruses have been implicated in various animal disorders, such as leukemia, immunodeficiency, and neurological dysfunction. HIV infection leads to progressive immunodeficiency as a result of persistent viral replication.[1-4] At present, there is no cure for infection with HIV and true longterm survival free of any demonstrable immune dysfunction is exceptional, if at all possible.[5] As immune function declines, the body becomes vulnerable to diverse infections and cancers responsible for the severe morbidity and mortality associated with AIDS. The loss of CD4 lymphocytes has a particularly severe impact on immune defense against viruses, fungi, parasites, and certain bacteria, particularly mycobacteria.

13.3 Transmission

HIV can be transmitted through blood, semen, vaginal fluid, and breast milk. Sharing needles during injection drug use and engaging in unprotected vaginal or anal intercourse are the activities that carry the highest risk of transmission. HIV-infected persons are capable of transmitting the virus at all stages of their disease. There is no evidence to suggest transmission occurs through exposure to food, fomites, tears, saliva, urine, insects, or casual contact. It is generally accepted that intact skin is an effective barrier to transmission. There are no documented cases of transmission through kissing or biting.

13.4 Epidemiology

The World Health Organization (WHO) Surveillance Program reports that the total number of AIDS cases globally as of the end of 1996 was in excess of 2 million. However, due to under-reporting, particularly in developing countries where the rates of AIDS are highest, the actual number of cases could be several-fold greater than this estimate. The number of reported cases world-wide has approximately doubled every year. WHO estimates that there will be 40 million people infected with HIV by the year 2000. Of these, 10 million are expected to be women and children.

13.5 Definition and classification

Developed in 1985 and revised in 1987, the CDC together with the WHO adopted a case definition and a classification of HIV infection for surveillance purposes in adults (Tables 1 and 2). Patients are assigned to hierarchical groups I to IV according to the highest group for which they meet the criteria and can only move to higher groups as they develop new signs and symptoms of HIV infection. There is a separate classification scheme for HIV

Table 1 Surveillance Case Definition for AIDS

Diseases diagnosed definitively without confirmation of HIV infection in patients without other causes of immunodeficiency:
    Candidiasis of the esophagus, trachea, bronchi, or lungs
    Cryptococcosis, extrapulmonary
    Cryptosporidiosis >1 month duration
    Cytomegalovirus (CMV) infection of any organ except the liver, spleen, or lymph nodes in
        patients > 1 month old
    Herpes simplex infection, mucocutaneous (>1 month duration) or of the bronchi, lungs, or
        esophagus in patients >1 month old
    Kaposi's sarcoma in patients <60 years old
    Primary CNS lymphoma in patients <60 years old
    Lymphoid interstitial pneumonitis (LIP) and/or pulmonary lymphoid hyperplasia (PLH) in
        patients <13 years old
    Mycobacterium avium complex or disseminated *M. kansasii*
    Pneumocystis carinii pneumonia
    Progressive multifocal leukoencephalopathy
    Toxoplasmosis of the brain in patients >1 month old
Diseases diagnosed definitively with confirmation of HIV infection:
    Multiple or recurrent pyogenic bacterial infections in patients <13 years old
    Invasive cervical cancer
    Coccidioidomycosis, disseminated
    Histoplasmosis, disseminated
    Isosporiasis >1 month duration
    Kaposi's sarcoma, any age
    Primary CNS lymphoma, any age
    Non-Hodgkin's lymphoma (small, non-cleaved lymphoma, Burkitt or non-Burkitt type, or
        immunoblastic sarcoma)
    Bacterial pneumonia, recurrent
    Mycobacterial disease other than *M. tuberculosis*, disseminated
    M. tuberculosis, extrapulmonary
    Pulmonary tuberculosis
    Salmonella septicemia, recurrent
Diseases diagnosed presumptively with confirmation of HIV infection:
    Candidiasis of the esophagus
    CMV retinitis
    Kaposi's sarcoma
    LIP/PLH in patients <13 years old
    Disseminated mycobacterial disease (without culture)
    Pneumocystis carinii pneumonia
    Toxoplasmosis of the brain in patients >1 month old
    HIV encephalopathy
    HIV wasting syndrome

infection in children under 13 (Table 3), as the clinical presentation of HIV infection in children often differs substantially from that in adults.

    Recently, the CDC revised the adult case definition (Table 4) to include all HIV infected persons with a CD4 lymphocyte count less than 200 cells/mm^3. While not adopting this particular revision, Canada, Australia, and the European community have added three more indicator diseases to the AIDS case definition, as also recommended by the CDC in their revised classification, that apply when persons are HIV antibody positive: recurrent bacterial pneumonia, pulmonary tuberculosis, and invasive cervical cancer in women. The term "AIDS-Related Complex" or "ARC," although never part of the CDC definition, was commonly used to describe conditions indicating immune system failure which fell short

Table 2   Classification System for HIV Infection in Adults

Group I Acute Infection
Group II Asymptomatic Infection
Group III Persistent Generalized Lymphadenopathy
Group IV Other diseases
  Subgroup A Constitutional disease
    • fever lasting more than 1 month
    • involuntary weight loss of at least 10%
    • diarrhea lasting more than 1 month
  Subgroup B Neurological disease
    • dementia
    • myelopathy
    • peripheral neuropathy
  Subgroup C Secondary infectious diseases
    Category C-1 Specified
    Category C-2 Others
  Subgroup D Secondary cancers
    • Kaposi's sarcoma
    • primary CNS lymphoma
    • other specified non-Hodgkin's lymphoma
  Subgroup E Other conditions
    • suggestive of immunodeficiency
    • not listed above

Table 3   Classification System for HIV Infection in Children Under 13 Years of Age

Class P-0 Indeterminate infection
Class P-1 Asymptomatic infection
  Subclass A Normal immune function
  Subclass B Abnormal immune function
  Subclass C Immune function not tested
Class P-2 Symptomatic infection
  Subclass A Nonspecific findings
  Subclass B Progressive neurologic disease including HIV encephalopathy in the CDC surveillance definition for AIDS
  Subclass C Lymphoid interstitial pneumonitis in the CDC surveillance definition for AIDS
  Subclass D Secondary infectious diseases
    Category D-1 Specified secondary infectious diseases in the CDC surveillance definition for AIDS
    Category D-2 Recurrent serious bacterial infections in the CDC surveillance definition for AIDS
    Category D-3 Other specified secondary infectious diseases
  Subclass E Secondary cancers
    Category E-1 Specified secondary cancers in the CDC surveillance definition for AIDS
    Category E-2 Other cancers possibly secondary to HIV infection
  Subclass F Other diseases possibly due to HIV infection

of the CDC criteria for AIDS. Some of these conditions are now included in the revised definition, Group IV, subgroup A. The term "ARC" is no longer used.

Although the CDC/WHO classification for HIV infection and disease is often interpreted as suggesting that patients progress sequentially through the groups, this is not necessarily so. It is not uncommon, for example, for infected individuals to remain asymptomatic for long periods and then to present suddenly with an episode of *Pneumocystis carinii* pneumonia (PCP), a direct transition from Group II to Group IV-C1. It must be emphasized that this classification was originally intended for epidemiological surveillance

Table 4 CDC Revised Classification System for HIV Infection and Expanded AIDS Surveillance Case Definition for Adolescents and Adults

CD4 cell categories	Clinical Categories		
	(A) Asymptomatic or PGL	(B) Symptomatic, not (A) or (C) conditions	(C) AIDS-indicator conditions
≥500	A1	B1	C1
200–499	A2	B2	C2
<200 (AIDS-indicator cell count)	A3	B3	C3

Description of Clinical Categories:

A One or more of the conditions listed below, with documented HIV infection. Conditions listed in categories B and C must not have occurred.

- asymptomatic HIV infection
- persistent generalized lymphadenopathy (PGL)
- acute (primary) HIV infection with accompanying illness or history of acute infection

B Symptomatic conditions that meet at least one of the following criteria: (a) the conditions are attributed to HIV infection and/or are indicative of a defect in cell-mediated immunity; or (b) the conditions are considered by physicians to have a clinical course or management that is complicated by HIV infection. Examples of conditions in clinical category B include, but are not limited to:

- bacterial endocarditis, meningitis, pneumonia, or sepsis
- vulvovaginal candidiasis that is persistent (greater than one month duration) or poorly responsive to therapy
- oropharyngeal candidiasis (thrush)
- severe cervical dysplasia or carcinoma
- constitutional symptoms, such as fever (38.4°C) or diarrhea lasting more than one month
- oral hairy leukoplakia
- herpes zoster (shingles), involving at least two distinct episodes or more than one dermatome
- idiopathic thrombocytopenic purpura
- listeriosis
- *Mycobacterium tuberculosis,* pulmonary
- nocardiosis
- pelvic inflammatory disease
- peripheral neuropathy

C Any condition listed in the 1987 surveillance case definition for AIDS. The conditions in clinical category C are strongly associated with severe immunodeficiency, occur frequently in HIV-infected individuals, and cause serious morbidity or mortality.

only. The CDC/WHO classification is merely a descriptive epidemiologic tool and offers little prognostic information, as most of the disease "activity" is contained in Group IV.

Obviously, a simple and widely available prognostic staging system for HIV disease would greatly contribute to the care of HIV-infected individuals, facilitating the development of guidelines for follow-up and management, including the indication for the use of specific therapeutic interventions. Such a system would also facilitate patient counselling and provide a prognostic standard with which new treatments could be gauged.

Recently, the WHO proposed a staging classification which is based on the recognition of four clinical groups and three laboratory strata (Table 5). The clinical groups are: asymptomatic, mildly symptomatic, moderately symptomatic, and severely symptomatic. These four clinical groups are stratified according to CD4 counts (0–199 cells/mm^3, 200–499 cells/mm^3, and ≥ 500 cells/mm^3) to create twelve distinct cells. A modification of the proposed WHO staging system described above has been developed to enhance its prognostic value by regrouping the original twelve cells into four stages, Stages I to IV,

Table 5 Modified WHO Staging System

Laboratory			Clinical group		
Lymph.	CD4	Asymp.	Mild	Mod.	Severe
>2000	>500	1A	2A	3A	4A
1000–2000	200–500	1B	2B	3B	4B
<1000	<200	1C	2C	3C	4C

Stage I   = 1A, 2A
Stage II   = 1B, 2B, 3A
Stage III = 1C, 2C, 3B
Stage IV   = 3C, 4A, 4B, 4C

Clinical Groups for the WHO Staging Classification

Group 1: Asymptomatic
- Asymptomatic
- PGL

Group 2: Mild
- Weight loss <10%
- Minor mucocutaneous symptoms or signs
- Herpes zoster
- Recurrent upper respiratory tract infections

Group 3: Moderate
- Progressive weight loss > 10%
- Oral candidiasis (thrush)
- Oral hairy leukoplakia
- Unexplained diarrhea >1 month
- Pulmonary TB
- Fever > 1month
- Severe bacterial infection (i.e., pneumonia, pyomyositis)
- Salmonella septicaemia (first episode)
- Isosporiasis with diarrhea persisting >1 month
- Herpes simplex
- Kaposi's sarcoma

Group 4: Severe
- Pneumocystis carinii pneumonia
- Toxoplasmosis (cerebral)
- Cryptosporidiosis with diarrhea persisting >1 month
- Cryptococcosis, extrapulmonary
- Cytomegalovirus disease other than liver, spleen, or lymph nodes
- Progressive Multifocal Leukoencephalopathy
- Any disseminated endemic mycosis
- Esophageal candidiasis
- Atypical mycobacteriosis (disseminated)
- Salmonella septicaemia (recurrent)
- Extrapulmonary tuberculosis
- Lymphoma
- Cachexia
- HIV encephalopathy
- Strongyloidiasis

according to their perceived individual prognosis. The proposed system provides four clinically relevant stages which correspond to our intuitive understanding of the natural history of HIV. This approach has been successfully validated in a number of cohorts in a variety of epidemiological settings.

13.6 Medical history and review of systems

The overall assessment of the HIV infected individual begins with a detailed history including a review of systems. The objective is to determine where the patient lies within the continuum of HIV disease. The history should specifically cover:

- *Date of infection:* Some patients may recall a mononucleosis-like illness shortly after a high-risk exposure, characteristic of the seroconversion illness. Alternatively, some patients may be able to identify the likely date of infection based on a review of past sexual contacts, period of needle sharing, or the availability of a prior negative HIV test. The duration of time elapsed since infection has prognostic significance, as the longer a person has been infected, the sooner the development of AIDS would be expected to occur.
- *Risk factors:* Detailed questions concerning sexual contacts, injection drug use, history of other sexually transmitted diseases, and blood transfusions will aid the physician in identifying behaviors and risk factors that increase the likelihood of additional medical problems.
- *Past medical history:* As immunodeficiency progresses, past illnesses such as tuberculosis (TB) may recur. History of previous TB, TB contacts, and tuberculin (PPD) skin tests, syphilis, herpes, hepatitis, and past immunizations should be documented. A travel history may identify patients at higher risk for particular infections with such organisms as *Coccidiodes immitis* or *Histoplasma capsulatum*. Conditions that may compromise future drug therapy should be specifically investigated (e.g., liver disease, inflamatory bowel disease, malabsorption, gout, seizures, kidney stones, renal disease, peripheral neuropathy, or chronic lung disease).
- *Systems review*: Constitutional symptoms, such as fever, night sweats, unexplained weight loss, or anorexia might represent progression of HIV disease but are also common presentations of opportunistic infections. Persisting or recurring constitutional symptoms should be investigated thoroughly. A past history of pneumonia, sinusitis, asthma, eczema, seborrheic dermatitis, onychomycosis, oral disease, shingles (HZV), among the many non-specific conditions that occur with increased frequency with HIV infection, should be explored. HIV infected women should also have a detailed gynecological (including frequency and results of Papanicolaou [PAP] smears) and obstetric history.
- *Allergies:* Allergies to environmental products, chemicals, and drugs are quite frequent among HIV-infected individuals. A detailed history of past drug intolerance or allergy should be thoroughly documented. Prior history of intolerance to sulfa-containing drugs should be specifically investigated.

13.7 Physical examination

The physical examination should focus on signs of immune dysfunction and any particular findings that might indicate the presence of an opportunistic disease. Special attention should be paid to any evidence of underlying conditions that may have an impact on management decisions at a later date, as described above. The patient's weight, vital signs, and temperature should be documented. Specific attention should be directed toward examination of the scalp and skin, visual fields and ocular fundi, sinuses, oral cavity, lymph nodes, abdomen, genital and rectal examination, as well as neurological exam and mental status.

- *Head and Neck:* Zoster scars, seborrheic rashes, red or purple nodules, mollusca, or warts are frequent manifestations of skin involvement in HIV infection. Sinusitis is likewise not uncommon. The oral examination in early disease may reveal cheilitis, aphthous ulcers, or periodontal disease. In later stages, hairy leukoplakia, herpes, and various presentations of oral candidiasis (thrush), may occur. Kaposi's sarcoma, also referred to as KS, and lymphoma can also be encountered on oral examination.
- *Chest:* Either "typical," lobar pneumonia with, in particular, encapsulated organisms such as *Streptococcus pneumoniae* and *Hemophilus influenzae* or "atypical," interstitial pneumonia due to *Pneumocystis carinii* may be detected upon examination of the chest. Wheezes secondary to obstructive airways disease may also be audible, as airways hyperreactivity is relatively common in this setting.
- *Abdomen:* Lymphoma or infection with *Mycobacterium avium* complex (MAC) may cause hepatosplenomegaly or abdominal tenderness. Epigastric tenderness may reflect distal esophageal disease with *Candida* species, *Cytomegalovirus* (CMV), or *Herpes* simplex virus (HSV). Peptic ulcer disease is also rather frequent in this setting.
- *Neurological System:* A mental status examination is a useful tool for the early recognition of cognitive impairment characteristic of AIDS dementia complex (ADC). Focal neurological findings suggest opportunistic infections such as toxoplasmosis or progressive multifocal leukoencephalopathy (PML). Similarly, focal findings are often the presenting complaint in patients with central nervous system lymphoma. Further examination of the nervous system may demonstrate peripheral neuropathy that can be secondary to HIV infection itself, nutritional deficits, or antiretroviral medications.
- *Genital System:* The genitals and perianal area should be closely examined for any evidence of sexually transmitted diseases, including genital warts, herpes, and molluscum. Anal carcinoma may also be evident.
- *Gynecological System:* Pelvic inflammatory disease and vaginal candidiasis are frequent. Furthermore, as many as 80% of women infected with HIV have evidence of cervical infection with human papilloma virus (HPV) making regular screening for cervical cancer with a PAP smear every six months necessary. Abnormal PAP smears should be followed by colposcopy.

13.8 General approach to the symptomatic patient

Not every illness in an HIV-infected patient is attributable to, or unique to, HIV infection or AIDS. HIV-infected patients, like everyone else, are susceptible to any usual illnesses. In fact, as a result of the immunodeficiency that is associated with HIV infection even before the development of overt AIDS, patients typically present with repeated bouts of common illnesses, such as seborrheic dermatitis, eczema, angular chelitis, shingles, onychomycosis, sinusitis, or asthma. When signs and symptoms appear, management should be the same as in non-HIV-infected individuals.

When CD4 cell counts are within the normal range, immune function is relatively normal and opportunistic infections are less likely. The work-up does not usually require any special initiatives. However, it should be noted that some conditions, such as tuberculosis, Kaposi's sarcoma, or lymphomas can occur despite normal CD4 counts. One should have a higher index of suspicion for opportunistic infections or malignancies as the CD4 count falls below normal and particularly once the CD4 count is below 200 cells/mm^3 or below a CD4 fraction of 15%.

Table 6

Viral load[a] HIV equivalents/ml	Progression to AIDS at 5 years	Median time to AIDS	Progression to death at 5 years	Median estimated survival
≤4,530	8%	>10 years	5%	>10 years
4,531–13,020	26%	7.7 years	10%	9.5 years
13,021–36,270	49%	5.3 years	25%	7.4 years
>36,270	62%	3.5 years	49%	5.1 years

[a] These thresholds specifically apply to the study group under the particular circumstances under which the study was conducted. Caution should be exercised when extrapolating to specific clinical situations. Current values, obtained according to present assay methodology on a real time basis are likely to be higher than those specified here.

Adapted from Mellors et al., *Science,* 272, 1167-1170, 1996.

13.9 Laboratory markers of disease progression

The CD4 lymphocyte count has traditionally been the key surrogate marker used for prognostic staging and therapeutic monitoring.[6] Recently, new molecular techniques have become available designed to detect circulating virion-associated HIV RNA in plasma. These studies have led to a major revision of our understanding of the natural history of HIV disease.[7] The notion of a prolonged phase of virologic latency antedating the symptomatic phase of the disease has been replaced by that of a continuous viral replication from the time of infection until the terminal phases of the illness.[8-12] It has now been clearly demonstrated that an ongoing high viral turnover is directly responsible for the ultimate destruction of the immune system.[13] The rate of CD4 lymphocyte loss will ultimately be dependent on the balance between viral replication, hence CD4 lymphocyte destruction, and CD4 lymphocyte production.

Three assays are currently available to measure plasma HIV-1 viral load. These are commonly referred to as RT-PCR (Roche Molecular Systems), bDNA (Chiron), and NASBA (Organon-Teknika). All three of these assays are generally comparable from a technical standpoint.[14] They are also comparable with regard to their reproducibility and physiological variability. The lower threshold of detection is in the 500 copies/ml range. The variability of the assays is approximately 0.3 $\log_{10}$ within the dynamic range of the test. As a result, a 0.5 $\log_{10}$ decrease in HIV-RNA level is generally regarded as a viral load decrease indicative of antiviral activity in the context of antiretroviral therapy. It should be noted that intercurrences (such as infections) or vaccinations can transiently but substantially increase plasma viral load.[15-17]

Levels of viral replication appear to be set at an early time point, following primary infection.[18,19] Mellors et al. recently reported on the correlation of plasma RNA viral load with disease progression and death in a seroprevalent cohort of gay men using archival samples.[20] As shown in Table 6, patients were divided into four equal groups (quartiles) based on their viral load levels.

The proportion of subjects who progressed to AIDS by 5 years were 8, 26, 49, and 62% for low to high viral load quartiles, respectively. The median times to development of AIDS for subjects in these viral load quartiles were >10, 7.7, 5.3, and 3.5 years, respectively. The proportion of subjects who died within 5 years were 5, 10, 25, and 49%, respectively. The median estimated survival times were >10, 9.5, 7.4, and 5.1 years, respectively. In contrast to the close relation between baseline viral load and outcome, baseline CD4 cell count failed to show a similar gradient among quartiles with respect to the risk of disease progression or death in these same subjects. Furthermore, among the three quartiles with the highest CD4 cell count no differences were observed with regard to these outcomes. These data also provide conclusive evidence of the independence of viral load from CD4 cell counts with regard to prognosis. Among subjects with CD4 cell count >500/mm³, there was a significant difference in time to death based on whether the baseline viral load was above or below the median (10,190 copies/ml). The 10 year survival was 70% and 20%, for the low and high viral load groups, respectively; noting that both groups had a median CD4 count of approximately 780/mm³. Similarly, among those with baseline CD4 count <500/mm³ a significantly shorter survival was associated with a baseline HIV RNA greater than the median (17,320 copies/ml), despite similar baseline CD4 counts among the groups.

Despite the increased interest on plasma viral load determinations, the CD4 count continues to be an important and useful aid to monitor HIV-infected individuals. It could be said that the CD4 count helps to determine where a patient is on the continuum of HIV disease. In adults, a CD4 count range of 400 to 1400 cells/mm³ (0.40–1.40 Giga/liter or G/l) is considered normal in most laboratories. Counts below 200 cells/mm³ are associated with increased risk of opportunistic infection and rapid disease progression.

The CD4 count is usually reported as a fraction and an absolute count. Although the absolute CD4 count is usually sufficient to guide the clinical management of a given patient, it must be noted that under specific circumstances this may be misleading. For example, patients who have undergone a splenectomy typically have a high CD4 absolute count. In these cases the CD4 fraction is a more appropriate reflection of the immunological status of the patient. It is therefore advisable to monitor the CD4 fraction in tandem with the CD4 count at all times to ensure that these are in general agreement.

CD4 counts show diurnal variation, being lowest in the morning and highest in the evening. In normal individuals the evening CD4 cell count can be nearly double what it is in the morning. Although the normal physiological variation may be reduced in HIV-infected patients, it is still recommended that specimens for CD4 counting in HIV-infected patients be collected in the morning. Patients should be advised to avoid alcohol, smoking, and excessive exercise prior to the collection of the specimen. Other factors that may affect the count include acute infections such as common viral illnesses, certain pharmaceutical agents such as corticosteroids, vaccinations, and stress. The results may also be influenced by differing laboratory methodologies. Despite controlling the time of collection, HIV-infected individuals who are clinically stable will still show considerable biologic variation in CD4 counts.[21,22] Fluctuations of up to 30% may occur which are not attributable to a change in disease status. As well, correlation between CD4 count and clinical status can be quite different from one patient to the next. Overall, it is important to monitor the trends in CD4 counts over time rather than placing too much emphasis on one specific reading.

From a practical stand point it is useful to consider the CD4 count as indicative of the level of immunosuppression or better yet "the immunological damage that has already occurred." On the other hand, the plasma viral load better illustrates disease activity and therefore "the damage that is about to occur." The prognostic contribution of viral load determinations at any level of CD4 counts is illustrated in Figure 1.

Recent data from several clinical trials conclusively demonstrated that a treatment reduction in plasma HIV-1 RNA viral load is associated with a decrease in the rate of disease progression.[23-25] In this context, a treatment-induced 10-fold (approximately 1 $\log_{10}$) reduction in HIV-1 RNA concentration in plasma was associated with approximately 50% decrease in the relative risk of death. Based on these data, the prognostic staging and therapeutic monitoring of HIV-infected patients has been extensively revised. Plasma viral load and CD4 counts determinations are to be measured at least quarterly in stable HIV-infected adults as part of their routine evaluation. More frequent determinations are warranted under special circumstances, such as when introducing antiretroviral therapy. Other surrogate markers such as beta 2 microglobulin, C1Q or immunecomplexes, ESR, triglycerides, and neopterin are no longer recommended in clinical practice.

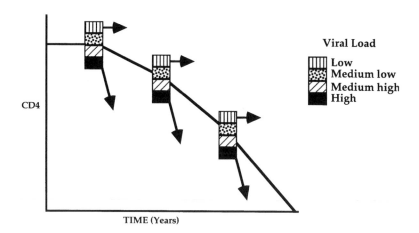

Figure 1 For a given CD4 count, individuals with high viral loads will have a more rapid decline in CD4 count and therefore, a worse clinical prognosis.

13.10   Baseline laboratory investigations

Baseline investigations are important, particularly before starting a treatment program. These should include:

- *Plasma HIV RNA viral load.*
- *CD4 lymphocyte count and percentage.*
- *CBC, differential, and platelet count.* Anemia, neutropenia, and thrombocytopenia are common in patients with HIV infection. Absolute lymphopenia should raise suspicion of advanced disease.
- *Liver (AST, LDH, alkaline phosphatase, bilirubin) and renal (BUN, creatinine) profiles.*
- *Hepatitis B, Hepatitis C, syphilis, and toxoplasmosis serologies.*
- *Tuberculin skin test.* An induration of ≥5 mm in diameter following a 5TU-PPD test should be regarded as a positive response in an HIV infected individual; INH prophylaxis should therefore be considered. Be aware that a negative response in persons with advanced HIV disease does not rule out tuberculosis, as such individuals may be anergic.[11,25]
- *Cultures and smears for sexually transmitted diseases* as indicated by the patient's history and physical exam.
- *Sputum cultures and smears for mycobacteriae* as indicated by the patient's history and physical exam.
- *Chest X-ray.*

13.11   Follow-up assessment

The routine follow-up of a stable asymptomatic HIV positive patient should include a history and physical examination as well as plasma viral load and CD4 count every three to four months, if the patient remains stable. Counseling should take place at each visit. Patients should also have an opportunity to discuss the most recent changes in management and therapy at each visit.

Symptomatic patients and those with AIDS should be seen at least monthly. More frequent and additional laboratory investigations may be warranted for patients receiving antiretroviral and other therapies. Further investigations will be done depending on clinical indication.

13.12 Prophylactic treatments and vaccinations

Preventive therapies play a major role in the management of HIV-infected individuals. The following interventions should be considered when evaluating a newly diagnosed patient:

- A tuberculin skin test should be performed. If there is induration of ≥5 mm in diameter, prophylaxis with isoniazid (INH) 5 mg/kg daily (maximum 300 mg/day) for 12 months should be initiated, along with pyridoxine to reduce the risk of INH toxicity. Prophylaxis may also be indicated in patients at high risk for tuberculosis who have cutaneous anergy, household contacts of an active tuberculosis case, patients with chest x-ray findings suggestive of previous tuberculosis who do not have a history of adequate treatment, or patients with a history of a positive PPD who have not previously received INH prophylaxis or tuberculosis treatment.

- While antigen recognition is still intact, it is essential to boost humoral immunity against certain common pathogens. Recommended vaccines include polyvalent vaccine against *Streptococcus pneumoniae* (Pneumovax) given once and Influenza vaccine given annually in the fall. The evidence in favor of the latter, however, remains controversial. Tetanus toxoid updates should be offered as necessary, and Hepatitis B vaccination should be encouraged for any susceptible patient at ongoing risk of acquiring hepatitis B virus. The inactivated polio vaccination should be given to a patient if traveling. Vaccines against Hemophilus influenzae type b and Neisseria meningitidis are not widely recommended at this time.

- As shown in Table 7, as HIV disease progresses prophylaxis and treatment of opportunistic infections become important. Recurrent genital herpes outbreaks may be dealt with using either intermittent treatment or regular suppressive therapy with oral acyclovir, depending on the frequency of the attacks. Mucosal candidiasis may be treated with topical agents or systemic azoles on an as needed basis. Systemic azole therapy is usually needed as the immunodeficiency progresses. In some cases intermittent or even continued suppressive therapy with systemic azoles may be warranted to control frequent relapses. Because more than 80% of patients with HIV infection will have at least one episode of PCP during their lifetime, timely prophylaxis of this condition should be offered consisting of one double strength tablet of trimethoprim-sulphamethoxasole daily. Alternatively, dapsone 100 mg/daily or aerosol pentamidine 300 mg once a month can be used. Prior to starting prophylaxis, patients should be assessed to rule out active pulmonary disease. Prophylaxis for toxoplasmosis is indicated for those patients who have positive serum serology for toxoplasma IgG and CD4 count less than 100 cells/mm^3, however trimethoprim-sulphamethoxasole daily, as indicated for PCP prophylaxis is also effective against toxoplasma. As disease progresses, prophylaxis for mycobacterium avium complex (MAC) with intermittent azithromycin or daily clarithromycin or rifabutin may also be considered. At CD4 <50/mm^3, screening by an ophthalmologist for CMV retinitis should be encouraged to be repeated at 3–6 month intervals thereafter.

13.13 Antiretroviral therapy

Over the last several months, the antiretroviral therapy armamentarium has increased substantially. Although availability of antiretrovirals vary regionally, we will include them in the following discussion. We will therefore consider the nucleoside analogues: zidovudine (AZT), didanosine (ddI), zalcitabine (ddC), lamivudine (3TC), and stavudine (d4T); the proteinase inhibitors: saquinavir (SQV), indinavir (IDV), ritonavir (RTV), and nelfi-

Table 7

CD4 count (cells/mm^3)	Management strategy
> 500	• General counseling (safer sex, nutrition, etc.) • History and physical examination every 3–6 months • Plasma viral load and CD4 count every 3–4 months • Pneumovax, annual influenza vaccinations • TB skin test and INH prophylaxis if indicated • Update DPT (dT for adults) and inactivated polio vaccinations • Hepatitis B vaccine if at risk • Syphilis serology
<500	• Antiretroviral therapy followed by plasma viral load a month after • Plasma viral load and CD4 count every 3-4 months • Candida and herpes suppression if frequent recurrences • Relevant history, physical, and laboratory investigations at least monthly if symptomatic, diagnosed with AIDS, or on antiretroviral therapy
<200	• Start prophylaxis for PCP
<100	• Plasma viral load and CD4 count every 3–4 months • Start prophylaxis for toxoplasmosis if seropositive and not on trimethoprim-sulfamethoxazole • At CD4 <75/mm^3, consider MAC prophylaxis • At CD4 <50/mm^3, screening by an ophthalmologist for CMV retinitis, repeated at 3–6 month intervals

navir (NFV); and the non-nucleoside reverse transcriptase inhibitors also known as NNR-TIs: nevirapine (NVP), delavirdine (DLV), and loviride (LOV).

13.14   The goal of antiretroviral therapy

The objective of antiretroviral therapy is to prevent clinical and laboratory progression of HIV disease. It is expected that longterm non-progression could be achieved by maintaining a "low" plasma viral load for prolonged periods of time, in the order of several, if not many, years.[26] The definition of a "low" viral load remains controversial at this time. However, most guidelines recommend levels below 5,000 copies/ml as reasonable and achievable.[27] Recent data suggests that the durability of antiviral response may be prolonged if plasma viral load is maintained below the level of detection of current assays (i.e., <500 copies/ml). For this reason a number of groups, including our own, would favor recommending levels below 500 copies/ml as the target of antiretroviral therapy.

13.15   When to start antiretroviral therapy

Based on the principles discussed above, it is recommended that antiretroviral therapy be offered to all HIV-infected individuals except those who have a normal CD4 count (>500/mm^3) <u>and</u> a very low and stable plasma RNA viral load (probably <5,000 copies/ml). This is to say that antiretroviral therapy should be offered if plasma RNA viral load is ≥5000 copies/ml or if the CD4 count is <500/mm^3.[28,29] If this approach is followed, clinical criteria will rarely play a significant role in the decision to initiate therapy as HIV-related clinical symptoms are exceptionally rare in individuals with normal CD4 counts and low plasma viral load.

13.16   *Relative potency of current antiretroviral therapy regimens*

At this time, monotherapy is no longer recommended. In contrast, the use of combination of antiretrovirals with no overlapping toxicity and demonstrated antiviral synergy is encouraged to maximize the length of the antiviral response.[30-33] Most of the commonly used two nucleoside regimens (AZT/ddI, AZT/ddC, AZT/3TC, d4T/3TC, and d4T/ddI) reliably achieve more than 1 log (90%) decrease in viral load for several months.[34,35] Triple drug combinations, including two nucleosides and nevirapine or a second generation protease inhibitor (ritonavir, indinavir, or nelfinavir) reliably reach 2 log (99%) sustained reductions in viral load.[36-38] More recently, preliminary data has been presented suggesting that the combination of saquinavir and ritonavir (even when used at the reduced dose of 400 mg twice daily for each drug) may achieve a 2 log reduction in plasma viral load in selected patients.[39]

13.16.1   *Initiating antiretroviral therapy*

Combinations of two nucleoside analogues have been recommended as first-line therapy in individuals who are antiretroviral therapy naive and have viral loads below 50,000 to 100,000 copies/ml, until recently. Although most of these patients are expected to achieve the stated goal of therapy with this approach, there is increasing concern that this effect is time limited. For this reason, most experts would currently recommend more powerful regimens, such as triple drug therapy including two nucleosides and either a non-nucleoside or a powerful protease inhibitor (indinavir, ritonavir, or nelfinavir).[40] There is no definitive evidence regarding the relative merits of a given combination over the others. Issues of availability, safety profile, cost, as well as patient and physician preference will influence this decision. It must be emphasized that over time patients are likely to resort to more than one combination, therefore it is always useful to consider to what extent a given choice has the potential of constraining future therapeutic options. Selected regimens are illustrated in Table 8.

Initiation of therapy should be followed with a determination of plasma RNA viral load and CD4 counts within 4–8 weeks to confirm that the expected drug-related effect has been achieved. These parameters should be monitored quarterly thereafter. It should be noted that at times the plasma RNA viral load may demonstrate the expected decrease without a typical reciprocal rise in CD4 count. This should not be necessarily interpreted as a therapeutic failure. Close monitoring under this circumstance may be warranted.

13.16.2   *When to change therapy*

Once antiretroviral therapy has been initiated, we often face the question of when and how treatment is to be changed. Obviously, the specific reasons leading to a change of therapy will often place severe constraints on the options available. In general, patients developing toxicity to a given agent should be advised to change to a second agent which has no overlapping toxicities. Similarly, when clinical or laboratory failure are the motivation for change, issues of cross resistance or the need to use combinations which are potentially synergistic become critically important.

The following provides a practical, though not necessarily all encompassing, clinical perspective on altering therapy under different circumstances assuming an environment where there is unrestricted access to AZT, ddI, ddC, d4T, 3TC, SQV, IDV, RTV, and NVP. Similar principles are to be extended to other drugs, such as the newer protease inhibitors (i.e., nelfinavir) and the newer non-nucleoside reverse transcriptase inhibitors (i.e., delavirdine and loviride).

Table 8

Selected antiretroviral therapy combinations	Proven clinical value	Proven antiviral effect	Comments
AZT/ddI	+		AZT/ddI/NVP or AZT/ddI/Pi are preferable.
AZT/ddC	+		AZT/ddC/NVP or AZT/ddC/Pi are preferable.
AZT/3TC	+		AZT/3TC/NVP or AZT/3TC/Pi are preferable.
d4T/3TC		+	D4T/3TC/NVP or D4T/3TC/Pi are preferable.
AZT/d4T			Contraindicated.
ddI/3TC			Not generally encouraged.
ddI/d4T		+	Monitor closely for sensory peripheral neuropathy.
One nucleoside & SQV			Not generally encouraged.
Two nucleosides & SQV		+	Not generally encouraged.
One nucleoside & IDV		+	Not generally encouraged.
One nucleoside & RTV		+	Not generally encouraged.
Two nucleosides & IDV		+	
Two nucleosides & RTV	+		
One nucleoside & NNRTI		+	Not generally encouraged.
Two nucleosides & NVP		+	
DLV		+	Limited experience to date precludes positioning.
LOV		+	Limited experience to date precludes positioning.
PI & NNRTI		+	Be aware of Pk interactions. Need for dose adjustments not clear yet.
RTV/SQV		+	Use reduced doses. +/– 3rd drug?

13.16.3 *Modifying therapy due to drug intolerance*

The development of intolerance often dictates an early change in the antiretroviral therapy regimen. Fortunately, there are a number of possible combinations of agents which do not have substantial overlapping toxicity. Nucleoside analogues can be divided into broad groups based on their safety profile.[41] On one hand, we recognize those drugs associated with potential bone marrow suppression, such as AZT and less frequently 3TC, which can produce anemia and neutropenia. On the other hand, we have drugs which are most commonly associated with peripheral neuropathy and occasionally pancreatitis, including ddC, d4T, and ddI. Other problems often leading to change in therapy include gastrointestinal intolerance (particularly common with AZT and ddI), poor palatability (ddI), abnormal liver function tests (AZT, d4T, protease inhibitors, and nevirapine), rash (AZT, nevirapine, and delavirdine), myositis (AZT), kidney stones (indinavir), and oral ulcers (ddC). The gastrointestinal intolerance and palatability problems associated with ddI have been substantially decreased with the recent introduction of the orange flavor-reduced mass formulation.

Drug interactions can also oblige a change in therapy.[42] This is particularly the case when other agents are required for treatment of other associated conditions. The known effect of protease inhibitors on cytochrome p450 is responsible for a fairly lengthy list of potential drug interactions that should be carefully reviewed before using these compounds.

Although this has been best characterized in the context of ritonavir use,[43] it is likely to also play a role when other protease inhibitors are used (i.e., indinavir).

It is also important to emphasize that intolerance in the distant past, even if due to a well documented adverse effect of an antiretroviral drug, does not necessarily preclude rechallenging if clinically indicated. Obviously this should always be done under controlled circumstances and in consultation with an experienced physician.

13.16.4 Modifying therapy due to treatment failure

Treatment failure (disease progression) has traditionally been defined in terms of the development of a new AIDS-defining illness or a minor opportunistic infection, development of HIV-related symptoms, or a decline in CD4 counts. However, based on our current understanding of the physiopathology of HIV disease and the goals of therapy discussed above, the antiretroviral therapy regimen should be changed prior to the development of clinical or immunological progression. This would imply that patients should be encouraged to reassess their antiretroviral regimen based on the results of ongoing plasma viral load monitoring. In general, changes in viral load are expected to precede CD4 declines. From a practical standpoint, if one month after initiating therapy the viral load has decreased within the expected range but short of the stated goal of therapy, one may consider either adding a third agent to a two drug regimen or switching to a novel triple drug regimen. If a patient has been chronically treated with a given combination therapy regimen and presents during follow-up with a viral load higher than 500 copies/ml, a change to a new triple drug regimen should be considered. Adding a single agent to a failing combination regimen should be strongly discouraged.

The decision of what to change to has typically been based on a thorough understanding of the past exposure to antiretroviral drugs and the possible cross resistance and potential for synergy of the available agents. The latter has been postulated, for example, as a possible rationale to avoid switching from a 3TC-based regimen to regimens containing ddC or possibly ddI. Again, the issue of drug-drug interaction can potentially place important constraints on the number of options available under these circumstances. The recent data suggesting that 3TC can re-establish AZT sensitivity among patients with established high levels of *in vitro* AZT resistance is of particular interest.[44] This feature of 3TC, as well as its favorable safety profile make this combination an attractive one, particularly among patients who have had prior AZT exposure.[45,46] It should be emphasized that changes in therapy be monitored with viral load immediately before and within the first 4–8 weeks of therapy so that the expected effect on viral load can be confirmed and therapy be adjusted if necessary.

Prior to the availability of viral load determinations, there have been clinical trials that demonstrated the benefit of a change in therapy in the absence of toxicity or overt disease progression, including CD4 decline.[47-50] The availability of plasma viral load determinations makes this strategy no longer desirable.

13.17   Specific antiretroviral agents

- *Zidovudine (ZDV, AZT, Retrovir®)*: This is a nucleoside analogue inhibitor of the reverse transcriptase. The recommended dose is 500 mg/day divided in 3 to 5 daily doses. Doses of 400 mg/day are generally regarded as clinically effective. If tolerability is compromised by side effects, the dose of ZDV is often reduced to 300 mg/day, particularly in the context of combination therapy. It should be noted that, while currently available data suggests 300 mg/day can have a favorable effect on surrogate markers, the clinical effectiveness of this dose has not been established. The main adverse reactions described in association with AZT therapy include nausea, headache, rash, anemia, leukopenia, liver dysfunction, and myositis with elevations of the CPK (elevated CPK).

- *Didanosine (ddI, Videx®):* This is a nucleoside analogue inhibitor of the reverse transcriptase. Dosing should be adjusted according to body weight:
  - 200 mg/day (two 50 mg tablets po bid) for body weight between 35 and 49 kg
  - 400 mg/day (two 100 mg tablets po bid) for body weight between 50 and 75 kg
  Although a dose of 600 mg/day was originally proposed for individuals weighing more than 75 kg, this dose is not generally encouraged. ddI must be taken on an empty stomach (i.e., two hours after or one hour before meals). However, it can be taken together with other antiretrovirals in the context of combination therapy regimens. The main adverse effect associated with ddI include gastrointestinal intolerance, diarrhea, emotional liability, hyperamylasemia, pancreatitis, peripheral neuropathy, hyperuricemia, gout, and hypertriglyceridemia. Although poor palatability has limited the use of ddI in the past, this issue has been ameliorated with the development of a new reduced mass orange-flavored formulation.

- *Zalcitabine (ddC, Hivid®):* This is a nucleoside analogue inhibitor of the reverse transcriptase. The recommended dose is 0.75 three times daily, for a total of 2.25 mg/day. It can be taken with food. The main adverse effects associated with ddC therapy include peripheral neuropathy and painful mouth ulcers. Less frequently, hyperamylasemia and pancreatitis have occurred in the context of ddC therapy.

- *Lamivudine (3TC, Epivir®):* This is a nucleoside analogue inhibitor of the reverse transcriptase. The recommended dose is 150 mg twice daily. It can be taken with food. The main adverse effect associated with 3TC therapy is reversible neutropenia. This can be exacerbated with ZDV use and advanced HIV disease.

- *Stavudine (d4T, Zerit®):* This is a nucleoside analogue inhibitor of the reverse transcriptase.[51] The recommended dose is 40 mg twice a day (30 mg twice a day if weight is less than 60 kg). It can be taken with food. The main adverse effect associated with d4T therapy is a reversible peripheral neuropathy.

- *Saquinavir (SQV-Invirase®):* SQV is the lead compound within the protease inhibitors.[52,53] SQV has a low bioavailability (approximately 4%). Recommended dosing is 600 mg orally tid. Reduced doses (400 mg bid of each) are recommended when SQV is used in combination with RTV. A new formulation, saquinavir-SGC (1200 mg po, tid) with enhanced bioavailability is currently under development.
  Diarrhea, abdominal discomfort/pain, headache, nausea, upset stomach, mouth ulcers, dizziness, numbness/tingling in limbs, rash, itching, muscle/bone pain, muscle aches, decreased appetite, and tiredness have been reported with increased frequency among patients taking SQV. Abnormal results on laboratory tests reported include: increased ALT, AST, bilirubin, and CPK; abnormal glucose, phosphorus, and potassium serum levels; and decreased white blood cells.

- *Ritonavir (RTV - Norvir®):* RTV is a new and potent protease inhibitor.[54] Recommended dose is 600 mg orally bid. It is generally recommended to escalate the dose progressively when initiating therapy. A regimen of 300 mg bid for 2 days, followed by 400 mg bid for 2 days, followed by 500 up bid for 2 to 10 days followed by 600 mg bid thereafter has been recommended. Reduced doses (400 mg bid of each) are recommended when RTV is used in combination with SQV.
  Circumoral paresthesias are frequent. Diarrhea, vomiting, headache, numbness and tingling, muscle weakness, fever, and lightheadedness have also been described. The most frequently reported laboratory abnormalities have been liver enzyme elevations and elevations in blood lipids.
  The following list represents a partial list of the drugs that are contraindicated in patients taking RTV: Meperidine, Propoxyphene, Piroxicam, Rifabutin, Cisapride, Amiodarone, Encainide, Flecainide, Propafenone, Quinidine, Bepridil, Astemizole,

Terfenadine, Clozapine, Pimozide, Alprazolam, Clorazepate, Diazepam, Estazolam, Flurazepam, Midazolam, Triazolam, and Zolpidem. Disulfiram (Antabuse®) must not be taken concomitantly due to possible interactions with alcohol containing formulations of RTV. Also, Clarithromycin (Biaxin®), at a dose of 500 mg once daily, should be substituted for Rifabutin (Mycobutin®) without dosage adjustment for patients with normal renal function. However, it should be adjusted for patients with impaired renal function. RTV should be used with extreme caution among patients at high risk for bleeding, such as hemophiliacs.

- *Indinavir (IDV - Crixivan®):* IDV is a newer protease inhibitor of similar potency to RTV.[55] IDV should be used in combination with other antiretrovirals. Recommended dosing is 800 mg tid orally.

  A laboratory side effect that has been frequently associated with indinavir sulfate is hyperbilirubinemia and at times jaundice. Nephrolithiasis as well as microscopic hematuria can occur in 10% of treated patients. Aggressive hydration appears to decrease this. The syndrome is due to the passage of IDV in the urine. Other side effects include nausea, vomiting, diarrhea, rash, fatigue, headache, blurred vision, dizziness, or lightheadedness.

- *Nevirapine (NVP, Viramune®):* This is the lead compound within the NNRTI.[56] Best results to date have been observed in combination with ZDV and ddI in full doses among antiretroviral therapy naive patients. Used in monotherapy or as add-on therapy it tends to have a time limited effect on plasma HIV-1 RNA load and CD4 count. There is *in vitro* evidence of NVP synergy with other nucleosides, such as 3TC. Recommended dosing is 200 mg orally once daily for the initial two weeks, to be increased to 200 mg twice a day thereafter.

  Skin rash is the most common adverse event. The majority of rashes occur during the first 4 weeks of therapy. Although approximately 30% of NVP-treated patients can experience rash by 24 weeks, 80% of NVP+ddI+ZDV-treated patients were able to complete 6 months of therapy in one study. Severe rashes occurred in under 5% of patients with no instances of Stevens Johnson's Syndrome. Headache, diarrhea, nausea, fatigue, drowsiness, fever, chills, joint and muscle aches, agitation, and coughing have also been reported, although they are rarely severe enough to warrant discontinuation of NVP therapy. Isolated transient increases in GGT and less frequently alkaline phosphatase have been described, however, these are most often without clinical consequences.

  Since NVP is similar in structure to valium (a frequently prescribed sleeping medication), it is possible that some of the side effects might include drowsiness, fatigue, and difficulty with movements. Caution should be exercised when sedation is prescribed to patients receiving NVP.

- *Delavirdine (DLV, Rescriptor®):* This is an experimental NNRTI, available only through a limited access program at this time. As with NVP, DLV should be used in combination with other (preferably two) nucleosides. Recommended dosing is 400 mg orally tid.

  Headache (47%), skin rash (39%), fatigue (20%), upset stomach (10%), change in body temperature (5%), increase in liver enzymes (1–3%), faintness/dizziness/lightheadedness (3%), changes in stools (3%), leg cramps (3%), changes in dreams (1%), and eye twitching (1%). Preliminary data suggest that DLV may (at least partially) reverse ZDV resistance.

- *Loviride (LOV):* This is an experimental NNRTI, only available through a limited access program at this time.[57] As with NVP, DLV should be used in combination with other (preferably two) nucleosides.[58] Recommended dosing is 100 mg orally tid.

The known side effects of LOV include diarrhea 10%, fatigue 10%, headache 9%, and nausea 1% as well as occasional skin rash and abnormalities in liver function tests.

13.17.1 Cerebrospinal fluid (CSF) penetration of antiretrovirals

Considerable attention has been paid over the last several years to the ability of antiretroviral drugs to penetrate the CSF. This has been previously felt to be an important contributor to the decrease in the frequency of neurological complications of HIV infection reported following the introduction of AZT in the late 1980s. Preliminary data from a study conducted in Amsterdam was recently presented. In this study d4T plus 3TC were able to decrease HIV levels in CSF to the same extent as AZT plus 3TC. There were comparable decreases in plasma HIV RNA between treatment arms 12 weeks into the therapy. The mean HIV RNA in the CSF was 3.57 $\log_{10}$ at the baseline, and it decreased to below the levels of quantitation of the assay in all patients by month three. The mean absolute CSF concentration 5 hours after oral administration of the study drugs was 41 ng/ml, 56 ng/ml, and 67 ng/ml for AZT, d4T, and 3TC, respectively, in these ten patients. Contrary to previous studies, these results suggest that d4T and 3TC, in addition to AZT have substantial CSF penetration. We also know that NVP has excellent CSF penetration. In contrast, the PIs, in general, penetrate the CSF poorly.

13.17.2 Newer antiretrovirals

The list of newer antiretroviral agents currently under investigation continues to grow at a rapid pace. Among them, 1592 and lobucavir represent very promising new nucleoside analogues which have demonstrated rather exceptional antiretroviral power in preliminary human testing. Adefovir, a new nucleotide agent, is also of interest in that it has a broad antiviral spectrum, including anti-HIV effect. Preliminary testing of this compound indicates that it would be suitable for once daily administration. This will undoubtedly become a critical priority as we try to enhance compliance to available medications. Among the new protease inhibitors, nelfinavir, the soft gel formulation of saquinavir, and 141 appear rather promising. Of note, a pharmacokinetic interaction between nelfinavir and saquinavir has been confirmed, demonstrating that nelfinavir can increase the area under the curve for SQV, although not quite as dramatically as seen with RTV/SQV. Among the newer non-nucleoside reverse transcriptase inhibitors DMP-266 has entered advanced clinical testing with promising results. Of note, this agent decreases the area under the curve of IDV and possibly other protease inhibitors. A similar drug-to-drug interaction has now been confirmed for NVP, which can decrease the area under the curve for IDV and SQV by up to 30%. A lesser interaction between NVP and RTV has been described. In contrast, DLV, another NNRTI undergoing clinical investigation, has been shown to have a potentially beneficial interaction with IDV in that it can reduce the peak and increase the trough of this agent. Further evaluation of this combination therapy approach will be necessary to clarify its clinical role.

Our understanding of HIV infection and antiretroviral therapy in particular continues to evolve at a very rapid pace. The overall management of the patient with HIV infection is dictated by the level of disease activity, as indicated by the plasma viral load, and by the degree of immune deficiency, best characterized — in the absence of symptoms — by the CD4 count. As with any chronic disease, the primary care physician is best suited to coordinate care in an ongoing fashion in close collaboration with experienced specialists. As signs and symptoms of specific diseases appear, referral for special investigation and treatment should be encouraged.

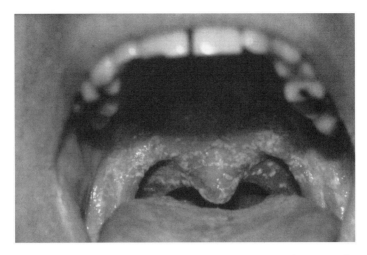

Severe case of thrush in an AIDS patient. (Photo courtesy of A.W. Hoke, M.D.)

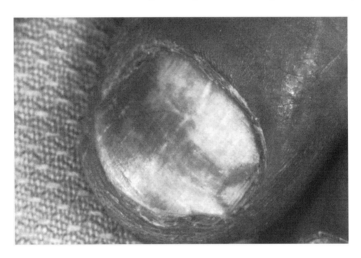

Onychomycosis. (Photo courtesy of A.W. Hoke, M.D.)

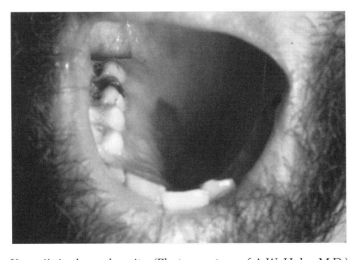

Kaposi's in the oral cavity. (Photo courtesy of A.W. Hoke, M.D.)

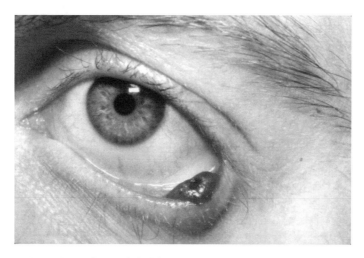

Kaposi's on the eyelid. (Photo courtesy of A.W. Hoke, M.D.)

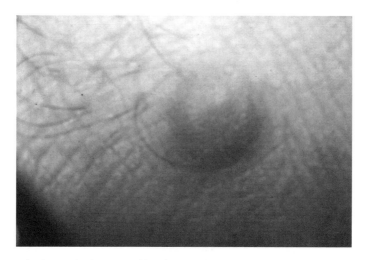

Kaposi's on the right foot which was differentiated from a histiocytoma. (Photo courtesy of A.W. Hoke, M.D.)

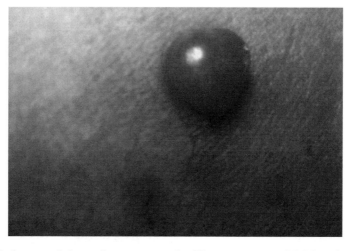

A single large nodule on the upper trunk. (Photo courtesy of A.W. Hoke, M.D.)

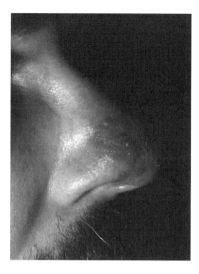

Kaposi's on the nose. (Photo courtesy of A.W. Hoke, M.D.)

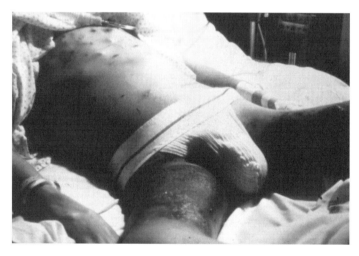

An advanced stage of Kaposi's sarcoma. (Photo courtesy of A.W. Hoke, M.D.)

References

1. Ho, D.D., Neumann, A.U., Perelson, A.S., Chen, W., Leonard, J.M., and Markowitz, M., Rapid turnover of plasma virions and CD4 lymphocytes in HIV-1 infection, *Nature*, 373, 123–126, 1995.
2. Wei, X., Ghosh, S.K., Taylor, M.E., et al., Viral dynamics in human immunodeficiency virus type 1 infection, *Nature*, 373, 117, 1995.
3. Perelson, A.S., Neumann, A.U., Markowitz, M., Leonard, J. M., and Ho, D.D., HIV-1 dynamics *in vivo*: virion clearance rate, infected cell life-span, and viral generation time, *Science*, 271, 1582–1586, 1996.
4. Coffin, J.M., HIV population dynamics *in vivo*: implications for genetic variation, pathogenesis, and therapy, *Science*, 267, 483–489, 1966.
5. Strathdee, S.A., Craib, K.J.P., Hogg, R.S., O'Shaughnessy, M.V., Montane, J.S.G., and Schechter, M.T., Long-term non-progression in HIV-infection: a cautionary note, *Lancet*, 346, 1372, 1995.
6. Stein, D.S., Korvick, J.A., and Vermud, S.H., CD4 lymphocyte cell enumeration for prediction of clinical course of human immunodeficiency virus disease: a review, *J. Infect. Dis.*, 165, 352–363, 1992.

7. Lafeuillade, A., Poggi, C., Profizi, N., Tamalet, C., and Thiebaut, C., Similar kinetics of HIV-1 replication in lymphoid organs and plasma, in Program and abstracts of the 3rd Conference on Retroviruses and Opportunistic Infections; January 28–February 1, 1996; Washington, D.C., 255.

8. Pantaleo, G., Graziosi, C., Demarest, J.M., et al., HIV infection is active and progressive in lymphoid tissue during the clinically latent stage of disease, *Nature*, 362, 355–358, 1993.

9. Piatak, M.I., Saag, M.S., Yang, L.C., et al., High levels of HIV- in plasma during all stages of infection determined by competitive PCR, *Science*, 259, 1749–1754, 1993.

10. Embretson, J., Zupancic, M., Ribas, J.L., et al., Massive covert infection of helper T lymphocytes and macrophages by HIV during the incubation period of AIDS, *Nature*, 362, 359, 1993.

11. Coombs, R.W., Welles, S.L., Hooper, C., et al., Association of plasma human immunodeficiency virus type-1 RNA level with risk of clinical progression in patients with advanced infection, *J. Infect. Dis.*, (in press) 1996.

12. Piatak, M., Saag, M.S., Yang, L.C., et al., High levels of HIV-1 in plasma during all stages of infection determined by competitive PCR, *Science*, 259, 1749–1754, 1993.

13. Havlir, D. and Richman, D.D., Viral dynamics of HIV: implications for drug development and therapeutic strategies, *Ann. Intern. Med.*, 124, 984–994, 1996.

14. Revets, H., Marissens, D., De Wit, S., et al., Comparative evaluation of NASBA HIV-RNA QT, AMPLICOR-HIV Monitor and QUANTIPLEX HIV RNA assay, three methods for quantification of Human Immunodeficiency Virus type 1 RNA in plasma, *J. Clin. Microbiol.*, 1058–1064, 1996.

15. Staprans, S.I., Hamilton, B.I., Follansbee, S.E., et al., Activation of virus replication after vaccination of HIV 1-infected individuals, *J. Exp. Med.*, 182, 1727–1737, 1995.

16. O'Brien, W.A., Grovit-Ferbas, K., Namazi, A., et al., Human immunodeficiency virus-type 1 replication can be increased in peripheral blood of seropositive patients after influenza vaccination, *Blood*, 86, 1082–1089, 1995.

17. Sharilyn, K.S., Ostrowsky, M.A., Justement, J.S., et al., Effect of immunization with a common recall antigen on viral expression in patients infected with Human Immunodeficiency Virus type 1, *N. Engl. J. Med.*, 334, 1222–1230, 1996.

18. Mellors, J.W., Kinsley, L. A., Rinaldo, C.R.J., et al., Quantitation of HIV-1 RNA in plasma predicts outcome after seroconversion, *Ann. Intern. Med.*, 122, 573–579, 1995.

19. Henrard, D.R., Phillips, J.F., Muenz, L.R., et al., Natural history of HIV-1 cell-free viremia, *JAMA*, 274, 554–558, 1995.

20. Mellors, J.W., Rinaldo, C.R., Jr., Gupta, P., et al., Prognosis in HIV-1 infection predicted by the quantity of virus in plasma, *Science*, 272, 1167, 1996.

21. Raboud, J.M., Haley, L., Mpntaner, J.S.G., et al., Quantification of the variation due to laboratory and physiologic sources in CD4 lymphocyte counts of clinically stable HIV-infected individuals, *J. Acquir. Immune Defic. Syndr.*, 10 (Suppl 2), S67–S73, 1995.

22. Hughes, M.D., Stein, D.S., Gundacker, H.M., Valentine, F.T., Phair, J.P., and Volberding, P.A., Within-subject variation in CD4 lymphocyte count in asymptomatic human immunodeficiency virus infection: implications for patients monitoring, *J. Infect. Dis.*, 169, 28–36, 1994.

23. Hammer, S.M., Katzenstein, D.A., Hughes, M.D., Hirsch, M.S., and Merigan, T.C., for the ACTG 175 Virology Substudy Team, Virologic markers and outcome in ACTG 175, in Program and abstracts of the 3rd Conference on Retroviruses and Opportunistic Infections; January 28–Febrguary 1, 1996; Washington, D.C., S24.

24. Gazzard, B., on behalf of the International Coordinating Committee, Chelsea and Westminster Hospital, London, United Kingdom, Further results from European/Australian Delta Trial, in Program and abstracts of the 3rd Conference on Retroviruses and Opportunistic Infections; January 28–February 1, 1996; Washington, D.C., LB5a.

25. O'Brien, W.A., Hartigan, P.M., Martin, D., and Esinhart, J., Changes in plasma HIV-1 RNA and CD4+ lymphocyte count relative to treatment and progression to AIDS, *N. Engl. J. Med.*, 334, 426–431, 1996.

26. Cao, Y., Qin, L., Zhang, L., Safrit, J., and Ho, D.D., Virologic and immunologic characterization of long-term survivors of human immunodeficiency virus type 1 infection, *N. Engl. J. Med.*, 332, 201–208, 1995.

27. Saag, M.S., Holodniy, M., Kuritzkes, D.R., et al., HIV viral load markers in clinical practice: recommendations of an International AIDS Society-USA Expert Panel, *Nat. Med.*, 2, 625–629, 1996.

28. Carpenter, C.C.J., Fischl, M.A., Hammer, S.M., Hirsch, M.S., Jacobsen, D.M., Katzenstein, D.A., Montaner, J.S.G., Richman, D.D., Saag, M.S., Schooley, R.T., Thompson, M.A., Vella, S., Yeni, P.G., and Volberding, P.A., Antiretroviral therapy for HIV infection in 1996. Recommendations of an international panel, *JAMA*, 276(2), 146–154, 1996.

29. BC Centre for Excellence in HIV/AIDS. Therapeutic Guidelines for the Treatment of HIV/AIDS and related conditions, 1996.

30. Schooley, R.T., Ramirez-Ronda, C., Lange, J.M.A., et al., Virologic and immunologic benefits of initial combination therapy with zidovudine and zalcitabine or didanosine compared to zidovudine monotherapy, *J. Infect. Dis.*, (in press), 1996.

31. The Delta Coordinating Committee, Delta: a randomized double-blind controlled trial comparing combinations of zidovudine plus didanosine or zalcitabine with zidovudine alone in HIV-infected individuals, *Lancet*, 348, 283–291, 1996.

32. Hammer, S.M., Katzenstein, D.A., Hughes, M.D., et al., A trial comparing nucleoside monotherapy with combination therapy in HIV-infected adults with CD4 cell counts from 200 to 500 per cubic milimeter, *N. Engl. J. Med.*, 335, 1081–1090, 1996.

33. Eron, J.I., Benoit, S.L., Jemsek, J., and MacArthur, R.D., Tretment with lamivudine, zidovudine, or both in HIV-positive patients with 200 to 500 CD4+ cells per cubic millimeter, *N. Engl. J. Med.*, 333, 1662–1669, 1995.

34. Pollard, R., Peterson, D., Hardy, D., et al., Antiviral effect and safety of stavudine (d4T) and didanosine (ddI) combination therapy in HIV-infected subjects in an ongoing pilot randomized double-blind trial, in Program and abstracts of the 3rd Conference on Retroviruses and Opportunistic Infections; January 28–February 1, 1996; Washington, D.C., 197.

35. Rouleau, D., Conway, B., Raboud, J., Patenaude, P., Schechter, M.T., O'Shaughnessy, M., and Montaner, J.S.G., A pilot open laber study of the antiviral effect of stavudine (d4T) and lamivudine (3TC) in advanced HIV disease, in Program and abstracts of the XI International Conference on AIDS; July 7–12, 1996; Vancouver, We.B.3137.

36. Montaner, J.S.G., et al., A Randomized, Double-blinded, Comparative Trial of the Effects of Zidovudine, Didanosine and nevirapine Combinations in Antiviral-naive, AIDS-free, HIV-infected Patients with CD4 Counts 200–600/mm³, in Program and abstracts of the XI International Conference on AIDS; July 7–12 1996; Vancouver.

37. Gulick, R., Mellors, J., Havlir, D., et al., Potent and sustained antiretroviral activity of indinavir (IDV) in combination with zidovudine (ZDV) and lamivudine (3TC), in Program and abstracts of the 3rd Conference on Retroviruses and Opportunistic Infections; January 28–February 1, 1996; Washington, D.C., LB7.

38. Mathez, D., De Truchis, P., Gorin, I., et al., Ritonavir, AZT, DDC, as a triple combination in AIDS patients, in Program and abstracts of the 3rd Conference on Retroviruses and opportunistic Infections; January 28–February 1, 1996; Washington, D.C., 285.

39. Cohen, C., Sun, E., Cameron, D., et al., Ritonavir-Saquinavir combination treatment in HIV-infected patients, in Program and abstracts of the 36th Interscience Conference on Antimicrobial Agents and Chemotherapy, American Society for Microbiology; September 17–20, 1996; New Orleans, LB7b.

40. Carpenter, C.C.J., Fischl, M.A., Hammer, S.M., Hirsch, M.S., Jacobsen, D.M., Katzenstein, D.A., Montaner, J.S.G., Richman, D.D., Saag, M.S., Schooley, R.T., Thompson, M.A., Vella, S., Yeni, P.G., and Volberding, P.A., Antiretroviral therapy for HIV infection in 1997. Updated recommendations of an international panel, *JAMA*, submitted, 1997.

41. Styrt, B.A., Piazza-Hepp, T.D., and Chikami, G.K., Clinical toxicity of antiretroviral nucleoside analogs, *Antiviral Res.*, 31, 121–135, 1996.

42. Piscitelli, S.C., Flexner, C., Minor, J.R., et al., Drug interactions in patients with human immunodeficiency virus, *Clin. Infect. Dis.*, 23, 685–693, 1996l.

43. Lea, A.P. and Faulds, D., Ritonavir, *Drugs*, 52, 541–546, 1996.

44. Larder, B.A., Kemp, S.D., and Harrigan, R., Potential mechanism for sustained antiretroviral efficacy of AZT-3TC combination therapy, *Science*, 269, 696–699, 1995.

45. Bartlett, J.A., Benoit, S.L., Johnson, V., et al., Lamivudine (LMV) plus zidovudine (ZDV) compared with zalcitabine (ddC) plus ZDV in patients with HIV infection, *Ann. Intern. Med.,* 124, 161–172, 1996.

46. Staszewski, S., Combination 3TC/ZDV vs. ZDV monotherapy in ZDV experienced HIV-1 positive patients with a CD4 of 100–400 cells/mm^3, in Program and abstracts of the 2nd Conference on Retroviruses and Opportunistic Infections; January 29–February 2, 1995; Washington, D.C., LB32.

47. Kahn, J.O., Lagakos, S.W., Richman, D.D., et al., A controlled trial comparing continued zidovudine with didanosine in human immunodeficiency virus infection, *N. Engl. J. Med.,* 327, 581–587, 1992.

48. Fischl, M.A., Olson, R.M., Follansbee, S.E., et al., Zalcitabine compared with zidovudine in patients with advanced HIV-1 infection who received previous zidovudine therapy, *Ann. Intern. Med.,* 762–769, 1993.

49. Spruance, S.L., Pavia, A.T., Peterson, D., et al., Didanosine compared with continuation of zidovudine in HIV-infected patients with signs of clinical deterioration while receiving zidovudine, *Ann. Intern. Med.,* 120, 360–368, 1994.

50. Montaner, J.S.G., Schechter, M.T., Rachlis, A., et al., Didanosine compared with continued zidovudine therapy for HIV-infected patients with 200 to 500 CD4 cells/mm^3. A double-blind, randomized, controlled trial, *Ann. Intern. Med.,* 123, 561–571, 1995.

51. Skowron, G., Biological effects and safety of stavudine: overview of phase I and II clinical trials, *J. Infect. Dis.,* 171(Suppl 2), S113–7, 1995.

52. Kitchen, V.S., Skinner, C., Ariyoshi, K., et al., Safety and activity of saquinavir in HIV infection, *Lancet,* 45, 952–955, 1995.

53. Vella, S., Clinical experience with saquinavir, *AIDS,* 9, 21–25, 1996.

54. Danner, S.A., Carr, A., Leonard, J.M., et al., A short-term study of the safety, pharmacokinetics, and efficacy of ritonavir, an inhibitor of HIV-1 protease, *N. Engl. J. Med.,* 333, 1528–1533, 1995.

55. Emini, E.A., Protease inhibitors, in Program and abstracts of the 3rd Conference on Retroviruses and Opportunistic Infections; January 28–February 1, 1996; Washington, D.C., L1.

56. Murphy, R. and Montaner, J., Nevirapine: a review of its development, pharmacological profile and potential for clinical use, *Exp. Opin. Invest. Drugs,* 5(9), 1183–1189, 1996.

57. Pauwels, R., Andries, K., Debyser, Z., et al., Potent and highly selective human immunodeficiency virus type 1 (HIV-1) inhibition by a series of alfa-anilinophenylacetamide derivates targeted at HIV-1 reverse transcriptase, *Proc. Natl. Acad. Sci. U.S.A.,* 90, 1711–1715, 1993.

58. Montaner, J., Cooper, D., Katlama, C., et al., CAESAR: Confirmation of the clinical benefit of 3TC (Epivir) in HIV-1 disease: Preliminary results, in Program and abstracts of the 36th International Conference on Antimicrobial agents and Chemotherapy; September 15–18, 1996; New Orleans, LB6.

Note added in Proof:

- *Nelfinavir (NFV, Viracept®):* This is a new protean inhibitor. NFV should be used in combination with other antiretrovirals. Recommended dosing is 750 mg tid orally with food. It has been associated with GI upset, particularly diarrhea. Otherwise NFV is generally very well tolerated.

chapter fourteen

Condyloma acuminatum

Michael Z. Zhang, Kenneth A. Borchardt, and Zhijiang Li

14.1   Introduction..272
14.2   Epidemiology...272
14.3   Clinical diseases..273
14.4   Clinical manifestations 273
      14.4.1   Exophytic condylomata acuminata...273
      14.4.2   HPV-associated intraepithelial neoplasia of external genitalia.................274
      14.4.3   HPV-induced cervical disease...274
      14.4.4   Urethral condylomata...274
      14.4.5   Perianal condylomata...274
      14.4.6   Condylomata acuminata of the urinary bladder..274
      14.4.7   HPV infection of the oral mucosa..275
      14.4.8   Laryngeal condyloma acuminata..275
      14.4.9   HPV associations with cancer...275
      14.4.10 Condylomata as a sign of child abuse 275
14.5   Diagnosis 275
      14.5.1   Clinical observation methods..275
      14.5.2   Cytologic (the Pap smear) and histologic methods 276
      14.5.3   DNA hybridization methods..276
14.6   Treatment...276
      14.6.1   Podophyllin..277
      14.6.2   Trichloroacetic acid 277
      14.6.3   Cryotherapy 277
      14.6.4   Surgical excision 277
      14.6.5   Chemotherapy 277
      14.6.6   Interferon 278
             14.6.6.1   Intralesional administration of IFN 278
             14.6.6.2   Systemic administration of IFN..278
             14.6.6.3   Topical administration of IFN...278
      14.6.7   Dinitrochlorobenzene (DNCB), levamisole, and BCG.................................278
      14.6.8   Vaccines...279
References...282

14.1   Introduction

Genital or venereal warts have been observed for centuries and described in outbreaks of syphilis in Europe in the late 15th century. Initially venereal warts were believed to be associated with syphilis and gonorrhea. The viral etiology of genital warts and its identification as the human papillomavirus (HPV) has been recent.[1] Genital warts or condyloma acuminata were not initially considered an important sexually transmitted disease (STD). This was the result of failure in determining the number of infections, the inability to recognize the presence or importance of subclinical infections, and an inadequate understanding of the potential carcinogenic capabilities produced by some HPV infections.[1]

Genital infections caused by HPV are becoming one of the the most prevalent STDs in the United States.[2,3] HPV is a double-stranded DNA virus. More than 70 types of HPV have been identified with similar patterns of DNA homology.[4,5] HPV-infected lesions are located in areas of sexual contact: the perineum, genitalia, crural folds, anus, or internally on the cervix and urethra.[6] The most common clinical expression of genital HPV infection is condyloma acuminatum. The incidence of condyloma acuminata has increased markedly in the last decade. Because of the development of molecular techniques, remarkable advances in HPV research have been made. Increasing evidence shows that HPVs are involved in the development of epithelial malignancies in both sexes.

The diagnosis of condyloma acuminata has been advanced by the development of molecular biological techniques. The clinical spectrum of HPV-induced lesions now includes many subclinical infections.

14.2   Epidemiology

The number of HPV infections has increased significantly in the last decade. Presently genital wart infections are recognized as the most common viral STD in the U.S., and one of the three most frequently identified STDs. HPV infections are frequent in patients with other STDs such as chlamydia, gonorrhea, syphilis, and trichomoniasis.[1] Most infections occur in sexually active populations, particularly those between the ages of 20–24. Body warmth, moist mucosal areas, and pregnancy hastens growth of genital warts. Patients with subclinical infections and either immunosuppressed by drugs or infected with human immunodeficiency virus (HIV) are susceptible to significant clinical infections.[1]

Condyloma acuminata is a disease introduced by an HPV infection. The restriction enzyme cleavage pattern of HPV DNA defines the type or subtype. A new HPV type shares less than 50% DNA homology with known types and a new subtype shares more than 50% of DNA homology with an existing type, but they differ in their restriction endonuclease cleavage patterns.[7,8] HPV particles are circular, double-stranded DNA with a diameter of 45–55 mn and contain 72 capsomeres, approximately 7900 base pairs with a molecular weight of almost 5×10^6 Dal.[8,9] HPV infections are species specific and diseases are correlated with specific HPV types. HPV types 6 and 11 have been shown to be the predominant viral types in classical condylomata acuminata warts.[3] The types involved in condyloma acuminatum have increased to sixteen: 1–6, 10, 11, 16, 18, 31, 33, 35, 39, 41, and 42.[7] HPV types 16, 18, 31, 33, 35, 39, 45, 51, and 52 have demonstrated the most significant oncogenic potential.[2,9]

Because HPV infections are not reportable and may be difficult to diagnose, an accurate incidence rate is unavailable. Between 1975 to 1978 the average incidence rate of condyloma acuminatum in all age groups was 0.1%.[3] The majority of patients were between the ages of 15–30 years with infection more frequent in women than men.

According to the Centers for Disease Control (CDC) data nationwide, 65% of patients were between 15–29 years with the greatest incidence rate in the age group between 20–24.[3] Male sexual partners of women with visible vulvar condylomata acuminata or abnormal Papanicolaou (Pap) smears were at a higher risk for acquiring HPV infection. The incubation period for the development of a clinically apparent HPV infection varied from 3 weeks to 8 months.[2] The sexual transmission of HPV infection presented problems with eradication and reinfection. Most HPV infections remained at a subclinical level, providing a reservoir for the transmission of the virus.[3]

14.3 Clinical diseases

The pathogenesis of HPV infection occurs with the entry of HPV into the basal cells of the epithelium. HPV DNA then replicates in synchrony with cellular DNA and is partitioned between dividing cells. Productive infection requires differentiation of epithelial cells, and viral structural proteins are expressed only in the fully differentiated superficial epithelial layers. Viral replication is associated with proliferation of all layers of the epithelium except the basal layer, producing acanthosis, parakeratosis, and hyperkeratosis. Animal models for HPV infection have been developed to assist defining the relationships between viral replication and the formation of characteristic HPV-induced lesions. First, human foreskin is inoculated with a condylomatous extract and implanted under the renal capsule of an athymic nude mouse. Three to four months later, condylomatous cysts develop. The mechanism of host defense to HPV infection is not defined, but clinical observations indicate that the immune system is important. Patients with both primary and an acquired immunodeficiency syndrome are susceptible to frequent and severe infections.[9] Anal warts are more frequent than penile warts in homosexual males.[10]

Women with vulvar condylomata are usually infected with HPV at multiple sites within the lower genital tract. Those with condylomata of the external genitalia may have concomitant vaginal as well as cervical infections.[2] Clinical signs such as vulvar itching, burning, and dyspareunia may be indicative of infection.[3]

14.4 Clinical manifestations

14.4.1 Exophytic condylomata acuminata

Anogenital warts have an incubation period of 1–8 months and are transmitted in approximately two thirds of sexual contacts with infected patients. The most frequent sites of infections in men are the penis, urethral meatus, and perianal area. In women the infections frequently appear in the vulva, vaginal, and cervical areas.[9] Classical exophytic condyloma presents in three forms: the hyperplastic, flat, or verrucous types. The hyperplastic condyloma is a large, moist, filiform lesion frequently present on the glans penis or the labia. A flat condyloma consists of small discrete lesions, which resemble large flat warts, and are frequently located on the glans penis. In women this condyloma appears as small flesh-colored papules studding the labia and surrounding tissue. The verrucous condyloma appears as a plain verruca vulgaris, involving the keratinized skin of the perineum.[11] A biopsy specimen of classic condyloma acuminata frequently demonstrates koilocytosis, acanthosis, and some cytologic atypia.

Anogenital warts may produce bleeding and local discomfort. Common symptoms in men are non-healing penile lesions, penile pruritus, urethral discharge, or a bloody ejaculate.[10,12] Itching, vulvar pain, and vaginal discharge can be associated with HPV infections in women.[3] Condylomata rapidly enlarge during pregnancy to produce an obstruction of the birth canal, which may develop into squamous cell carcinomas.[9] Laryngeal condyloma acuminata have been diagnosed more frequently in infants from a mother with an HPV-infected birth canal.[13] Either type 6 or 11 are reported in most cases.[11]

14.4.2   *HPV-associated intraepithelial neoplasia of external genitalia*

Recently this cluster has been called the Bowenoid papulosis (BP) group to describe its benign-appearing clinical lesions with malignant histopathology. BP is a cutaneous condition of the external genitalia primarily present in sexually active adults. Clinical evidence indicates that HPV type 16 is the etiologic agent in BP. This infection increases the risk for a higher grade cervical intraepithelial neoplasia (CIN) and invasive carcinoma.[14] BP demonstrates three growth types: flat, endophytic, and papillary exophytic. When the flat growth pattern occurs on the vulva, it may be diagnosed as vulvar intraepithelial neoplasia (VIN). One third of the patients present symptoms of pruritus. Diagnosis of VIN requires a histologic evaluation. The grading of cytologic atypia has been suggested: VIN I produces a mild atypia limited to the lower third of the vulvar squamous epithelium; VIN II involves the middle third of the epithelium with a moderate atypia; and VIN III results in a severe atypia appearing on the upper third of the epithelium.[11]

14.4.3   *HPV-induced cervical disease*

Three growth patterns are described in cervical HPV infections: flat, endophytic, and exophytic. The flat and macroscopically invisible epithelial hyperplasia of the cervix was first described in 1977. These subclinical lesions are normal in appearance, but the cytology, histology, and colposcopic features are indistinguishable from CIN. Histologic evaluation of exophytic cervical condyloma reveals marked koilocytosis. Often flat or endophytic lesions demonstrate minimum koilocytosis with dysplastic changes. CIN is graded according to the presence of cellular atypia. CIN I involves the lower one third of the epithelium with mild atypia. CIN II results in a moderate atypia involving the middle third of the epithelium, while CIN III produces a thickened epithelial atypia.[11,14] Borderline CIN indicates a diagnostic uncertainty as to whether CIN I is superimposed on a flat condyloma.[15] HPV viral DNA isolation is required to establish HPV infection.[11] Mild atypia may be produced by types 6, 11, 42, 43 or 44. Moderate or severe atypia is represented by types 16, 18, 31, 35, 45, 51, 52, and 56.[11,15]

14.4.4   *Urethral condylomata*

Condyloma frequently infect the urethral meatus or the first 4 mm of the proximal urethra. By applying a 3% acetic acid solution on the lesions, colposcopy with magnification is more effective then urinary cytology in diagnosing this urethral infection.[11]

14.4.5   *Perianal condylomata*

Perianal condylomata are observed as extensions of vulvar lesions in 80% of women with vulvar condylomata. Increasing numbers of rectal condylomata have been reported in homosexual men.[11]

14.4.6   *Condylomata acuminata of the urinary bladder*

Most lesions of condyloma occur on the external genitalia and the mucous membranes of the female urethra. An HPV infection involving the urinary bladder is rare; only 13 cases have been reported and many of these involved immunosuppressed patients.[16] Bilateral uretheral obstruction may require surgical removal of the lesions.

14.4.7   HPV infection of the oral mucosa

The lesions involving oral mucosa are classified into benign, pre-malignant, or malignant. Benign oral lesions include squamous cell papilloma, verruca vulgaris, condyloma acuminatum, and focal epithelial hyperplasia. Pre-malignant and malignant oral lesions include leukoplakia and squamous cell carcinoma. Koilocytosis is the most common cytopathic effect in both types of lesions. The benign oral lesions are associated with types 2, 4, 6, 11, 13, and 32, while the malignant oral lesions are associated with types 16 and 18. Immunocompromised patients have demonstrated unusual oral lesions associated with HPV infection.[17]

14.4.8   Laryngeal condyloma acuminata

HPV types 2, 6, and 11 are involved in this disease. Most cases reported occur in infants from an HPV-infected birth canal. There appears to be a relationship between genital warts in infected mothers and laryngeal condyloma acuminata in infants.[7]

14.4.9   HPV associations with cancer

HPV, particularly types 16, 18 31, 33, 35, and 39 are frequently observed in genital cancers.[7,10] The HPV virus has an extended latent period between exposure to the virus and the development of the malignant tumor. There is substantial clinical evidence to associate HPV with cancer. Squamous cell carcinomas are frequently observed in patients with epidermodysplasia verruciformis, which is a verrucous condition associated with specific HPV types. Also, HPV DNA has been recovered in malignancies such as epidermodysplasia verruciformis. In animal experiments HPV has produced malignant tumors both in rabbits and cattle. Finally, human HPV DNA has been discovered in certain malignancies, such as vulvar carcinoma *in situ*, cervical carcinoma *in situ*, BP, verrucous carcinoma, and squamous cell neoplasms. Clinical studies have indicated that significant numbers of patients with subclinical HPV infections may be at increased risk for cancer.[11] Recent research has demonstrated that the unexplained proliferation of cells may be associated with the interaction of the proteins transcribed by HPV viral genes E6 and E7, and the cellular proteins transcribed by two recently identified tumor suppressor genes, P53 and RB.[10]

14.4.10   Condylomata as a sign of child abuse

Condyloma acuminata in infants and children may indicate sexual abuse.[11] A clinician should be cognizant of the posibility of sexual abuse when examining a child with condylomata acuminata.

14.5   Diagnosis

Visible genital warts constitute only a minority of HPV infections. Specialized testing is required to detect other evidence of HPV infection, particularly those subclinical. The majority of subclinical infections are undetectable by routine examination.[2]

14.5.1   Clinical observation methods

Condylomata are readily recognized either as cauliflower-like projections or flat papular lesions. Molluscum contagiosum may be confused with anogenital warts. Identification of subclinical HPV infections requires the application of acetic acid which increases the sensitivity of the examination. This procedure involves soaking the skin of the genital area with vinegar or 3% acetic acid for 5 min, and then examining the skin either directly or under magnification. The skin will appear a shiny white as the result of the acetic acid. The lesions of intraepithelial neoplasia appear either dull gray or dull white after the application of the acetic acid.[12] Three types of subclinical lesions have been defined: vestibular papillae, fused papillae, or aceto-white epithelium. Vestibular papillae lesions appear as multiple small villous projections of mucous membranes of the vulva. Fused papillae refer to fused vulvar skin, which demonstrates a granular rather than villous appearance. Aceto-white epithelium is a normal-appearing vular epithelium, which has had acetic acid applied. HPV DNA are isolated from all three types of subclinical lesions.[12]

Androscopy is an effective method for examination of male genitals with a colposcope after applying a vinegar solution to the skin. This may identify lesions that are inapparent on gross inspection. Any male who has had sexual contact with a partner diagnosed with condyloma acuminatum, dysplasia, or cancer of the genital tract should be examined by androscopy.[18]

14.5.2 Cytologic (the Pap smear) and histologic methods

Koilocytosis is the cytopathic effect induced by a HPV infection in epithelium, which results in a large cell with a hyperchromatic nucleus and a perinuclear clear ring in the cytoplasm. Electron microscopy has been used to identify HPV-sized particles in some tissue specimens because many HPV-infected tissues fail to exhibit koilocytosis.[8] Immuno-staining is a more sensitive and useful method, which employs specific antibodies reacting with HPV within the infected tissue. Antibodies are coupled with horseradish peroxidase or biotin for tissue staining.[12]

14.5.3 DNA hybridization methods

This is the most frequently employed method for detecting HPV infections and differentiating HPV types in research laboratories. The principle of DNA hybridization requires a DNA molecule containing a radioactive label. It is introduced in a reaction that will bind to either an identical DNA molecule or a closely related one. The binding is then detected and analyzed.

The Southern blot test is the most commonly employed test to detect and type HPV. DNA is extracted from the specimen, cut into specific fragments, and then separated according to size. Then the separated fragments are transferred to a solid membrane support which is exposed to the HPV DNA of a labeled, cloned type. In a positive test, the labeled probe binds to the membrane. This test is highly specific and sensitive — it can detect one HPV DNA molecule per 10 cells or less. The major disadvantages of the test are its labor intensity and the period required before reading.

One frequently employed method is the filter *in situ* hybridization assay, which detects HPV in cells collected by cervical scrapes. Another commonly used technique is the tissue *in situ* hybridization assay that identifies HPV in tissue sections.

Presently, the most sensitive test is the polymerase chain reaction (PCR) technique. It has the potential for significant future inplementation. This test requires only a small segment of HPV DNA to be amplified and identified. PCR has been reported to detect as little as one viral genome in 10^5 cells.[12]

14.6 Treatment

None of the treatment modalities available for HPV infection are specific. The major treatments are either cytotoxic or destructive.[6] The purpose of treatment includes the eradication of condylomata or dysplastic tissues, the reduction of symptoms, and preventing subsequent transmission.[11] Recrudescence is a predominant problem and there may be reinfection by sexual partners, therefore, use of condoms should be recommended to all patients. Sexual partners should be examined and effectively treated when necessary.

14.6.1   Podophyllin

The resin from the North American *Podophyllin peltatum* and Indian *Podophyllin emodi* plants is a cytotoxic agent. Podophyllin is used ubiquitously as an initial treatment for condyloma acuminatum.[19] Podophyllotoxin is the active agent, which binds to tubulin, the protein subunit of the spindle microtubules. This prevents normal spindle assembly and arrests mitosis in the metaphase, which results in subsequent epithelial cell death. Podophyllin is typically applied as a 10–25% solution in a tincture of benzoin and is washed off after 2–4 h. Protection of surrounding normal tissue with petrolatum or collodion is recommended to decrease the systemic absorption and local irritation. The CDC has recommended that condylomata acuminata be treated with a 10% solution of podophyllin resin once or twice weekly. When there is no response after four applications, alternative therapy should be initiated. Podophyllum is not recommended for treating either mucous membrane tissue or pregnant women because of potential local or systemic toxicity. Localized pain, burning, edema, and erosions are found in 10–15% of patients treated with podophyllin. Acute systemic toxicity produces nausea, vomiting, abdominal pain, and diarrhea. Delayed systemic reactions include bone marrow suppression, central nervous system effects, renal failure, and death. Early studies indicated that the cure rates for podophyllin were greater than 90%.[11]

14.6.2   Trichloroacetic acid

Trichloroacetic acid, as a 50–85% solution in 70% alcohol, may be substituted when podophyllin is ineffective.[19] Topical application may produce an intense skin irritation lasting for 3–5 min. The solution is applied to the affected area with a cotton swab every other day for 3–4 weeks.[10]

14.6.3   Cryotherapy

This was the initial therapy recommended by CDC STD Treatment Guidelines in 1985.[19] Liquid nitrogen cryotherapy is commonly used. The precision of laser treatment affords destruction of condylomata with the preservation of normal tissue.[12] A 91% cure rate has been reported in condylomata previously treated unsuccessfully with podophyllin. Because treatment with nitrogen may be painful when applied to mucous membranes, anesthesia is recommended for both adults and children.[11]

14.6.4   Surgical excision

After surgical removal there is a significant rate of recurrence. Because of the extended latency in normal surrounding skin of HPV infections, it is difficult to extirpate all HPV-infected tissue.

14.6.5   Chemotherapy

A topical 5% 5-fluorouracil (5-FU) has been used for the treatment of condyloma acuminata. It inhibits DNA and RNA synthesis and prevents cellular proliferation. Adverse effects include erosive vulvitis, vulvar irritation, and vaginal discharge. Topical 5-FU is not recommended in treating pregnant women because of its teratogenic effects.[11,12]

14.6.6   Interferon

Interferons (IFNs) are a group of biologically active glycoproteins with antiviral, antipro-liferative, and immunomodulatory properties.[5,10] IFNs are classified into three types: alpha, beta, and gamma. Alpha originate from leukocytes or lymphoblasts infected with virus, beta are derived from fibroblasts exposed to double-stranded RNA and gamma develop from lymphocytes stimulated by mitogens or by an antigen to which they have been sensitized.[11,12,20,21] The natural available IFN is alpha, which can be derived from pooled, stimulated leukocytes. Recombinant alpha, beta, and gamma IFNs have been developed. IFNs affect viral infections by various mechanisms by inducing the production of enzymes against viral replication. IFNs may act on host defenses by: increasing lymphocytotoxic activity of natural killer lymphocytes; enhancing IgE-mediated histamine release from basophils; increasing macrophage phagocytosis or antibody-dependent cell-mediated cytotoxicity; and either suppressing or stimulating antibody responses.

14.6.6.1   Intralesional administration of IFN
This produces a relatively high local concentration of IFN in the injected wart. Clinical studies have demonstrated the effectiveness of the intralesional administration of IFN in the treatment of condyloma acuminata. A 10^6 IU dosage of alpha-2 IFN has been employed 3 times a week for 3 weeks on patients unsuccessfully treated with podophyllin.[20,21]

14.6.6.2   Systemic administration of IFN
This regimen may be used to treat both clinical and subclinical infections. Unfortunately the problems of systemic toxicity and inadequate delivery to infected tissue has limited its effectiveness.[20]

14.6.6.3   Topical administration of IFN
Early studies reported successful treatment in 90% of patients, but subsequent studies have not confirmed these results.[11]

   A recombinant alpha IFN and a natural alpha IFN have been approved for the treat-ment of condylomata acuminata in the U.S. Recombinant IFN differs from natural INF by one amino acid substitution.[6] The recombinant alpha IFN is available in vials with various quantities, but only the 10 million IU vial is used for condylomata. It is reconstituted with 1 ml of bacteriostatic water for injection. Once reconstituted, the resulting solution is stable for 1 month at 5°C. A dose of 0.1 ml is injected into the base of each lesion three times per week and on alternate days for 3 weeks. A tuberculin or 1-ml syringe is used with a 30-gauge needle. As many as five lesions may be treated simultaneously and additional lesions subsequently. The natural alpha IFN injection is available in 5 million IU vials containing 1 ml of fluid per vial. It does not require dilution and can be stored at 5°C for more than 6 months. A dose of 0.1 ml is injected into the base of each lesion using a tuberculin or 1-ml syringe with a 30-gauge needle twice per week for 8 weeks. The most common sequelae for either local or parenteral IFN administration are flu-like symptoms, such as myalgias, fever, chills, headache, nausea, and fatigue.[6,11] Acetaminophen can be added to the IFN solution to alleviate flu-like symptoms. A blood count and blood chem-istry are recommended before treatment with IFN and at regular intervals following treatment.[20]

14.6.7   Dinitrochlorobenzene (DNCB), levamisole, and BCG

DNCB is a nonspecific stimuli to cell-mediated immunity and has been used with success for treating condyloma acuminata. Local tissue response and absorption results in high serum levels which restrict its use. Neither levamisole or BCG are frequently used in treatment because of ineffective results.[11]

14.6.8   Vaccines

A specific HPV vaccine would be the most effective therapeutic regimen, unfortunately none is available. Problems with purity, preparation, and potential side effects have prevented the employment of autogenous vaccines in the U.S. A significant void exists because of this.[11]

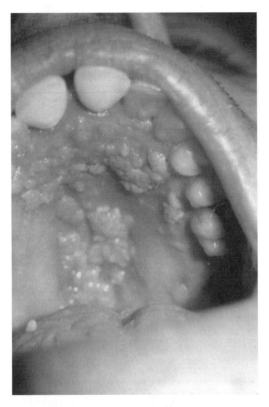

Oral warts in HIV patient. (Photo courtesy of A.W. Hoke, M.D.)

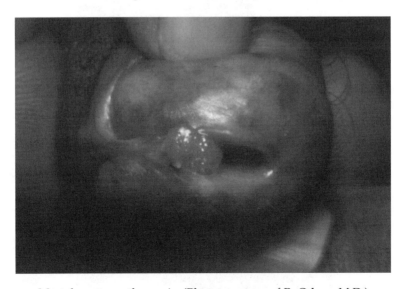

Meatal warts on the penis. (Photo courtesy of R. Odom, M.D.)

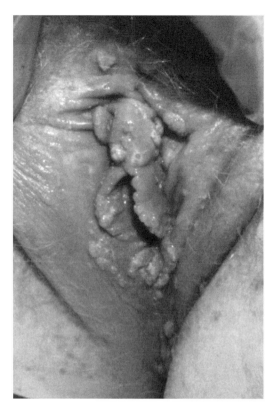

Vaginal warts. (Photo courtesy of A.W. Hoke, M.D.)

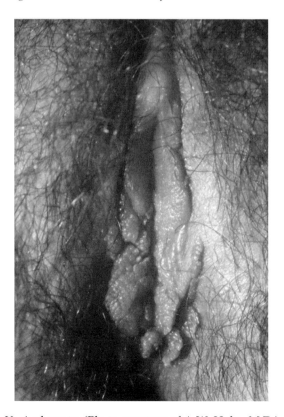

Vaginal warts. (Photo courtesy of A.W. Hoke, M.D.)

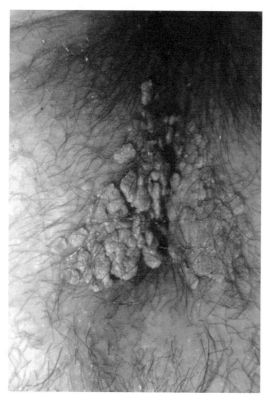

Anal warts. (Photo courtesy of A.W. Hoke, M.D.)

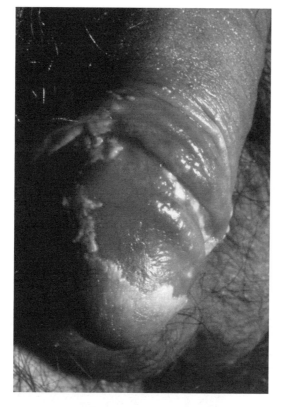

Irritation reaction to patient treated with podophyllin (Photo courtesy of A.W. Hoke, M.D.)

References

1. Horn, J., Genital human papillomavirus infection: new challenges from an old STD culprit, *STB Bull.*, 9, 3, 1989.
2. Krowchuk, D.P., Anglin, T.M., Genital human papillomavirus infections in adomescents: implications for evaluation and management, *Semin. Dermatol.*, 11, 24, 1992.
3. Deitch, K.V., Smith, J.E., Symptoms of chronic vaginal infection and microscopic condyloma in women, *J. Obst., Gynecol., Neonat. Nurs.*, 19(2), 133, 1990.
4. Franco, E.L., Human papillomavirus and the natural history of cervical cancer, *Infect. Med.*, 57, 1993.
5. Moscicki, A.-B., Genital human papillomavirus infections, *Adolesc. Med.*, 1, 451, 1990.
6. Browder, J.F., Araujo, O.E., Myer, N.A., Flowers, F.P., The interferons and their use in condyloma acuminata, *Ann. Pharmacother.*, 26(1), 42, 1992.
7. Chuang, T.-Y., Condylomata acuminata (genital warts), an epidemiologic view, *J. Am. Acad. Dermatol.*, 16, 376, 1987.
8. Syrjanen, K.J., Human papillomavirus (HPV) infections of the female genital tract and their associations with intraepithelial neoplasia and squamous cell carcinoma, *Pathol. Ann.*, 1, 53, 1986.
9. Reichman, R.C., Strike, D.G., Pathogenesis and treatment of human genital papillomavirus infections: a review, *Antiviral Res.*, 11(3), 109, 1989.
10. Maymon, R., Shulman, A., Maymon, B., Bekerman, A., Werchow, M., Faktor, J.H., Altaras, M., Penile condylomata: a gynecological epidemic disease: a review of the current approach and management aspects, *Obstet. Gynecol. Sur.*, 49(11), 790, 1994.
11. Clark, D.P., Condyloma acuminata, *Dermatol. Clin.*, 5(4), 779, 1987.
12. Brown, D.R., Fife, K.H., Human papillomavirus infection of the genital tract, *Med. Clin. N. Am.*, 74(6), 1455, 1990.
13. Kalter, D.C., Rosen, T., Sexually transmitted diseases, *Emer. Med. Clin. N. Am.*, 3(4), 693, 1985.
14. Stafford, E.M., Greenberg, H., Miles, P.A., Cervical intraepithelial neoplasia III in an adolescent with Bowenoid papulosis. *J. Adolescent Health Care*, 11(6), 523, 1990.
15. Fox, H., Buckley, C.H., Current problems in the pathology of intraepithelial lesions of the uterine cervix, *Histpathology*, 17(1), 1, 1990.
16. Ginsberg, P.C., Williams, J.J., Klaus, R.L., Bilateral ureteral obstruction secondary to condylomata acuminata of the urinary bladder, *J. Am. Osteopath. Assoc.*, 89(1), 69, 1989.
17. Garlick, J.A., Taichman, L.B., Human papillomavirus infection of the oral mucosa, *Am. J. Dermatopathol.*, 13(4), 386, 1991.
18. Epperson, W.J., Preventing cervical cancer by treating genital warts in men. Why male sex partners need androscopy, *Postgrad. Med.*, 88(5), 229, 1990.
19. Marcus, J., Camisa, C., Podophyllin therapy for condyloma acuminatum, *Int. J. Dermatol.*, 29(10), 693, 1990.
20. Lebwohl, M., Contard, P., Interferon and condylomata acuminata, *Int. J. Dermatol.*, 29(10), 699, 1990.
21. Finter, N.B., Chapman, S., Dowd, P., Johnston, J.M., Manna, V., Sarantis, N., Sheron, N., Scott, G., Phua, S., Tutum, P.B., The use of interferon-alpha in virus infections, *Drugs*, 42(5), 749, 1991.

chapter fifteen

Molluscum contagiosum

Zhijian Li, Kenneth A. Borchardt, and Michael Z. Zhang

15.1 Introduction..283
15.2 Etiology..283
15.3 Epidemiology...284
15.4 Pathogenesis..285
15.5 Clinical manifestations 285
15.6 Diagnosis 286
15.7 Treatment...287
References..289

15.1 Introduction

The characteristic appearance of molluscum contagiosum (MC) was first described by Bateman in 1817.[1] In his treatise, the disorder was called *molluscum*, which was a common term for pedunculated lesions. It was identified as *contagiosum* to signify its transmissibility, which he believed was due to "milky fluid" that could be expressed from the lesion. MC is a benign papular lesion of the skin and mucous membranes which is sexually transmitted in adults. It is caused by the *Molluscum contagiosum* virus (MCV), a member of the poxvirus family. A significant increase in the frequency of MCV has occurred in the sexually active adult society in the United States in recent years, primarily as a sexually transmitted disease (STDs) and in HIV-infected individuals.[2-4]

15.2 Etiology

MCV has been purified from skin lesions and is considered to be a poxvirus on the basis of size, structure, chemical composition, physical characteristics, and behavior.[5-8] Ultrastructural studies of MCV revealed a brick-shaped particle, approximately $300 \times 200 \times 100$ nm in dimension, consisting of a biconcave viral core enclosed by an inner membrane and an outer envelope. The viral genome consists of a single molecule of linear double-stranded DNA, with terminal or near-terminal intrastrand covalent links; its molecular weight is 118 M (178 kb).[9] Characteristic of the poxvirus family, MCV replicates in the cytoplasm in discrete electron-dense areas described as "viral factories."[5,10,11] However, MCV lacks serologic cross-reactivity with other family members and is unable to rescue other types of heat-inactivated poxviruses in mixed infection by the process known as nongenetic reactivation.[5,12]

Attempts at experimental cultivation of MCV have been unsuccessful. There is currently no *in vitro* system for cultivation of MCV. Electron microscopic studies indicate that the virus particles penetrate the cell by phagocytosis, undergo envelope uncoating, then progress to the stage of free virus cores within 8 to 12 h. The cytopathic changes of cell swelling, rounding, and clumping appear within 24 h and appear to require early viral gene function since they can be blocked by inhibitors of RNA and protein synthesis. The characteristic cytopathic effect is transitory, however, regressing within 4 days and disappearing during serial propagation of cell lines after three to four passages.[5,11,13]

An evaluation of virions from skin lesions by SDS-PAGE identified seven major polypeptides and showed variability between patients, suggesting a potential for use in strain evaluation.[14] The evaluation of viral DNA may be a more powerful tool for molecular analysis. Limited studies reported a similar restriction endonuclease pattern among epidemiologically related lesions,[15] the cloning of MCV DNA, and its use in restriction enzyme analysis.[9] Based on restriction endonuclease analysis of MCV DNA, there appear to be two major strains, MCV-1 and MCV-2, although the two strains cannot apparently be differentiated by gross pathology of the lesions.[7-9,16-19]

15.3   *Epidemiology*

Characterization of the epidemiology of infection with MCV has been limited by several factors. In most patients, the lesions cause few problems and are self-limited.[5,20] It is likely that many infected patients do not seek medical attention, and there are few population-based data on those patients who do since MC is usually not reportable. Furthermore, there is currently no *in vitro* system for cultivation of MCV, which has restricted studies of virus transmission, asymptomatic infections, and seroprevalence and limited epidemiologic studies of detection of characteristic clinical lesions by physical examination.[5,9]

MC has a worldwide distribution with reports ranging from Alaska,[21] New Guinea,[22] and Scotland.[12] The disorder mainly affects children, sexually active adults, and immunocompromised individuals. Epidemiologic studies suggest that transmission may be related to factors such as warmth and humidity of climate[23] and poor hygiene.[12,24] But another study indicated that close contact with the index case was more important than climate or hygiene. MC developed in 35% of exposed family members, and the majority of cases occurred in families with average to excellent hygienic standards.[21]

The range of ages was from 3 months to 57 years. Early epidemiologic studies supported the hypothesis of MC being primarily a disorder of children, with a peak incidence at 10–12 years of age.[12,22] The peak ages of occurrence (20–29 years) were similar to those of other STDs,[3,5,20,25] although the age of infections in women were younger than men.[25]

The incidence of MC is increasing in the sexually active populations. There has been a statistically significant increase in the number of patient visits for MC over a 17-year period, increasing from 10,600 in 1966 to 113,800 in 1983. The proportion of patient visits attributable to MC increased from 1.2 per 100,000 visits in 1966 to 11.0 per 100,000 visits in 1983. In the U.S. the increase in cases occurred uniformly. Men were diagnosed only slightly more frequently than women.[25]

Transmission of MC appears to occur by both sexual and nonsexual routes.[5,20,26] It has been diagnosed in wrestlers, masseurs, a surgeon, and after steam and sauna bathing.[12] In adults, lower abdominal, thigh, and genital lesions are more frequent than those in extragenital locations.[5,20]

The infection has been diagnosed in immunocompromised hosts. Most infected patients appear to have a deficiency in either the function or absolute numbers of T lymphocytes. A heterogeneous group of diseases has been described in association with disseminated MC, including atopic dermatitis,[27] epidermodysplasia verruciformis,[28] and selective IgM deficiency.[29] MC has been reported in patients with sarcoidosis,[30] chronic lymphocytic leukemia,[31] and treatment with prednisone and methotrexate.[32]

MC is a common cutaneous disorder seen in patients with HIV infection. The association was first reported in 1983 when it was noted in an autopsy study that 2 of 10 patients with AIDS had MC lesions.[33] Since 1983, there have been frequent reports of MC in patients with HIV infection.[34-41] The prevalence in this population may be as high as 5-18%.[42-46] Because the life expectancy of patients with HIV infection is now extended, the prevalence of MC in this population can be expected to increase. It also appears likely that MC will be seen in other groups of profoundly immunocompromised patients, such as those who have undergone organ transplantation and those maintained on immunosuppressive agents.

15.4 Pathogenesis

MCV is a natural pathogen of humans, especially children.[47] The pathologic changes induced by MCV infection are very characteristic and generally limited to the epidermis. MC lesions consist of focal areas of hyperplastic epidermis surrounding cyst-shaped lobules filled with keratinized debris and degenerating molluscum bodies. In the basal layer, the nuclei and cytoplasm of the keratinocytes are enlarged.

The cells by the spindle layer begin to display cytoplasmic vacuolation and enlargement and then replacement by eosinophilic compartmentalized globules, the molluscum bodies. These compress the nuclei to the cell periphery. In the granular layer, the molluscum bodies become more homogeneous with loss of their internal structural markings and are finally desquamated into the cystic lobules.[5,10,12]

The role of host immunity in the control of MCV infection has been poorly defined. Because of the greater prevalence of lesions in children than in adults,[22,48] host resistance may increase with age. The inflammatory reaction suggests evidence of a cell-mediated immune response to MCV antigens, because the appearance of inflammation often precedes the resolution of lesions.[49] Case reports of widespread lesions in patients with impaired T-cell function, especially those with AIDS, indicate the importance of cell-mediated immunity.[37,50] The role of humoral immunity remains unclear, but the presence of low levels of antibody in most patients, regardless of disease duration, suggests that it must be minor.[5,51]

15.5 Clinical manifestations

The incubation period for MC averages between 2–3 months, with a range from 1–6 months.[5,20,52] In most patients, the lesions are self-limited.[5,20] Lesions develop as tiny pinpoint papules which grow over several weeks to a diameter of 3–5 mm. Infrequently a lesion enlarges to 10–20 mm, producing the "giant molluscum."[20,34,53,54] Typically a lesion appears as a smooth-surfaced, firm, spherical papule, with an average diameter of 3–5 mm.[55] They usually appear white, translucent, or light yellow in color.[56]

In adults lesions most frequently occur on the thighs, inguinal region, buttocks, and lower abdominal wall. They usually are not present either on the external genitalia, perianal region, or mucosal surfaces. This pattern contrasts with the distribution of genital warts. Children typically develop lesions on the face, trunk, and extremities. Lesions on the palms, soles, and mucous membrane are rare. When a linear distribution of lesions occurs, it suggests autoinoculation by scratching.[20] MC may appear intraorally, periorally, intraocularly, and periocularly where it presents as trachoma or chronic follicular conjunctivitis associated with lesions of the lips.[57] In normal hosts, the number of lesions usually varies between 10–20, ranging from 1–100. A patient with impaired immunity can develop hundreds of lesions.[5,20,37,50] Patients with abnormal cell-mediated immunity are at risk of developing extensive outbreaks of lesions. MC has been observed in patients with sarcoidosis, Hodgkin's disease, AIDS, and in those receiving immuno-suppressive therapy.[5,27,37,50]

The most commonly noted complications associated with MC include irritation, inflammation, and secondary infection. Lesions on the eyelids may be associated with a follicular or papillary conjunctivitis, but superficial punctuate keratoses rarely result.[58] The most common complication of MC is bacterial superinfection, which occurs in approximately 40% of cases. Another sequelae is "molluscum dermatitis," which appears 1–15 months after the onset of skin lesions in approximately 10% of patients. The dermatitis consists of a sharply bordered eczematoid reaction 3–10 cm in diameter surrounding individual lesions. It may involve only a few lesions, and usually disappears as the lesion resolves.[5]

The average duration of an untreated MC infection is approximately 2 years, and ranges from 2 weeks to 4 years. Individual lesions usually resolve within 2 months. Recurrences of lesions after clearance have been noted in 15–35% of patients; whether these represent new infections or exacerbation of subclinical or latent infection is not clear.

15.6   Diagnosis

The clinical diagnosis of MC is apparently on the basis of its characteristic pearly, umbilicated papule with the caseous center. The papule appears on the face, trunk, extremities, or genital region. Lesions may be misdiagnosed either as genital warts or keratoacanthomas. Other considerations in the differential diagnosis include syringomas, plane warts, lichen planus, epithelial and intradermal nevi, seborrheic dermatitis, basal cell epithelioma, infection with herpes simplex and varicella-zoster virus, and atopic dermatitis.[5,20,59]

In atypical cases the diagnosis may be confirmed by demonstrating the pathognomonic enlarged epithelial cells with intracytoplasmic molluscum bodies in cytologic or histologic studies. Thinly spread smears of material expressed from lesion cores stained by Wright, Giemsa, or Gram stain will demonstrate sheets of infected cells. Hematoxylin eosin stained sections of punch biopsies will reveal the characteristic epidermal histopathologic changes.[5,20]

Other diagnostic techniques include detection of MCV antigen employing fluorescent antibody or visualization of the abundant viral particles by electron microscopy.[5] Antibodies to MC can be identified in lesions, regardless of duration. Serum antibodies are measurable by complement fixation, tissue culture neutralization, fluorescent antibody, and gel agar diffusion techniques.[58] The lack of standardization and extensive evaluation of serologic tests precludes their routine use.[60]

The differential diagnosis may be broad due to the usual clinical picture with which MC sometimes presents. In a study of 42 cases of MC diagnosed by skin biopsy, only 8 were correctly suspected by clinical examination.[61] The other clinical diagnoses included basal cell carcinoma, histiocytoma, keratoacanthoma, intradermal nevus, Darier's disease, nevoxanthoendothelioma, syringoma, epithelial nevi, sebaceous adenoma, atopic dermatitis, dermatitis herpetiformis, mycosis fungoides, and Jessner's lymphocytic infiltration.

MC has also been mistaken for leukemia cutis.[62] Several authors have reported cutaneous cryptococcus presenting as molluscum-like eruptions. *Cryptococcus neoformanus* is an encapsulated yeast present in soil, dust, and pigeon excreta. It typically induces pulmonary disease, but as many as 20% of patients with cryptococcosis have cutaneous involvement. Cutaneous cryptococcosis can precede systemic symptoms by 2–8 months, and may be the first sign of HIV infection.[63,64]

15.7   Treatment

In treatment of MC, it is important to utilize therapy that does not exacerbate the disease. Although MC may be self-limited and asymptomatic in healthy individuals, therapy is warranted to prevent autoinoculation or transmission of the virus to close contacts. In general, treatments have focused on removing the cutaneous lesion either by surgery or producing epidermal injury, with subsequent desquamation of the molluscum and surrounding uninvolved skin.

Curettage has been advocated as an effective treatment in children,[65,66] adults with genital lesions,[67] and in patients with advanced HIV disease.[68] Freezing with ethyl chloride before curettage and the use of caustic agents such as 1% tincture of iodine, podophyllin, or trichloroacetic acid are an effective combination therapy. Light electrodesiccation may be used after curettage.[67] Cryotherapy with liquid nitrogen spray has been successful.[69]

Cantharidin, prepared as a 0.9% solution in equal parts of acetone and flexible collodion, was successfully used to treat 12 patients with a total of 250 lesions. The preparation was effective in all patients after 1–3 treatments, with a 7-day interval between treatments. A 0.5% solution of cantharidin was ineffective. Tromovitch and Allen (1966) recommended using a 0.7% cantharidin mixture with an occlusive dressing of plastic tape.[70]

Successful therapy with topical vitamin A acid (tretinoin) has been described in two patients with genital lesions. Twice daily applications of 0.1% tretinoin was prescribed in one patient with resolution of the lesions after 11 days of therapy, although he experienced scrotal irritation. A similar result was obtained in the second patient using 0.05% tretinoin cream. Effective treatment has been observed with the highest tolerated concentration of tretinoin being applied nightly, which reduced the size and frequency of new lesions.[68,71]

Griseofulvin has been used orally in five patients with MC at dosages of 500 mg daily to patients over 14 years of age and 250 mg to younger patients. The patients had lesions for 15–30 days before treatment and treatment was given for 4–6 weeks. In all patients the lesions began to regress within 2 weeks and resolved within 6 weeks after therapy was initiated. No recurrence was seen in the 6–8 month follow-up period.[72]

Another treatment approach involves expressing the contents of the central lesion followed by application of a caustic agent or light electrodesiccation.[55] Caustic agents that have been used include silver nitrate, phenol, carbolic acid, tincture of iodine, podophyllin, cantharidin, tretinoin, and trichloroacetic acid. Treatment with any of these methods usually results in healing without scarring, as the viral replication is a superficial process limited to the epidermis. Unfortunately, recurrence is frequent even when using tretinoin, particularly among AIDS patients. Even persistent treatment may fail to prevent the rapid recurrence of MC.[2] Immunocompromised patients, particularly those infected with HIV, often have large and numerous MC, which do not resolve spontaneously and are refractory to treatment.[73]

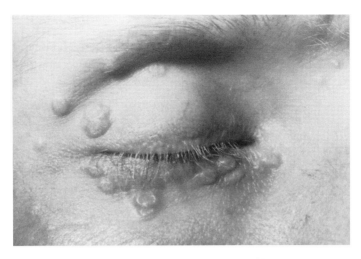

Atypical presentation of *Molluscum contagiosum* on the eyelids of an AIDS patient. (Photo courtesy of A.W. Hoke, M.D.)

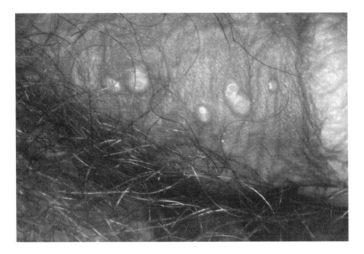

Molluscum contagiosum on the penis. (Photo courtesy of R. Odom, M.D.)

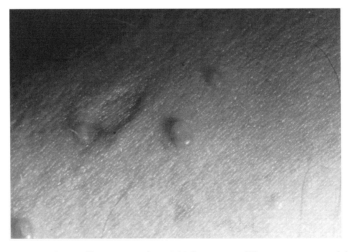

Molluscum contagiosum in the axillary area of an AIDS patient. (Photo courtesy of A.W. Hoke, M.D.)

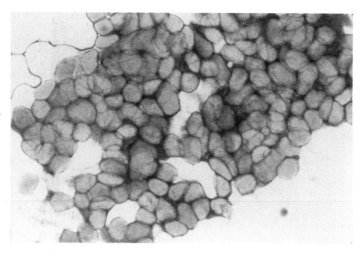

Molluscum contagiosum microscopic at 100×. (Photo courtesy of A.W. Hoke, M.D.)

References

1. Douglas, J.M., Molluscum contagiosum, in *Sexually Transmitted Diseases,* 2nd ed., Holmes, K.K., Mardh, P., Sparling, P.F., et al., eds., New York, 1990.
2. Lombardo, P.C., Molluscum contagiosum and the acquired immunodeficiency syndrome, *Arch. Dermatol.,* 121, 834, 1985.
3. Oriel, J.D., The increase in molluscum contagiosum, *Br. Med. J.,* 294, 74, 1987.
4. Penneys, N.S. and Hicks, B., Unusual cutaneous lesions associated with acquired immuno-deficiency syndrome, *J. Am. Acad. Dermatol.,* 13, 845, 1985.
5. Brown, S.T., et al., Molluscum contagiosum, *Sex.Trans. Dis.,* 8, 227, 1981.
6. Pierard-Frenchimont, C., Legrain, A., and Pierard, G.E., Growth and regression of molluscum contagiosum, *J. Am. Acad. Dermatol.,* 9, 669, 1983.
7. Porter, C.D. and Archard, L.C., Characterization and physical mapping of molluscum con-tagiosum virus DNA and location of a sequence capable of encoding a conserved domain of epidermal growth factor, *J. Gen. Virol.,* 68, 673, 1987.
8. Scholz, J., Rosen-Wolff, A., Bugert, J., Reisner, H., White, M.I., Darai, G., and Postlethwaite, R., Molecular epidemiology of molluscum contagiosum, *J. Infect. Dis.,* 158, 898, 1988.
9. Darai, G., Reisner, H., Scholz, J., et al., Analysis of the genome of molluscum contagiosum virus by restriction endonuclease analysis and molecular cloning, *J. Med. Virol.,* 18, 29, 1986.
10. Reed, R.J. and Parkinson, R.P., The histogensis of molluscum contagiosum, *Am. J. Surg. Pathol.,* 1, 161, 1977.
11. Epstein, W.L. and Fukuyama, K., Maturation of molluscum contagiosum virus (MCV) *in vivo*: Quantitative electron microscopic autoradiography, *J. Invest. Dermatol.,* 60, 73, 1973.
12. Postlethwaite, R., Molluscum contagiosum: a review, *Arch. Environ. Health,* 21, 432, 1970.
13. McFadden, G., et al., Biogenesis of pox-viruses: transitory expression of molluscum conta-giosum early functions, *Virology,* 94, 297, 1979.
14. Oda, H., et al., Structural polypeptides of molluscum contagiosum virus: their variability in various isolates and location within the virion, *J. Med. Virol.,* 9, 19, 1982.
15. Parr, R.P., Burnett, J.W., and Garon, C.F., Structural characterization of the molluscum con-tagiosum virus genome, *Virology,* 81, 247 1977.
16. Bugert, J.J. and Darai, G., Stability of molluscum contagiosum virus DNA among 184 patient isolates, *J. Med. Virol.,* 33, 211, 1991.
17. Porter, C.D., Blake, N.W., Archard, L.C., et al., Molluscum contagiosum virus types in genital and non-genital lesions, *Br. J. Dermatol.,* 12, 37, 1989.
18. Scholz, J., Rosen-Wolff, A., Bugert, J., et al., Epidemiology of molluscum contagiosum using genetic analysis of the viral DNA, *J. Med. Virol.,* 27, 87, 1989.

19. Thompaon, C.H., DeZwart-Steffe, R.T., and Briggs, I.M., Molecular epidemiology of Australian isolates of molluscum contagiosum, *J. Med. Virol.*, 32, 1, 1990.

20. Felman, Y.M. and Nikitas, J.A., Sexually transmitted molluscum contagiosum, *Dermatol. Clin.*, 1, 103, 1983.

21. Overfield, T.M. and Brody, J.A., An epidemiologic study of molluscum contagiosum in Anchorage, Alaska, *J. Pediatr.*, 69, 640, 1966.

22. Sturt, R.J., Muller, H.K., and Francis, G.D., Molluscum contagiosum in villages of the West Sepik district of New Guinea, *Med. J. Aust.*, 2, 751, 1971.

23. Mihara, M., Three-dimensional ultrastructural study of molluscum contagiosum in the skin using scanning-electron microscopy, *Br. J. Dermatol.*, 125, 557, 1991.

24. Pirie, G.D., Bishop, P.M., Burke, D.C., and Postlethwaite, R., Some properities of purified molluscum contagiosum virus, *J. Gen.Virol.*, 13, 311, 1971.

25. Becker, T.M., Blount, J.H., Douglas, J., and Judson, F.N., Trends in molluscum contagiosum in the United States, 1966–1983, *Sex. Trans. Dis.*, 13, 88, 1986.

26. Niizeki, K., et al., An epidemic study of molluscum contagiosum: relationship to swimming, *Dermatologica*, 169, 197, 1984.

27. Pauly, C.R., Artis, W.M., and Jones, H.E., Atopic dermatitis, impaired cellular immunity, and molluscum contagiosum, *Arch. Dermatol.*, 114, 391, 1978.

28. Slawsky L.D., Gilson, R.T., Hockley, A.J., and Libow, L.F., Epidermodysplasia verruciformis associated with severe immunodeficiency, *J. Am. Acad. Dermatol.*, 27, 448, 1992.

29. Mayumi, M., Yamoaka, K., Tsutsui, T., et al., Selective immunoglobulin M deficiency associated with disseminated molluscum contagiosum, *Eur. J. Pediatr.*, 145, 99, 1986.

30. Ganpule, M. and Garrets, M., Molluscum contagiosum and sarcoidosis: report of a case, *Br. J. Dermatol.*, 85, 587, 1971.

31. Cotton, D.W., Cooper, C., Barret, D.F., and Leppard, B.J., Serve atypical molluscum contagiosum infection in an immunocompromised host, *Br. J. Dermatol.*, 116, 871, 1987.

32. Rosenberg, E.W. and Yusk, J.W., Molluscum contagiosum: eruption following treatment with prednisone and methotrexate, *Arch. Dermatol.*, 101, 439, 1970.

33. Reichert, C.M., O'Leary T.J., Levens, D.L., et al., Autopsy pathology in the acquired immunodeficiency syndrome. *Am. J. Pathol.*, 112, 357, 1983.

34. Betloch, I., Pinazo, I., Mestre, F., and Altes, J., Molluscum contagiosum in human immunodeficiency virus infection: response to zidovudine, *Int. J. Dermatol.*, 28, 351, 1989.

35. Concus, A.P., Helfand, R.F., Imber, M.J., et al., Cutaneous cryptococcus mimicking molluscum contagiosum in a patient with AIDS, *J. Infect. Dis.*, 158, 897, 1988.

36. Hira S.K., Wadhawan, D., Kamanga, J., et al., Cutaneous manifestations of human immunodeficiency in Lusaks, Zamba, *J. Am. Acad. Dermatol.*, 19, 451, 1988.

37. Katzman, M., Carey, J.T., Elmets, C.A., et al., Molluscum contagiosum and the acquired immunodeficiency syndrome: clinical and immunologic details of two cases, *Br. J. Dermatol.*, 116, 131, 1987.

38. Katzman, M., Elmets, C.A., and Lederman, M.M., Molluscum contagiosum and the acquired immunodeficiency syndrome, *Ann. Intern. Med.*, 102, 413, 1985.

39. Kohn, S.R., Molluscum contagiosum in patients with acquired immunodeficiency syndrome, *Arch. Ophthalmol.*, 105, 458, 1987.

40. Charles, N.C. and Frieberg, D.N., Epibulbar molluscum contagiosum in acquired immunodeficiency syndrome, *Ophthalmology*, 99, 1123, 1992.

41. Sulica, R.L., Kelly, J., Berberian, B.J., and Glaun, R., Cutaneous cryptococcosis with molluscum contagiosum coinfection in a patient with acquired immunodeficiency syndrome, *Cutis*, 53, 88, 1994.

42. Goodman, D.S., Teplitz, E.D., Wishner, A., et al., Prevalence of cutaneous disease in patients with acquired immmunodeficiency syndrome (AIDS) or AIDS-related complex, *J. Am. Acad. Dermatol.*, 17, 210, 1987.

43. Matis, W.L., Triana, A., Shaoiro, R., et al., Dermatologic findings associated with human immunodeficiency virus infection, *J. Am. Acad. Dermatol.*, 17, 746, 1987.

44. Coldiron, B.M. and Bergstrasser, P.R., Prevalence and clinical spectrum of skin disease in patients infected with human immunodeficiency virus, *Arch. Dermatol.*, 125, 357, 1989.

45. Koopman, R.J.J., Van Merrienboer, F.C.J., Vreden, S.G.S., and Dolmans, W.M.V., Molluscum contagiosum: a marker for advanced HIV infection, *Br. J. Dermatol.*, 126, 528, 1992.

46. Schwartz, J.J. and Myskowski, P.L., Molluscum contagiosum in patients with human immunodeficiency virus infection: a review of twenty-seven patients, *J. Am. Acad. Dermatol.*, 27, 583, 1992.

47. Buller, R.M.L. and Palumbo, G.J., Poxvirus pathogenesis, *Microbiol. Rev.*, 55, 80,1991.

48. Murray, M.J., et al., Molluscum contagiosum and herpes simplex in Maasai pastoralists: Refeeding activation of virus infection following famine?, *Trans. R. Soc. Trop. Med. Hyg.*, 74, 371, 1980.

49. Kipping, H.F., Molluscum dermatitis, *Arch. Dermatol.*, 103, 106, 1971.

50. Redfield, R.R., James, W.D., Wright, D.C., et al., Severe molluscum contagiosum infection in a patient with human T cell lymphotrophic (HTLV-III) disease, *J. Am. Acad. Dermatol.*, 13, 821, 1985.

51. Shirodaria, P.V. and Matthews, R.S., Observation on the antibody responses in molluscum contagiosum, *Br. J. Dermatol.*, 96, 29, 1977.

52. Hawley, T.G., The natural history of molluscum contagiosum in Fijian children, *J. Hyg.*, 68, 631, 1970.

53. Fivenson, D.P., Weltman, R.E., and Gibson, S.H., Giant molluscum contagiosum presenting as basal cell carcinoma in an acquired immunodeficiency syndrome patient, *J. Am. Acad. Dermatol.*, 19, 912, 1988.

54. Linberg, J.V. and Blaylock, W.K., Giant molluscum contagiosum following splenectomy, *Arch. Ophthalmol.*, 108, 1076, 1990.

55. Felman, Y.M. and Nikitas, J.A., Genital molluscum contagiosum, *Cutis*, 26, 28, 1980.

56. Mroczkowski, T.F., Molluscum contagiosum, in *Sexually Transmitted Disease*, Mroczkowski, T.F., ed., Igakushoin, New York, 1990, 157.

57. Whitaker, S.B., Wiegand, S.E., and Budnick, S.D., Intraoral molluscum contagiosum, *Oral Surg. Oral Med. Pathol.*, 72, 334, 1991.

58. Felman, Y.M., Molluscum contagiosum, *Cutis*, 33, 113, 1984.

59. Dennis, J., et al., Molluscum contagiosum, another sexually transmitted disease: its impact on the clinical virology laboratory, *J. Infect. Dis.*, 151, 376, 1985.

60. Williams, L.R., and Webster, G., Warts and molluscum contagiosum, *Clin. Dermatol.*, 9, 87, 1991.

61. Mehregan, A.H., Molluscum contagiosum: a clinicopathologic study, *Arch. Dermatol.*, 81, 173, 1961.

62. Ackerman, A.B. and Tanski, E.V., Pseudoleukemia cutis, report of a case in association with molluscum contagiosum, *Cancer*, 40, 813, 1977.

63. Picon, L., Vaillant, L., Duong, T., et al., Cutaneous cryptococcosis resembling molluscum contagiosum: a first manifestation of SIDA, *Acta Derm. Vernereol. (Stockholm)*, 69, 365, 1989.

64. Schupbach, C.W., Wheeler C.E., Briggaman, R.A., et al., Cutaneous manifestations of disseminated cryptococcus, *Arch. Dermatol.*, 112, 1734, 1976.

65. Rosdahl, I., Edmar, B., Gisslen, H., et al., Curettage of molluscum contagiosum in children: analgesia by topical application of a lidocaine/prilocaine cream(EMLA), *Acta Derm. Venereol. (Stockholm)*, 68, 149, 1988.

66. de Waard-van der spek, F.B., Oranje, A.P., Lillieborg, S., et al., Treatment of molluscum contagiosum using a lidocaine/prilocaine cream (EMLA) for analgesia, *J. Am. Acad. Dermatol.*, 4, 685, 1990.

67. Olansky, S. and Clair, A., How we treat molluscum contagiosum, *Postgrad. Med.*, 47, 259, 1970.

68. Garrett, S.J., Robinson, J.K., and Roenogk, H.H., Trichloroacetic acid peel of molluscum contagiosum in immunocompromised patients, *J. Dermatol. Surg. Oncol.*, 18, 855, 1992.

69. Boulier, I.C., Myskowski, P.L., and Torre, D.P., Disposable attachments in cryosurgery: a useful adjunct in the treatment of HIV-associated neoplasma, *J. Dermatol. Surg. Oncol.*, 17, 277, 1991.

70. Tromovitch, T.A. and Allen, J.C., Molluscum contagiosum, *Cutis*, 2, 21, 1966.

71. Papa, C.M. and Berger, R.S., Veneral herpes-like molluscum contagiosum: treatment with tretinoin, *Cutis*, 18, 537, 1976.

72. Singh, O.P. and Kanwar, A.J., Griseofulvin therapy in molluscum contagiosum, *Arch. Dermatol.*, 113, 1615, 1977.

73. Beutner, K.R., Cutaneous viral infections, *Pediatr. Ann.*, 22, 247, 1993.

The gay bowel syndrome

chapter sixteen

The gay bowel syndrome: a 20-year retrospective

Walter F. Schlech III

16.1 Introduction...296
16.2 Epidemiology...296
    16.2.1 General epidemiologic features of the gay bowel syndrome....................296
    16.2.2 Epidemiologic features of specific infections associated with
    the gay bowel syndrome 297
        16.2.2.1 Viral infections...297
            16.2.2.1.1 Viral hepatitis..297
            16.2.2.1.2 Human herpes viruses 298
            16.2.2.1.3 Human papilloma virus.....................................298
            16.2.2.1.4 Human immunodeficiency virus.......................298
        16.2.2.2 Bacterial infections 299
            16.2.2.2.1 *N. gonorrhoeae* 299
            16.2.2.2.2 *T. pallidum* 299
            16.2.2.2.3 *Chlamydia trachomatis* 299
            16.2.2.2.4 Intestinal spirochetosis 299
            16.2.2.2.5 *Campylobacter* infections 300
            16.2.2.2.6 *Shigella* infections..300
            16.2.2.2.7 *Salmonella* infections.......................................300
            16.2.2.2.8 *Mycobacterium avium intracellulare* infection.............300
        16.2.2.3 Protozoal infections...300
            16.2.2.3.1 *Giardia lamblia*..300
            16.2.2.3.2 *Entamoeba histolytica* 301
            16.2.2.3.3 Other amebae..301
            16.2.2.3.4 *Cryptosporidium* species 301
            16.2.2.3.5 Microspordia 301
            16.2.2.3.6 *Isospora belli*...301
            16.2.2.3.7 Other parasites..301
16.3 Clinical features of the gay bowel syndrome...301
    16.3.1 Proctitis 302
    16.3.2 Proctocolitis 303
    16.3.3 Enteritis 304

0-8493-9476-7/97/$0.00+$.50
© 1997 by CRC Press LLC

16.4 Diagnostic studies in the gay bowel syndrome..304
    16.4.1 History and physical examination 304
    16.4.2 Microbiologic studies..305
    16.4.3 Endoscopic biopsy 305
    16.4.4 Serologic studies..305
16.5 Treatment...306
References 307

16.1 Introduction

The term "gay bowel syndrome" was coined in 1976 by Kazal and colleagues who had established a large proctologic practice among gay men. The focus in their original papers[1,2] was on sexually transmitted and traumatic conditions of the perianus and rectum confirmed by proctologic examination and evaluable by a limited number of visual and laboratory clues. While this description of the syndrome provided a valuable starting point for a prospective assessment, the data were largely anecdotal and subject to referral bias. Prospective studies spearheaded by the Seattle STD Clinic[3,4] using more sophisticated laboratory techniques, expanded the clinical concept from perianal and rectal disease to include proctitis, proctocolitis, and enteritis in this patient population. Useful diagnostic and treatment algorithms were developed to incorporate new information on the management of the condition. The gay bowel syndrome now included the classical sexually transmitted infectious diseases as well as a wide variety of traditional enteric infections.[5-7]

The last chapter in gay bowel syndrome may not have been written, but recognition of the gastrointestinal complications of HIV infection in the last decade has greatly expanded the number of pathogens broadly considered as part of the gay bowel syndrome.[8,9] In addition, the concept of opportunistic neoplasm of the gastrointestinal tract associated with oncogenic transmissible viral infection has been recognized.[10,11] Offsetting this expansion of diagnostic possibilities has been a decrease in the transmission of STDs through behaviorial change in the gay community directed at avoiding HIV transmission.[12,13]

16.2 Epidemiology

16.2.1 General epidemiologic features of the gay bowel syndrome

For the viral, bacterial, and protozoan pathogens responsible for the gay bowel syndrome two major modes of transmission have been described. In the first, contact exposure of the rectal mucosa to a variety of pathogens occurs through rectal intercourse. The source of the organism could be the skin of the penis or the ejaculate, depending on the site of infection in the initial host. The susceptibility of the rectal mucosa to infection is enhanced by the trauma associated with rectal intercourse.[14] Trauma itself in its most severe manifestations can lead to intestinal perforation and perineal sepsis.[15,16] The injury may be associated with unusual sexual practices such as "fisting" or the use of dildos or other objects for sexual gratification. These occurrences fortunately are rare and will not be further discussed as part of the gay bowel syndrome.

The second important mode of transmission is through the fecal-oral route. In this setting the lower bowel and rectum is colonized by the transmissible pathogen. The practice of anilingus ("rimming") or in extreme cases, coprophagy, may result in transmission to the sexual partner.[17,18] Transmission may also occur when fellatio follows rectal intercourse if sexual partners take both active and passive roles in anal intercourse. Judson has succinctly stated the important role of fecal-oral transmission in the spread of enteric disease:

> "... by providing direct fecal-oral contact, anilingus circumvents several thousand years of public health progress aimed at separating human excreta from food and water supplies ..."[19]

For some infections the specific contribution of sexual or fecal-oral transmission is difficult to ascertain and both may apply.

A number of factors have contributed to the high rates of enteritis, proctocolitis, and proctitis in the male homosexual population in comparison to heterosexual men and women. These risk factors have been extensively looked at, particularly in the study of HIV transmission, and include contact with a large number of different sexual partners, the relative anonymity of these sexual contacts, and the increased likelihood in gay men that rectal infection may be asymptomatic or not visibly apparent. It has also become clear that genital ulcer disease, which includes rectal ulcerative disease in men having sex with men, may predispose transmitting other pathogens such as HIV infection.[20] The incidence of rectal infection with the traditional sexually transmitted pathogens such as *Neisseria gonorrhoeae*[12] and *Treponema pallidum*[13] has decreased in recent years and suggests that educational efforts to mitigate these risk factors have been at least partially successful in the gay community. Recent increases in these infections in some studies do provide cause for concern, however.[21,22] Prospective data on the acquisition of enteric pathogens is not readily available, although outbreaks of hepatitis A continue to occur among gay men.[23,24]

If the use of the term "gay" also refers to lesbians, the little data that are available suggest that the gay bowel syndrome is no more common in this group than in heterosexual populations. The frequency of anal intercourse in heterosexual relationships also appears to be low. Rectal infection with *N. gonorrhoeae* in heterosexual women is frequent but probably reflects perineal colonization as a primary source rather than anal receptive intercourse.[25]

16.2.2   Epidemiologic features of specific infections associated with the gay bowel syndrome

16.2.2.1   Viral infections

16.2.2.1.1   Viral hepatitis.

Hepatitis A — Hepatitis A or "infectious hepatitis" is transmitted by the fecal-oral route and was one of the first enteric infections described as part of the gay bowel syndrome.[26] Serologic surveys of gay men have shown high seroprevalence rates for hepatitis A[27] and outbreaks of hepatitis A continue to occur in this population.[23,24] Both icteric and anicteric infections occur followed by lifelong protection from reinfection. Analysis of risk factors during epidemics of hepatitis A have demonstrated that anilingus and the number of sexual partners are independent risk factors for infection.[27,28]

Hepatitis B — Hepatitis B continues to be an important infection in gay men with seroprevalence rates for hepatitis B markers averaging 50–60%, ten times higher than would be expected in the general population even in areas where injection drug use is high.[29] Hepatitis B can be found in feces, but transmission is most associated with passive rectal intercourse and rectal mucosa injury.[30,31] Semen or blood are the transmitting vehicles. Anicteric infection is common and chronic hepatitis B carriage appears more common in homosexual than heterosexual populations who have acquired hepatitis B.[32] The prevalence of hepatitis e antigen, a marker for infectivity, is also higher in gay men.

Hepatitis C — Hepatitis C is more frequently found in gay men, although injection drug using populations are at highest risk.[33,34] As in hepatitis B, this parentally transmitted agent can be acquired through rectal intercourse and studies of predominantly HIV-infected populations of gay men have shown that anti-HCV antibodies are present at a

10-fold greater rate than in other populations.[35] A recent comparison of hepatitis C and hepatitis B infections in homosexual men from San Francisco demonstrated that HCV infection was associated with >50 sexual partners per year, >25 oral receptive partners per year, and >25 anal receptive partners per year.[36] HBV infection was more strongly associated with the same practices and rates of hepatitis C were only 4.6% in this population. Fecal-oral transmission is probably less important for hepatitis C transmission than direct inoculation by semen or blood.

16.2.2.1.2 Human herpes viruses.

Herpes simplex virus — Herpes simplex virus (HSV) is the most common cause of transmissible proctitis after *N. gonorrhoea* in gay men.[36] HSV 2 is most frequently found, but transmission of HSV 1 by oral-anal sexual activity does occur. Approximately 25% of gay men presenting with anal rectal pain will be experiencing a primary HIV infection of the rectum.[37] Serologic analyses suggest that only 20% are relapsing infections,[37] but in gay men with advanced HIV infection recurrent painful, indolent ulceration of the perianal and perianus and rectum is common.[38] Asymptomatic shedding of virus probably occurs in the same frequency as in heterosexual men and women.

Other human herpes viruses — Primary infection with human cytomegalovirus (CMV), Epstein-Barr virus (EBV), and HSV 6, and 7 does not cause primary disease of the intestinal tract. Some of these viruses, however, are more common in gay men and may be acquired through anal intercourse.[39-41] The primary risk factor for infection is the number of sexual partners. The role of local trauma to the rectum in transmission is uncertain.

Recently a new human herpes virus (HHV-8) has been described in association with Kaposi's sarcoma.[42] This opportunistic neoplasm is most frequently seen in gay men with advanced HIV infection and often involves the gastrointestinal tract. Kaposi's sarcoma is infrequent in other risk groups for HIV infection including transfusion recipients and injection drug users, suggesting that it is caused by a sexually transmitted agent. It is likely that passive rectal intercourse would contribute to transmission, although data are not yet available to confirm this. The emphasis on safer sexual practices which has resulted in a decrease in sexually transmitted infections in gay men in recent years has been paralleled by a decrease in the prevalence of Kaposi's sarcoma in men with HIV infection.[43]

16.2.2.1.3 Human papilloma virus.

Condyloma acuminatum or genital warts caused by the human papilloma virus (HPV) is the most frequent infection of the perianal and rectal area in gay men. Early series suggested that 50% of men presenting with perianal or rectal complaints had this infection.[1,2] Transmission of the virus is by direct inoculation and trauma is an important contributing factor.[44] Perirectal disease is also found in heterosexual men and women not engaging in rectal intercourse, but condylomata present above the anal verge in these groups are rare.

Molecular techniques have allowed identification of many different strains of HPV.[45] These different types are responsible for phenotypic variation in the appearance of the warts. More importantly, some types which are responsible for cervical cancer in women may also be associated with atypia of the anal mucosa and frank anal carcinoma in gay men.[46] Anal carcinoma is considered an opportunistic neoplasm in men with advanced HIV infection,[49] as is cervical carcinoma in HIV-infected women.

16.2.2.1.4 Human immunodeficiency virus.

HIV infection has become an integral part of the gay bowel syndrome in the last decade. Primary HIV infection has been associated with gastrointestinal ulceration primarily involving the oropharynx and esophagus.[49] It is a self-limited condition. Subsequently, the immunosuppression associated with HIV infection modifies the presentation of other STDs such as syphilis[49] and enteric diseases.[48] Advanced HIV infection has also led to the description of a new generation of bacterial and protozoan pathogens responsible for the gay bowel syndrome. Finally, HIV itself has been described as a cause of "HIV enteropathy," a wasting syndrome associated with diarrhea and malabsorption.[51]

16.2.2.2   Bacterial infections

16.2.2.2.1   N. gonorrhoeae.   Until recently, *N. gonorrhoeae* has been the most common cause of proctitis in gay men.[4] While the contribution of passive rectal intercourse to acquisition of gonorrhoeae in heterosexual women is uncertain, anal rectal intercourse is the primary mode of transmission in gay men.[25] Studies carried out twenty years ago in several STD clinics demonstrated prevalence rates of 28–44%.[25,52-54] However, with the recognition of the role of rectal intercourse in the transmission of HIV infection, significant decreases in the rates of anorectal gonorrhea have occurred.[55,56] Clinic studies in the 1980s have therefore demonstrated lower rates of infection in the range of 8–10%.[57] Prospective studies, however, have found increases in rates of rectal gonorrhoeae, particularly among young gay men in the 1990s suggesting that preventative messages about condom use are not being reinforced in this population.[22]

16.2.2.2.2   T. pallidum.   Anorectal syphilis is transmitted by direct contact of primary and secondary lesions of the penis with the rectal mucosa or the reverse. Perianal chancres can also develop and occasionally the organism may be transmitted from an oral infection by anilingus. Prospective studies have shown that about half the cases of newly diagnosed primary and secondary syphilis occur in gay men[58, 59] and 1–5% of gay men presenting to an STD clinic have evidence of primary or secondary syphilis. Intuitively, anal intercourse would be responsible for a majority of these cases, but because asymptomatic disease is common in syphilis this risk factor has not been fully studied. Genital ulcer disease including syphilis is associated with a higher risk of HIV acquisition in heterosexual women and in homosexual men.[58,59] While rates of syphilis, like gonorrhea, have decreased among gay men, recent data suggest that new infections continue to occur in this population despite the threat of acquiring HIV infection.[22]

16.2.2.2.3   Chlamydia trachomatis.   Rectal *C. trachomatis* infections are common in gay men and approach the frequency of gonococcal infection.[5] Coinfection with *N. gonorrhoeae* in the rectum occurs but not with the same frequency (15–20%) as seen in gonococcal urethritis. Direct inoculation of the mucosa by contaminated ejaculate is the presumed mode of transmission. The clinical syndrome associated with rectal *Chlamydia* infection is dependent on the serotype; the lymphogranuloma venereum serovars (L1, 2, and 3),[5,60] while much rarer, cause more severe illness. Serovars D-K are associated with asymptomatic carriage or milder forms of proctitis. Rates of 3-10% in various studies of gay men have been found.[61] Some differences in the distribution of serovars causing rectal infection in men and cervical infection in women have been found,[62] but the clinical significance of these differences is uncertain. Certain serovars may survive better at the rectal mucosa interface, a phenomenon that has been documented for *N. gonorrhoeae* strains.[63]

16.2.2.2.4   Intestinal spirochetosis.   Anaerobic intestinal spirochetes cause dysentery in swine,[64] and intestinal spirochetes have been isolated in a high proportion of homosexual men (30–40%) with and without symptoms[65,66] in comparison to heterosexual populations. The genus *Brachyspira aalborgii* has been used to describe these organisms.[67] In a comparative study of rectal biopsies from 130 symptomatic and asymptomatic gay men, intestinal spirochetosis was found in 30%.[66] Most of these men had gastrointestinal symptoms but no correlation of the histologic features of spirochetosis with symptoms was found. Intestinal spirochetosis has also been found in HIV-infected men with persistent diarrhea,[68] but the contribution of this organism to symptomatic disease is still undetermined. The mode of transmission is similarly uncertain but may involve fecal-oral transmission.

16.2.2.2.5   Campylobacter infections.   *Campylobacter jejuni* causes proctocolitis in gay men and occurs in 5–10% of men presenting with gastrointestinal symptoms.[7] Approximately half this number may carry the organism asymptomatically, a prevalence rate similar to that found in heterosexual populations. A larger proportion of gay men with and without symptoms carry *Campylobacter*-like organisms when stools or rectal swabs are screened using selective media for *Campylobacter* sp.[7] Taxonomic studies are incomplete. The species names *C. cinaedi* and *C. fenneliae* were originally described,[69] but these organisms are now considered to be in the *Helicobacter* genus. *C. jejuni*, *C. fetus*, and these two "new" *Campylobacter* species have also been isolated from the bloodstream in immunocompromised HIV-infected patients with a sepsis syndrome.[70]

16.2.2.2.6   Shigella infections.   Shigellosis causes 3–4% of symptomatic proctitis in gay men and is a much less common enteric infection than *Campylobacter*.[3,4,71] Transmission is by direct contact or indirectly from fecal-oral contamination. *Shigella flexneri* appears to be the most common cause of shigellosis in gay men followed by *S. sonniae*.[72] Surveillance for *Shigella* infection in a number of cities with large gay populations have demonstrated substantially more cases in males than females, in some cases representing 70% of reports. Recent data in the AIDS era are not available for enteric infections in general and *Shigella* specifically, but infection rates for enteric infections may not have decreased to the same extent as routes for gonorrhea or syphilis. Sepsis with *Shigella* is extraordinarily rare but has been described in patients with advanced HIV infection.[73]

16.2.2.2.7   Salmonella infections.   *Salmonella* infections are primarily foodborne in gay men as well as in heterosexual populations, but fecal-oral transmission of the typhoidal and non-typhoidal strains has been described anecdotally in gay men.[74,75] It is more commonly described in heterosexual patients in the developing world then in gay men, emphasizing the minor contribution of *Salmonella* to the gay bowel syndrome. *Salmonella* sepsis occurs in HIV and non-HIV-infected men and women, but recurrent *Salmonella* sepsis is an AIDS-defining condition.

16.2.2.2.8   Mycobacterium avium intracellulare infection.   Gastrointestinal infection with this pathogen has only been described with the onset of the AIDS epidemic. Disseminated *M. avium intracellulare* (MAI) infection, which includes infiltration of the gastrointestinal subepithelium and lymphatics with malabsorption and diarrhea, is an AIDS-defining diagnosis.[76] Some studies suggest that 40% of patients with AIDS may develops disseminated MAI infection.[77] The risk of MAI infection increases dramatically when CD4 cell counts are less than 100 cm/mm. Sexual transmission and fecal-oral transmission probably do not play a role in this infection which is acquired from the environment and possibly from potable water.[78]

16.2.2.3   Protozoal infections

16.2.2.3.1   Giardia lamblia.   Giardiasis was one of the earliest recognized causes of enteritis in gay men which was discovered when disproportionate number of cases occurred in single men in New York who had not traveled.[79,80] Prospective studies of the gay bowel syndrome have confirmed these earlier observations and rates of *Giardia* infections have been found in 5–20% of gay men presenting to STD clinics with gastrointestinal symptoms.[81,82]

16.2.2.3.2 Entamoeba histolytica. *Entamoeba histolytica* can be identified in the stool of gay men with and without diarrhea.[81,82] However, invasive amebiasis and liver abscess is generally not seen in gay men and the proportion of *Entamoeba* strains capable of causing invasive disease is not clear. Prospective studies have suggested that nonpathogenic xynodemes are responsible for most of the organisms found in the stool[83] and are not responsible for gastrointestinal symptoms. Sexual transmission of amebae appears likely because of the high carriage rates in gay men in comparison to heterosexual populations and is probably secondary to fecal-oral transmission rather than fecal contamination of water sources in the developing world.

16.2.2.3.3 Other amebae. Mixed protozoa infections are extremely common in gay men with prospective studies identifying colonization rates of 50–60%. Nonpathogenic amebae make up approximately 50% of this group.[84] Species found on stool examination include *Entamoeba coli, Entamoeba nana, Iodamoeba butschlii, Entamoeba hartmanni, Dientamoeba fragilis,* and *Blastocystis hominis.*[18] The contribution of these agents to diarrheal syndromes in gay men is very uncertain as is the specific mode of transmission for most of these agents.

16.2.2.3.4 Cryptosporidium species. Cryptosporidiosis owes its recognition as a gastrointestinal pathogen to the AIDS epidemic.[85] Initial descriptions of profuse chronic watery diarrhea in gay men with advanced immunosuppression caused by this organism were followed by its identification as a cause of sporadic self-limited diarrhea in noncompromised populations.[86,87] While animal exposure has been identified as a risk factor in some outbreaks of cryptosporidiosis in healthy patients, the source of *Cryptosporidia* in gay men is unclear. Fecal-oral transmission may be important, but an environmental source is probably responsible for most infections, even in this population.[86,87,92]

16.2.2.3.5 Microsporidia. Electron microscopic studies in AIDS patients with diarrhea and malabsorption have identified several small noninvasive parasites collectively called microsporidia, infecting the gastrointestinal mucosa. Five genus designations have been determined — *Nosema* sp., *Encephalitozoon* sp., *Pleistophora* sp., *Enterocytozoon bieneusi,* and *Septata intestinalis.*[88] Like cryptosporidiosis and isosporiasis this infection has been primarily described in gay men with advanced HIV infection. The mode of transmission and the environmental source remain unknown but sexual transmission seems unlikely.

16.2.2.3.6 Isospora belli. The gastrointestinal syndrome caused by *Isospora belli* is identical to cryptosporidiosis in patients with advanced HIV infection.[89] The relative frequency of isosporiasis, in comparison to cryptosporidiosis and microsporidiosis, has not been determined in prospective studies of men with advanced HIV infection. It appears less common than cryptosporidiosis but more common than microsporidiosis according to anecdotal reports.

16.2.2.3.7 Other parasites. Description of other parasitic infections in gay men have been primarily anecdotal but include *Enterobius vermicularis,*[90] *Trichuris* sp.,[91] and strongyloidiasis (*Strongyloides stercoralis*).[92] Fecal-oral transmission may be possible with these agents, particularly when anilingus is a risk factor. Disseminated strongyloidiasis has been described in patients with AIDS but the mode of transmission is uncertain.[92]

16.3   Clinical features of the gay bowel syndrome

Initial descriptions of the gay bowel syndrome focused on perianal, anal, and rectal abnormalities in gay men including the various traumatic conditions, anal fistula, and

Table 1   Microorganisms Associated with the Gay Bowel Syndrome

Syndrome	Organism
Asymptomatic/local lesion[a]	HPV
	T. pallidum
	E. histolytica
	N. gonorrhoea
	Helicobacter sp.
	B. aalborgi
	Nonpathogenic amebae
	C. trachomatis (non-LGV)
Proctitis	HSV-1 and HSV-2
	N. gonorrhoea
	C. trachomatis
	T. pallidum
Proctocolitis	CMV[b]
	C. trachomatis (LGV variants)
	Shigella sp.
	E. histolytica
	B. aalborgi
	Campylobacter sp.
	Salmonella sp.
Enteritis	CMV[b]
	HIV
	Campylobacter sp.
	Salmonella sp.
	M. avium intracellulare
	Cryptosporidia sp.
	Isospora belli[b]
	Microsporidia[b]
	Giardia lamblia
	Strongyloides stereoralis

[a] The organisms noted may cause symptomatic disease as well.

[b] In advanced HIV infection.

abscesses.[1] In expanding the syndrome, Quinn et al. divided cases into three entities based on their clinical features and microbial cause.[3] These included proctitis, proctocolitis, and enteritis as well as asymptomatic conditions of the lower gastrointestinal tract as determined by examination, biopsy, or other laboratory studies. The organisms associated with each syndrome are summarized in Table 1.

16.3.1   Proctitis

Proctitis is defined by the presence of abnormalities in the distal 15 cm of the gastrointestinal tract. Primary clinical features include constipation, anorectal discharge, and rectal pain or tenesmus.

Prospective studies carried out by Quinn et al. suggest that *N. gonorrhoeae*, HSV, *C. trachomatis*, and *T. pallidum* are responsible for 75% of cases of proctitis. *E. histolytica*, *C. jejuni*, and *G. lamblia* are also associated with proctitis, but multiple pathogens are present in a number of cases.[3,4] *N. gonorrhoeae*, HSV, and *Chlamydia* (LGV variant) were statistically associated with proctitis symptoms.

N. gonorrhoeae proctitis is characterized by mucopurulent discharge, although asymptomatic carriage is present in 30–40% of cases screened.[25] The presence of pain correlates with the degree of inflammation. *C. trachomatis* infection with serovars D through K causes

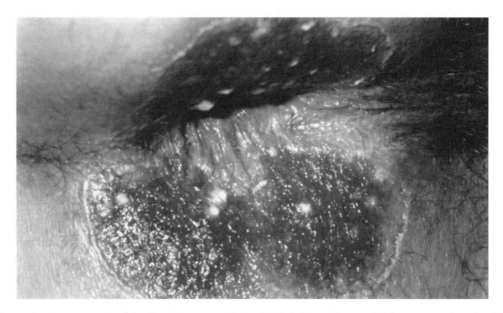

Figure 1   Severe perirectal ulceration caused by HSV 2 in a 45-year-old homosexual male. The ulceration persisted for six weeks and was initially responsive to acyclovir. Resistance subsequently developed with relapse and was treated successfully with foscarnet.

a mild form of proctitis with no characteristic sigmoidoscopic features.[5] Primary *T. pallidum* infection is characterized by the presence of a chancre which can be of any size and either painful or painless.[93,94] Large chancres may mimic rectal carcinoma in appearance. Secondary syphilis (condyloma lata) can be confused with rectal condyloma acuminatum caused by HPV, which are also frequently present in patients with proctitis symptoms.

Proctitis associated with primary HSV infection is a distinctive clinical entity.[6] HSV proctitis is more likely than other infections to cause severe pain and constipation. Neurologic abnormalities are a feature of this infection and also distinguish it from other causes of proctitis.[95] These symptoms and signs include paresthesias, neuralgia, difficulty with urination, and impotence and are thought to be either due to pain or sacral radiculopathy. Systemic symptoms such as fever, chills, and headache are also common and may be associated with a mild pleocytosis on CSF examination when a lumbar puncture is carried out because of the neurologic features. In patients with advanced HIV infection deep, chronic, recurrent ulceration involving the anal and perianal area is a major feature[38] (Figure 1). Unlike the self-limited primary and recurrent infections in immunocompetent gay men, these ulcerations will persist unless specifically treated and are considered an AIDS-defining opportunistic infection in HIV-infected individuals.

16.3.2   Proctocolitis

Proctocolitis is defined by pathologic abnormalities found beyond 15 cm from the anal verge and additional clinical symptoms not usually associated with proctitis are found such as: diarrhea, cramps, and bloating. Enteric pathogens such as the *Campylobacter* species, *Shigella*, and *E. histolytica* are often responsible for this syndrome. Of the traditionally sexually transmitted pathogens the most important is the LGV variant of *C. trachomatis* infection.[5] The prototypic infectious proctocolitis is shigellosis which is often accompanied by diarrhea, fever, and tenesmus.[96] Blood and mucopus may be present and sigmoidoscopic exam usually shows a highly inflamed mucosa which bleeds easily. *C. jejuni* and *Campylobacter*-like organisms are associated with diarrhea and bloating but local rectal pain is less common.[7] Mucosal inflammation is often present but asymptomatic carriage with normal sigmoidoscopic findings does occur. Infection with *E. histolytica* is similar in presentation, although characteristic ulcerations of amebic colitis may sometimes be found[97] and dysenteric symptoms may occasionally predominate over local pain.

Proctocolitis caused by LGV serovars of *C. trachomatis* has several more distinctive features.[5,60] Severe pain and cramping, mucopurulent discharge, and painful inguinal or femoral adenopathy are characteristic of this *Chlamydia* infection. The appearance on sigmoidoscopic exam suggests idiopathic inflammatory bowel disease. Biopsy of rectal mucosa may demonstrate granulomatous change such as is seen in Crohn's colitis, which can further confuse the clinician if a history of rectal intercourse or sexual orientation has not been obtained.[97,98]

16.3.3   Enteritis

Enteritis is defined by normal sigmoidoscopic finding in the lower bowel, the absence of proctitis symptoms, and the presence of diarrhea, abdominal pain, bloating, or nausea. In early studies the only pathogen associated with an enteric presentation in the gay bowel syndrome was *G. lamblia*.[3,80] Subsequent studies have suggested that *E. histolytica*, *Campylobacter* sp., *Salmonella* sp., and perhaps other amebae may cause a primarily enteric syndrome.[79] In HIV-infected patients these enteric symptoms may be severe and accompanied by sepsis.

Enteric features are also the primary distinguishing characteristic of newer AIDS-associated pathogens — *Cryptosporidia* sp., *Isopora* sp., microsporidia, and *M. avium intracellulare*. Infections with these pathogens are characterized by watery diarrhea and malabsorption and their presentation may also mimic inflammatory bowel disease. CMV infection of the gastrointestinal tract can occur anywhere from the oropharynx to the rectum but most characteristically causes an enterocolitis. Bloody diarrhea may occur and is more characteristic of CMV colitis than intestinal disease associated with other pathogens. Megacolon and secondary perforation requiring colectomy may occur with CMV colitis but are rare in cases of enteritis caused by *Cryptosporidia* sp. or microsporidia.[86-89]

16.4   Diagnostic studies in the gay bowel syndrome

16.4.1   History and physical examination

Several useful algorithms have been developed to assist physicians in the diagnosis and management of these syndromes.[99] A starting point is a careful, detailed sexual history. The history also should include potential environmental exposures to enteric pathogens such as food and recent travel. The cardinal symptoms of gastrointestinal disease should be explored to allow categorization of the patient into one of the three major syndromes: proctitis, proctocolitis, or enteritis.

Although the presenting complaint may be gastrointestinal, a general physical examination searching for systemic features of HIV infection is important. These include an examination of the oropharynx for thrush, oral hairy leukoplakia, or lesions suggestive of Kaposi's sarcoma. The presence of adenopathy, particularly painful adenopathy in the inguinal and femoral lymph nodes, is important to note. Abdominal exam may reveal hepatosplenomegaly or an abdominal mass suggestive of gastrointestinal lymphoma or *M. avium* infection of the mesenteric or paraortic lymph nodes. The genitourinary examination should focus on evidence of primary or secondary syphilis, herpetic ulceration, urethritis, or epididymitis.

A careful external exam of the perianal area is important. Fissures, ulceration, and hemorrhoidal inflammation should be identified. Ulcerations or vesicles characteristic of HSV infection may be present. Mucopurulent discharge at the anal verge should be noted.

A thorough external exam should be followed by anoscopy and, if enteric symptoms are present, flexible sigmoidoscopy. The presence of inflammation, purulence, ulceration, and bleeding are important to note on endoscopy.

16.4.2   Microbiologic studies

A Gram stain of any mucopurulent discharge in or from the rectum accompanied by cultures for *N. gonorrhoeae* should be obtained. A Gram stain of the discharge is more sensitive and specific in detecting gonococcal infection than a rectal swab taken blindly, but it is still a less sensitive test then culture on selective media.[100] Culture for *C. trachomatis* can also be carried out on purulent material or from a swab taken from visibly inflamed mucosa.[5] Stool cultures are not recommended for the isolation of *N. gonorrhoeae* or *C. trachomatis* and direct detection by noncultural techniques are not useful. Biopsy of any ulcerated areas should be carried out, although the usefulness of randomly taken mucosal biopsies has not been determined.[65,101] Intestinal spirochetosis is identified by biopsy and hematoxylin-eosin stain of mucosa.[66] Ulcerations either at the anal verge or in the rectum should be examined by darkfield microscopy to rule out *T. pallidum* infection. However, because of the presence of non-treponemal spirochetes in the lower bowel, interpretation of darkfield microscopy may be difficult. Most clinicians depend on serologic studies for the diagnosis of syphilis. Culture of vesicular fluid or the bed of an ulceration should also be done for HSV. For patients with advanced HIV infection, CMV culture should also be performed as CMV ulceration in the perirectal area has a similar appearance to HSV infection.

Examination of a diarrheal stool is also an important component of the laboratory diagnosis for the gay bowel syndrome. The specimens should be cultured on specialized media for *Shigella*, *Salmonella*, and *Campylobacter* species. The examination of stool for parasites is threefold: (1) fresh stool should be examined for motile *G. lamblia* and trophozoites of *E. histolytica*; (2) preserved specimens may be studied for cysts and trophozoites of pathogenic and nonpathogenic ameba as well as for the eggs of nematodes; and (3) a modified acid-fast stain should be carried out in patients with HIV infection to detect *Cryptosporidia*, *Microsporidium*, and *Isospora* species. Stool exam for MAI infection is rarely useful and MAI colitis is diagnosed by histologic exam of mucosal biopsies or a positive blood culture in the presence of a compatible clinical syndrome.

16.4.3   Endoscopic biopsy

The role of routine rectal biopsy is uncertain but biopsy of any ulceration or mass lesions may be important in defining the etiology of the gay bowel syndrome. Biopsy is diagnostic for anal carcinoma or Kaposi's sarcoma in the immunocompromised male. Condyloma acuminata generally have a characteristic macroscopic appearance, although some confusion with condyloma lata may occur and biopsy may be appropriate. Upper gastrointestinal endoscopy is warranted when malabsorption is present and is a more sensitive technique in the diagnosis of *G. lamblia* infection than stool examination. The "Entero test" for the diagnosis of giardiasis has been largely replaced by endoscopy and examination of directly obtained duodenal mucosal smears. Electron microscopic study of gastrointestinal mucosa biopsies are usually limited to upper intestinal endoscopy when cryptosporidiosis or microsporidiosis is suspected.

16.4.4   Serologic studies

Serologic studies for the LGV serovars of *C. trachomatis* should be carried out in patients with proctocolitis. Serologic studies for the diagnosis of HSV infection have improved and

Table 2 Recommended Therapeutic Agents for Microorganisms Associated with the Gay Bowel Syndrome

Organism	Drug	Alternates
Viruses		
HSV 1, 2	Acyclovir	Famciclovir, valacyclovir, foscarnet
CMV	Ganciclovir	Foscarnet, cidofovir
HPV	Podophyllin (topical)	5-fluorouracil (topical)
Bacteria		
N. gonorrheae	Ceftriaxone	Cefixime, ciprofloxacin
C. trachomatis	Doxycycline	Azithromycin, erythromycin
Shigella sp.	Ciprofloxacin	Ofloxacin
Salmonella[a] sp.	Ciprofloxacin	TMP-SMX
Campylobacter sp.[a]	Erythromycin	TMP-SMX
Spirochetosis[b]	—	Ciprofloxacin
Helicobacter sp.	Ampicillin/gentamicin	Ciprofloxacin
M. avium intracellulare	Clarithromycin + ethambutol + rifabutin	Ciprofloxacin, amikacin
Parasites		
G. lambia	Metronidazole	Quinacrine
E. histolytica		
symptomatic	Metronidazole	Tinidazole
asymptomatic	Iodoquinol	Paromomycin
Nonpathogenic amoeba	Metronidazole	
Cryptosporidia sp.[b]	Paromomycin	Azithromycin
Microsporidia[b]	Albendazole	

[a] No treatment necessary for mild disease.
[b] No standard treatment and effectiveness uncertain.

seroconversion in primary infection in men with herpetic proctitis can aid in diagnosis. However, a viral culture for HSV I or II is sensitive and specific and remains the "gold standard" of diagnosis. On the other hand, a serologic test is the mainstay in the diagnosis of *T. pallidum* infection of the lower bowel or rectum as darkfield examination of gastrointestinal ulceration is problematic. In men with a previous history of syphilis and a positive RPR an increase in the titer of antibody suggests reinfection. A negative RPR does not rule out syphilis in the primary stage and a repeat test should be carried out two to three weeks following the initial test if it is negative.

A screening test for HIV infection should always be carried out. A positive HIV test expands the spectrum of diseases associated with the gay bowel syndrome and may modify the clinical presentation of more traditional pathogens, either sexually or enterically transmitted.

16.5 Treatment

The current drug regimens for management of the specific infections associated with the gay bowel syndrome are presented in Table 2. In general treatment should be directed toward the specific pathogen identified by the clinical examination and accompanying laboratory studies. It is important to recognize that multiple pathogens may be present in 30–50% of patients with this syndrome and that treatment failure should prompt further diagnostic studies if treatment for a single pathogen appears to fail.

For some clinical syndromes, such as proctitis, an empiric approach has been suggested. Rampalo et al. in a study of 129 homosexual men with proctitis compared treatment with penicillin G and doxycycline *prior* to the availability of a specific laboratory diagnosis to *delayed* therapy directed at specific infecting microorganisms found by the laboratory studies.[37] More rapid resolution of symptoms and signs of proctitis occurred in the group treated empirically, however, 25% of the total group had HSV proctitis and did not respond to the antibacterial agents. The authors caution that an empiric approach to treatment that covers the traditional sexually transmitted pathogens as well as many enteric bacteria would seem appropriate but would be inappropriate in HIV-infected patients. An empiric approach to management of enteritis and proctocolitis is also not appropriate as the pathogens causing these two syndromes are more diverse.

While ampicillin-probenecid regimens are still useful in the management of cervical and urethral *N. gonorrhoeae* infections in regions where penicillinase-producing *N. gonorrhoeae* are not common, this regimen is inappropriate for rectal gonorrhea in gay men. The current drug recommended, ceftriaxone, is as advantageous as it is effective at all three sites commonly infected in gay men — the pharynx, urethra, and rectum. The quinolones remain an alternative treatment for gonococcal infections of the rectum. For *C. trachomatis* infection doxycycline is the most appropriate choice. Prolonged therapy is used in LGV proctocolitis in comparison to non-LGV strains. The usefulness of azithromycin, currently available for urethral chlamydial infection, has not been studied in rectal chlamydia infection, whether caused by urethral or LGV serovars. Metronidazole continues to be the recommended therapy for parasitic infection caused by *G. lamblia* or *E. histolytica*. There is continued debate about the necessity of treating carriage of *E. histolytica* cysts in gay men but most clinicians would treat symptomatic patients with metronidazole, followed by the luminal amebacide, iodoquinol. The treatment of nonpathogenic amebae or *B. hominis* infections has not been standardized and asymptomatic infection should not be treated.

The management of opportunistic protozoal pathogens in advanced HIV infections remains difficult. No consistently beneficial results have been obtained with any drug regimen in cryptosporidiosis, although paromomycin may be useful. Albendazole has been helpful in some cases of microsporidiosis but management of both these conditions usually involves nonspecific symptomatic treatment with Imodium or Lomotil, somatostatic analogs, parenteral nutrition, and careful fluid management. Several options are available for the management of CMV infection including ganciclovir, foscarnet, and cidofovir. Only ganciclovir has enough anecdotal evidence to suggest efficacy in gastrointestinal CMV infection, while all these drugs appear active in CMV retinitis. Regimens for *M. avium* infection of the bowel are similarly undefined but combination therapy with clarithromycin, ethambutol, and rifabutin may result in improvement in symptoms and an improved quality of life.[102]

References

1. Kazal, H. L., Sohn, N., Carrasco, J. I., Robilotti, J. G. Jr., Delaney W. E., The "gay bowel syndrome": clinico-pathologic correlation in 260 cases, *Ann. Clin. Lab. Sci.*, 6, 184, 1976.
2. Sohn, N., Robilotti, J. G. Jr., The "gay bowel syndrome": a review of colonic and rectal conditions in 200 male homosexuals, *Am. J. Gastroenterol.*, 67, 478, 1977.
3. Quinn, T. C., Stamm, W. E, Goodell, S. E., Mturtichian, E., Benedetti, J., Corey, L., Schuffler, M. D., Holmes, K. K., The polymicrobial origin of intestinal infections in homosexual men, *N. Engl. J. Med.*, 309, 576, 1983.
4. Quinn, T. C., Corey, L., Chafee, R. G., Schuffler, M. D., Brancato, F. P., Holmes, K. K., The etiology of anorectal infections in homosexual men, *Am. J. Med.*, 71, 395, 1981.
5. Quinn, T. C., Goodell, S. E., Mturtichian, E., Schuffler, M. D., Wang, S.-P., Stamm, W. E., Holmes, K. K., *Chlamydia trachomatis* proctitis, *N. Engl. J. Med.*, 305, 195, 1981.
6. Goodell, S. E., Quinn, T. C., Mturtichian, E., Schuffler, M. D., Holmes, K. K., Corey, L., Herpes simplex virus proctitis in homosexual men: clinical, sigmoidoscopic and histopathologic features, *N. Engl. J. Med.*, 308, 868, 1983.

7. Quinn, T. C., Goodell, S. E., Fennell, C. L., Wang, S.-P., Schuffler, M. D., Holmes, K. K., Stamm, W. E., Infections with *Campylobacter jejuni* and *Campylobacter*-like organisms in homosexual men, *Ann. Intern. Med.*, 101, 187, 1984.

8. Yee, J., Wall, S. D., Gastrointestinal manifestations of AIDS, *Gasteroenterol. Clin. N. Am.*, 24, 413, 1995.

9. Kotler, D. P., Gastrointestinal manifestations of human immunodeficiency virus infection, *Adv. Intern. Med.*, 40, 197, 1995.

10. Stern, J. O., Dieterich, D., Faust, M., Disseminated Kaposi's sarcoma: involvement of the GI tract among a group of homosexual men, *Gastroenterology*, 82, 1184, 1982.

11. Daling, J. R., Weiss, N. S., Kolpfenstein, L. L., Cochran, L. E., Chow, W. H., Daifuku, R., Correlates of homosexual behaviour and the incidence of anal cancer, *JAMA*, 247, 1988, 1982.

12. Judson, F. N., Fear of AIDS and gonorrhoea rates in homosexual men, *Lancet*, 2, 159, 1983.

13. Centers for Disease Control and Prevention. Declining rates of rectal and pharyngeal gonorrhea among males — New York City, *MMWR*, 33, 295, 1984.

14. Baker, R. W., Peppercorn, M. A., Enteric diseases of homosexual men, *Pharmacotherapy*, 2, 32, 1982.

15. Sohn, N., Weinstein, M. A., Gonchar, J., Social injuries of the rectum, *Am. J. Surg.*, 134, 611, 1977.

16. Kreutzer, E., Hansbrough, J., Superimposed traumatic and gonococcal proctitis: report of two cases, *Sex. Trans. Dis.*, 6, 75, 1979.

17. Law, C. L, Grierson, J. M., Stephens, S. M., Rectal spirochetosis in homosexual men: the association with sexual practices, HIV infection and enteric flora, *Genitourin. Med.*, 70, 26, 1994.

18. Bienzle, U., Coester, C. H., Knobloch, J., Guggenmoos-Holzmann, I., Protozoal enteric infections in homosexual men, *Klin. Wochenschr.*, 62, 323, 1984.

19. Judson, F. N., Sexually transmitted viral hepatitis and enteric pathogens, *Urol. Clin. N. Am.*, 11, 177, 1984.

20. Stamm, W. E., Handsfield, H., Rompalo, A. M., Ashley, R. L., Roberts, P. L., Corey, L., The association between genital ulcer disease and acquisition of HIV infection in homosexual men, *JAMA*, 260, 1429, 1988.

21. Centers for Disease Control. Trends in gonorrhoea in homosexually active men — King County, Washington 1989, *MMWR*, 38, 762, 1989.

22. Evans, B. G., Catchpole, M. A., Heptonstall, J., Mortimer, J. Y., McCarrigle, C. A., Nicoll, H. E., Waight, P., Gill, O. N., Swan, A. V., Sexually transmitted diseases and HIV-1 infection among homosexual men in England and Wales, *BMJ*, 306, 426, 1993.

23. Desenclos, J. C., MacLafferty, L., Community wide outbreak of hepatitis A linked to children in daycare centres and with increased transmission in young adult men in Florida 1988–1989, *J. Epidemiol. Commun. Health*, 47, 269, 1993.

24. Stewart, T., Crofts, N., An outbreak of hepatitis A among homosexual men in Melbourne, *Med. J. Aust.*, 158, 519, 1993.

25. Klein, E. J., Fisher, L. S., Chow, A. W., Guze, L. B., Anorectal gonococcal infection, *Ann. Intern. Med.*, 86, 340, 1977.

26. Owen, R. L., Dritz, S. K., Wibbelsman, C. J., Venereal aspects of gastroenterology, *W. J. Med.*, 130, 236, 1979.

27. Corey, L., Holmes, K. K., Sexual transmission of hepatitis A in homosexual men: incidence and mechanism, *N. Engl. J. Med.*, 302, 435, 1980.

28. Christenson, B., Brostrom, C., Bottiger, M., Hermanson, J., An epidemic outbreak of hepatitis A among homosexual men in Stockholm, *Am. J. Epidemiol.*, 116, 599, 1982.

29. Schreeder, M. T., Thompson, S. E., Hadler, S. C., Hepatitis B in homosexual men: prevalence of infection and factors related to its transmission, *JID*, 146, 7, 1982.

30. Reiner, N. E., Judson, F. N., Bond, W. W., Francis, D. P., Petersen, N. J., Detection of asymptomatic rectal mucosal lesions and hepatitis B surface antigen at sites of sexual contact in homosexual men with persistent hepatitis B virus infection: evidence for defacto parenteral transmission, *Ann. Intern. Med.*, 96, 170, 1982.

31. Villarejos, V. M., Visona, K. A., Guitierrez, A., Rodriguez, A., Role of saliva, urine, and feces in the transmission of type B hepatitis, *N. Engl. J. Med.*, 291, 1375, 1974.

32. Szmuness, W., Much, W. M., Prince, A. M., On the role of sexual behaviour in the spread of hepatitis B infection, *Ann. Intern. Med.,* 83, 489, 1975.

33. West, H. H., Worm, A. M., Jensen, B. L., Kroon, S., Hepatitis C virus antibodies in homosexual men and intravenous drug users in Denmark, *Infection,* 21, 115, 1993.

34. Van Beek, I., Buckley, R., Stewart, M., MacDonald, M., Kaldor, J., Risk factors for hepatitis C virus infection among injecting drug users in Sydney, *Genitourin. Med.,* 70, 321, 1994.

35. Van Ameijden, E. J., Van Den Hoek, J. A., Mientjes, G. H., Coutinho, R. A., A longitudinal study on the incidence and transmission patterns of HIV, HBV and HCV infection among drug users in Amsterdam, *Eur. J. Epidemiol.,* 9, 255, 1993.

36. Osmond, D. H., Charlebois, E., Sheppard, H. W., Page, K., Comparison of risk factors for hepatitis C and hepatitis B virus infection in homosexual men, *J. Infect. Dis.,* 167, 66, 1993.

37. Rompalo, A. M., Roberts, P., Johnson, K., Stamm, W. E., Empirical therapy for the management of acute proctitis in homosexual men, *JAMA,* 260, 348, 1988.

38. Siegal, F. P., Lopez, C., Hammer, G. S., Brown, A. E., Cunningham-Rundles, R., Severe acquired immunodeficiency in male homosexuals manifested by chronic perianal ulcerative herpes simplex lesions, *N. Engl. J. Med.,* 305, 1439, 1981.

39. Ho, M., Epidemiology of cytomegalovirus infections, *Rev. Infect. Dis.,* 12, S701, 1990.

40. Embil, J. A., Pereira, L. H., MacNeil, J. P., Manley, K. M., Haase, D. A., Levels of cytomegalovirus seropositivity in homosexual and heterosexual men, *Sex. Trans. Dis.,* 15, 85, 1988.

41. Buimovici-Klein, E., Lange, M., Ong, K. R., Grieco, M. H., Cooper, L. Z., Virus isolation and immune studies in a cohort of homosexual men, *J. Med. Virol.,* 25, 371, 1988.

42. Moore, P. S., Chang, Y., Detection of herpes virus-like DNA sequences in Kaposi's sarcoma in patients with and without HIV infection, *N. Engl. J. Med.,* 332, 1181, 1995.

43. Drew, W. L., Mills, J., Hauer, L. B., Miner, R. C., Rutherford, G. W., Declining prevalence of Kaposi's sarcoma in homosexual AIDS patients paralleled by fall in cytomegalovirus transmission, *Lancet,* 1, 66, 1988.

44. Koutsky, L. A., Galloway, D. A., Holmes, K. K., Epidemiology of genital human papilloma virus infection, *Epidemiol. Rev.,* 10, 122, 1988.

45. Zurhausen H., ed., Human pathogenic papilloma viruses in *Current Topics in Microbiology and Immunology,* Ed., V., 186, New York: Springer-Verlag, 1994.

46. Frazer, I. H., Medley, G., Crapper, R. M., Brown, T. C., Mackay, J. R., Association between anorectal dysplasia, human papillomavirus and human immunodeficiency virus infection in homosexual men, *Lancet,* 2, 657, 1986.

47. Centers for Disease Control and Prevention, 1993 revised classification system for HIV infection and expanded surveillance case definition for AIDS among adolescents and adults, *MMWR,* 41, 1, 1992.

48. Gaines, H., Vonsydow, M., Pehrson, P. O., Lundberg, H. P., Clinical picture of primary HIV infection presenting as a glandular fever-like illness, *BMJ,* 297, 1363, 1988.

49. Johns, D. R., Tierney, M., Felsenstein, D., Alteration in the natural history of neurosyphillis by concurrent infection with the human immunodefiency virus, *NEJM,* 316, 1569, 1987.

50. Fischl, M. A., Dickinson, G. M., Sinave, C., Pitchenik, A. E., Cleary, T. J., Salmonella bacteremia as manifestation of acquired immunodeficiency syndrome, *Arch. Intern. Med.,* 146, 113, 1986.

51. Greenson, J. K., Belitsos, P. C., Yardley, J. H., Bartlett, J. G., AIDS enteropathy: occult enteric infection in duodenal mucosal alterations in chronic diarrhea, *Ann. Intern. Med.,* 114, 366, 1991.

52. McMillan, A., Young, H., Gonorrhea in homosexual men, *Sex. Trans. Dis.,* 5, 146, 1978.

53. Judson, F. N., Penley, K. A., Robinson, M. E., Smith, J. K., Comparative prevalence rates of sexually transmitted diseases in heterosexual and homosexual men, *Am. J. Epidemiol.,* 112, 836, 1980.

54. Owen, R. L., Hill, J. L., Rectal and pharyngeal gonorrhea in homosexual men, *JAMA,* 220, 1315, 1972.

55. Vandelaar, M. J. W., Pickering, J., Vanderhoek, J. A. R., Vangriensven, G. J. P., Coutinho, R. A., Vandewater, H. P. A., Declining gonorrhea rates in the Netherlands, 1976-88; consequences for the AIDS epidemic, *Genitourin. Med.,* 66, 148, 1990.

56. British Cooperative Clinical Group, Homosexuality and venereal disease in the United Kingdom: a second study, *Br. J. Vener. Dis.,* 56, 6, 1980.

57. Judson, F. N., Sexually transmitted disease in gay men, *Sex. Trans. Dis.,* 4, 76, 1977.

58. Greenblatt, R. M., Lukehart, S. A., Plummer, F. A., Quinn, T. C., Genital ulceration is a risk factor for human immunodefiency virus infection, *AIDS*, 2, 47, 1988.
59. Hutchinson, C. M., Rompalo, A. M., Reichart, C. A., Hook, E. W., 3rd Characteristics of patients with syphilis attending Baltimore STD clinics. Multiple high risk subgroups and interactions with human immunodeficiency virus, *Arch. Int. Med.*, 151, 511, 1991.
60. Levine, J. S., Smith, P. D., Brugge, W. R., Chronic proctitis in male homosexuals due to lymphogranuloma venereum, *Gastroenterology*, 79, 563, 1980.
61. Rompalo, A. M., Price, C. B., Roberts, P. L., Stamm, W. E., Potential value of rectal-screening cultures for *Chlamydia trachomatous* in homosexual men, *JID*, 153, 888, 1986.
62. Barnes, R. C., Rompalo, A. M., Stamm, W. E., Comparison of *Chlamydia trachomatis* serovars causing rectal and cervical infections, *JID*, 156, 953, 1987.
63. Morse, S. A., Lysko, P. G., McFarland, L., Knapp, J. S., Sandstrom, E., Critchlow, C., Holmes, K. K., Gonococcal strains from homosexual men have outer membranes with reduced permeability to hydrophobic molecules, *Infect. Immun.*, 37, 432, 1982.
64. Harris, D. L., Kinun, J. N., Significance of anaerobic spirochetes in the intestines of animals, *Am. J. Clin. Nutr.*, 27, 1297, 1974.
65. McMillan, A., Lee, F. D., Sigmoidoscopic and microscopic appearance of the rectal mucosa in homosexual men, *Gut*, 22, 1035, 1981.
66. Surawicz, C. M., Roberts, P. L., Rompalo, A., Quinn, T. C., Holmes, K. K., Stamm, W. E., Intestinal spirochetosis in homosexual men, *Am. J. Med.*, 82, 587, 1987.
67. Hovind-Hougen, K., Birch-Anderson, A., Henrik-Neilsen, R., Intestinal spirochetosis: morphology characterization and cultivation of the spirochete *Brachyspira aalborgi* (gen.nov.,sp.nov), *J. Clin. Microbiol.*, 16, 1127, 1982.
68. Lafeuillade, A., Quilichini, R., Benderitter, T., Delbeke, E., Dhiver, C., Gastant, J. A., Intestinal spirochetosis in HIV infected homosexual men, *Postgrad. Med.*, 66, 253, 1990.
69. Totten, P. A., Fennell, C. L., Tenover, F. C., Wezenberg, J. M., Perine, P. L., Stamm, W. E., Holmes, K. K., *Campylobacter cinaedi* (sp. nov.) and *Campylobacter fennelliae* (sp. nov.): two new *Campylobacter* species associated with enteric disease in homosexual men, *JID*, 151, 131, 1985.
70. Ng, V. L., Hadley, W. K., Fennell, C. L., Flores, B. M., Stamm, W. E., Successive bacteremias with "*Campylobacter cinaedi*" and *Campylobacter fennelliae*" in a bisexual male, *J. Clin. Microbiol.*, 25, 2008, 1987.
71. Dritz, S. K., Ainsworth, T. E., Back, A, Boucher, L. A., Patterns of sexually transmitted enteric diseases in a city, *Lancet*, 2, 3, 1977.
72. Dritz, S. K., Back, A. F., *Shigella* enteritis venereally transmitted, *N. Engl. J. Med.*, 291, 1194, 1974.
73. Blaser, M. J., Hale, T. L., Formal, S. B., Recurrent shigellosis complicating human immunodefiency virus infection: failure of preexisting antibodies to confer protection, *Am. J. Med.*, 86, 105, 1989.
74. Dritz, S. K., Braff, E. H., Sexually transmitted typhoid fever, *N. Engl. J. Med.*, 296, 1359, 1977.
75. Smith, P. D., Macher, A. M., Bookman, M. A., Boccia, R. V., *Salmonella typhimurium* enteritis and bacteremia in the acquired immunodeficiency syndrome, *Ann. Intern. Med.*, 102, 207, 1985.
76. Gray, J. R., Rabeneck, L., Atypical mycobacterial infection of the gastrointestinal tract of AIDS patients, *Am. J. Gastroenterol.*, 84, 1521, 1989.
77. Nightingale, S. D., Byrd, L. T., Southern, P. M., Jockusch, J. D., Cal, S. X., Wynne, B. A., Incidence of *Mycobacterium avium intracellulare* complex bacteremia in human immunodefiency virus positive patients, *J. Infect. Dis.*, 165, 1082, 1992.
78. DuMoulin, G. C., Stottmeier, K. D., Pelletier, P. A., Tsang, A. Y., Hedley-White, J., Concentration of *Mycobacterium avium* by hospital hot water systems, *JAMA*, 260, 1599, 1988.
79. Phillips, S. C., Mildvan, D., William, D. C., Gelb, A. M., White, M. C., Sexual transmission of enteric protozoa and helminths in a venereal disease clinic population, *N. Engl. J. Med.*, 305, 603, 1981.
80. Most, H., Manhattan: "a tropical isle"?, *Am. J. Trop. Med. Hyg.*, 17, 333, 1968.
81. Markell, E. K., Havens, R. F., Kuritsubo, R. A., Wingerd, J., Intestinal protozoa in homosexual men of the San Francisco Bay area: prevalence and correlates of infection, *Am. J. Trop. Med. Hyg.*, 32, 239, 1984.

82. William, D. C., Shookhoff, H. B., Felman, W. M., Deramos, S. W., High rates of enteric protozoal infections in selected homosexual men attending a venereal disease clinic, *Sex. Trans. Dis.*, 5, 155, 1978.

83. Sargenaunt, P. G., Oates, J. K., MacLellan, I., Oriel, J. D., Goldmeier, D., *Entamoeba histolytica* in male homosexuals, *Br. J. Vener. Dis.*, 59, 193, 1983.

84. Peters, C. S., Sable, R., Janda, W. M., Chitton, A. L., Kocka, F. E., Problems of enteric parasites in homosexual patients attending an outpatient clinic, *J. Clin. Microbiol.*, 24, 684, 1986.

85. Centers for Disease Control and Prevention, Cryptosporidiosis: an assessment of chemotherapy of males with acquired immune deficiency syndrome (AIDS), *MMWR*, 31, 589, 1982.

86. Fayer, R., Unger, B. L. P., *Cryptosporidium* spp. and cryptosporidiosis, *Microbiol. Rev.*, 50, 458, 1986.

87. Current, W. L., Garcia, L. S., Cryptosporidiosis, *Clin. Microbiol. Rev.*, 4, 325, 1991.

88. Weber, R., Bryan, R. T., Schwartz, D. A., Owen, R. L., Human microsporidial infections, *Clin. Microbiol. Rev.*, 7, 424, 1994.

89. Soave, R., Johnson, W. D. Jr., Cryptosporidium and *Isospora belli* infections, *J. Infect. Dis.*, 157, 225, 1988.

90. McMillan, A., Threadworms in homosexual males, *Br. Med. J.*, 1, 367, 1978.

91. Waugh, M. A., Sexual transmission of intestinal parasites, *Br. J. Vener. Dis.*, 50, 157, 1974.

92. Gompels, M. M., Todd, J., Peters, B. S., Maire, J., Pinching, A. J., Disseminated strongyloidisis in AIDS: uncommon but important, *AIDS*, 5, 329, 1991.

93. Gouckman, J. B., Kleinman, M. S., May, A. G., Primary syphillis of rectum, *N.Y. State Med. J.*, 74, 220, 1974.

94. Quinn, T. C., Lukehart, S. A., Goodell, S., Mturtichian, E., Rectal mass caused by *Treponema pallidum*: confirmation by immunofluorescence staining, *Gastroenterology*, 82, 135, 1982.

95. Samarasinghe, P. L., Oates, J. K., MacLennan, I. P. B., Herpetic proctitis and sacral radiculomyelopathy — a hazard for homosexual men, *Br. Med. J.*, 2, 365, 1979.

96. Dritz, S. K., Back, A. F., *Shigella* enteritis venereally transmitted, *N. Engl. J. Med.*, 291, 1194, 1974.

97. McMillan, A., Gilmour, H. M., McNeillage, G., Scott, G. R., Amoebiasis in homosexual men, *Gut*, 25, 356, 1984.

98. Boland, R. K., Sands, M., Schachter, J., et al., Lyphogranuloma venereum and acute ulcerative proctitis, *Am. J. Med.*, 72, 703, 1982.

99. Rompalo, A. M., Quinn, T. C., Sexually transmitted enteric and rectal infections in homosexual men, *Infect. Dis. Clin. N. Am.*, 1, 235, 1987.

100. Deheragoda, P., Diagnosis of rectal gonnorhea by blind anorectal swabs compared with direct vision swabs taken by a proctoscope, *Br. J. Vener. Dis.*, 53, 311, 1977.

101. Surawicz, C. M., Goodell, S. E., Quinn, T. C., Roberts, P., Corey, L., Holmes, K. K., Schuffler, M. D., Stamm, W. E., Spectrum of rectal biopsy abnormalities in homosexual men with intestinal symptoms, *Gastroenterology*, 91, 651, 1986.

102. Shafran, S. D., Singer, J., Zarowny, D. P., Phillips, P., Salit, I., Walmsley, S. L., Fong, I. W., Gill, M. J., Rachlis, A. R., Lalonde, R. C., Fanning, M. M., Tsoukas, C. M., Turgeon, F., Aoki, F. Y., A comparison of two regimens for the treatment of *Mycobacterium avium* complex bacteremia in AIDS: rifabutin, ethambutol, and clarithromycin versus rifampin, ethambutol, clofazamine, and ciprofloxacin. Canadian HIV Trials Network Protocol 010 Study Group, *NEJM*, 335, 377, 1996.

Ectoparasites

chapter seventeen

Scabies

Kenneth A. Borchardt, Axel W. Hoke, Nino Maida, and Michael Z. Zhang

17.1   Introduction...315
17.2   Epidemiology..315
17.3   Anatomical features...316
17.4   Life cycle...316
17.5   Clinical disease 316
17.6   Diagnosis 319
17.7   Treatment..320
References...321

17.1   Introduction

Scabies is derived from the Latin word, scabera, meaning to scratch. The etiologic agent for this mite infestation is *Sarcoptes scabiei* variety *hominis*. Various species produce infestations in 40 different species of animals. Mite infestations have been associated with humans for thousands of years. They were described by Aristotle in 384–323 B.C. as "lice of the flesh" that produced vesicles. It was not until 1100 A.D. that Averroes identified the scabies mite, but he failed to establish its relationship with scabies. Although the mite and eggs were identified microscopically and proven to be the cause of scabies by Bonoma (1663–1696), the information was not disseminated because of political and religious opposition.[1] The scabies mite was rediscovered by Raspail and Renucci in 1834, who described the relationship between the mite and the disease.[2] Von Hebra in 1868 demonstrated in volunteers that human scabies was produced by *S. scabiei*.[1]

17.2   Epidemiology

Each year an estimated 300 million cases of scabies occur world wide.[3] The prevalence of scabies in rural areas of Africa and developing countries ranges between 2–19%.[4,5] In some rural island communities it varies between 30–70%, and in specific villages as many as 50–100% of children may be infested.[6] In industrialized countries sexual contact is the most significant mode of transmission. Children 2 years of age have a higher prevalence than those over the age of 10, while women have a 50% higher prevalence rate than men.[7] Not every individual exposed to an infested individual, irrespective of either the proximity, duration, or the severity of the infestation will develop scabies. Approximately 50–66% become infested after exposure.[8]

Decreased immunologic competence in debilitated elderly patients often reduces itching leading to misdiagnosis such as dry skin or eczema. Atypical presentations with eczematous lesions of the face, breasts, palms, and soles, often with thick crusting of finger webs and paronychial areas as seen in crusted or "Norwegian" scabies, is usually initially confused with other dematoses. Failure to recognize this rare form of scabies, in which thousands of mites are shed from the patient, results in mini-epidemics in nursing homes. This form of scabies appears in hospitals when there are patients immunocomprimised by chemotherapy or chronic steroid usage. This is essentially a problem in patients on immunosuppressive medications preceding or following transplants, such as renal transplants. Finally, crusted scabies is frequently seen in mental illness, especially in patients with severe mongolism.[9,10]

Mites have demonstrated an ability to maintain their viability for up to three days on a variety of surfaces such as sofas, chairs, and floors. These sites could serve as possible sources of infestation.[11]

Herd immunity has been proposed to explain cyclical prevalence of scabies. But the data from well reported groups indicate that herd immunity to scabies does not occur, and epidemics continue until eliminated by systemic treatment.[8]

17.3   Anatomical features

The *S. scabiei hominis* mite appears eyeless, with a translucent, white body. Its body surface is irregular with transverse corrugations. The body of the female is approximately $1/3$ mm in length, while the male's is usually smaller. The mite presents a head, though the mouth part or "jaws" which extend beyond the anterior edge of the body are often erroneously called the head. It has four pairs of legs, two short pairs in front ending in small "suckers," and two long pairs posteriorly with fine bristles. The suckers appear to help the mite walk, which it can do as rapidly as one inch per minute.

17.4   Life cycle

The male has a shorter life span than the female and permanently resides on the skin's surface. Shortly after contact with the skin, the adult female burrows partially into it and awaits fertilization. The male then dies.[12] *In vitro* studies have demonstrated that male mites have no preferential attraction to females at any stage of their life cycle, suggesting the lack of sex pheromone.[13] The female is fertile for life after mating. Egg laying begins approximately 40 h after fertilization. She then she departs from the partial burrow and continues to burrow 2–4 mm per day until reaching the upper dermis.[8] Mites require living dermis for both fluids and nutrients. They fail to ingest blood because of the absence of capillaries in the epidermal layers. Sycbala or fecal pellets are deposited within the burrow, which may be an irritant that produces itching.[14] A mite scratched from its burrow may begin another if not injured.

The female burrows approximately 0.5–5 mm a day laying 2–4 eggs. These are secured to the burrow's floor by a sticky substance. Of the 40–50 eggs produced, less then 10% survive to become adults. The period from fertilization to adulthood is approximately 14 days and involves 5 stages in development to the adult. Larva move to the skin surface and feed until they become immature mites and make their own burrows[11] (Figure 1).

17.5   Clinical disease

Fewer than 10 mites are present in a typical scabies patient.[15] Mites may burrow into the skin in any area of the body. Rarely is the face or scalp involved except in infants and

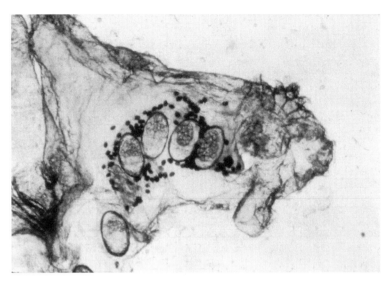

Figure 1   Adult female with ava and sycabala. (Photo courtesy of A.W. Hoke, M.D.)

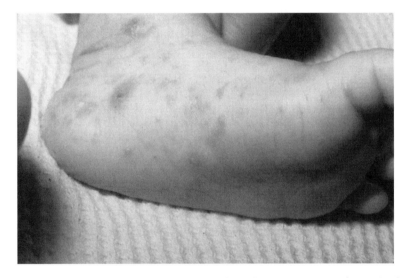

Figure 2   Scabies infestation on the foot of an infant. (Photo courtesy of A.W. Hoke, M.D.)

immunocompromised patients. Sparing of the face and scalp in adults is thought to be due to the large number of pilosebaceous glands in these sites.[16]

In infants the greatest number of burrows are found in the insteps of the soles, the palms, finger webs, sides of the hands, and volar wrists. In this age group, lesions of the palms and soles often present as vesicles or vesiculopustules resembling bullous impetigo (Figures 2–6). Dry scaly lesions of the cheeks and trunk may be interpreted as eczema and mistreated with topical steroids. Such therapy may reduce symptoms and signs of scabies delaying proper diagnosis and treatment. Because friends and family all want to cuddle these cute infants, this close contact may lead to extensive spread of scabies among family and friends.

In adult males the important sites are the penis and the scrotum (Figure 7). The most frequent sites in both males and females are the finger webs, side of the hands, volar wrists, peri-axillary area, elbows, knees, ankles, trunk, unbilicus, and breast.[12]

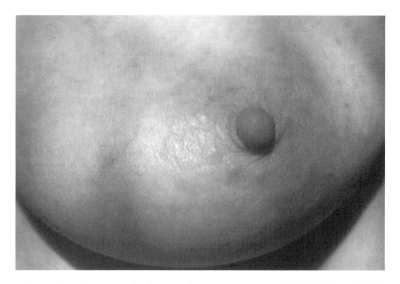

Figure 3　Scabies on the breast. (Photo courtesy of A.W. Hoke, M.D.)

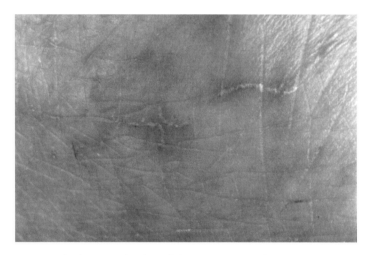

Figure 4　Scabies on the foot. (Photo courtesy of A.W. Hoke, M.D.)

Scabies may present atypically as either crusted or anergic when the helper T-cell count is less than 200. Anergic scabies appear as a diffuse papular eruption in which each papule is a burrow[17] (Figure 8).

Elderly or debilitated patients may demonstrate only nonspecific pruritic eruptions. This may be misdiagnosed as either eczema, dry skin, or generalized itching and scratching due to anxiety. But the single most significant symptom of scabies in the elderly is pruritis, especially at night. In response to the pruritis, the patient may produce erythema and scaling which masks the appearance of the burrows.[18,19]

In patients with HIV/AIDS scabies should be suspected when either an atypical itching or nonitching rash occurs. The appearance of the infestation can be misleading because of the diffuse papular or psoriasiform presentation. Keratotic scabies is most frequently found in AIDS patients. A scabies infestation in AIDS may permit a mite transmission of HIV when scratching produces blood that is ingested. Hemoglobin has been detected in mites.[20]

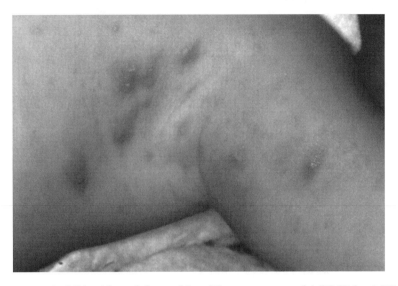

Figure 5   A child with nodular scabies. (Photo courtesy of A.W. Hoke, M.D.)

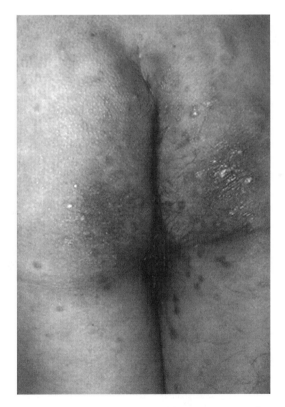

Figure 6   Nodular scabies on the buttocks. (Photo courtesy of A.W. Hoke, M.D.)

17.6   *Diagnosis*

It is important to employ good magnification and lighting when searching for a burrow in the most appropriate site. The burrow appears as a serpeginous tract, pale gray to white, approximately 1–5 mm in length, and ending with a small erythematous papule.[8]

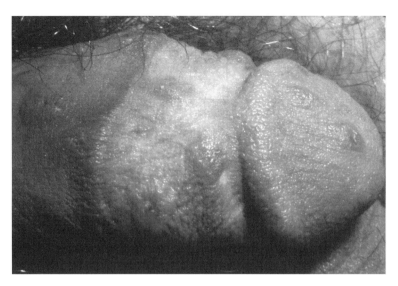

Figure 7   Scabies on the penis. (Photo courtesy of A.W. Hoke, M.D.)

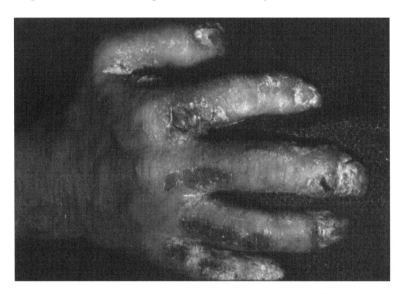

Figure 8   Norwegian scabies. (Photo courtesy of F. Hubler, M.D.)

Once the burrow has been located, a number 15 Bard-Parker blade should be dipped into immersion oil before carefully scraping the burrow at a right angle. This keeps the scraped material on the blade. It is best to scrape several burrows, which increases the possibility of a positive diagnosis. One should be careful not to produce bleeding in performing this procedure since it indicates an excessive or too deep scraping. The material can be examined microscopically at 10× for fecal pellets. These appear as small pale brown to golden, round to oval, singularly or in groups, and approximately the size of the female mite. It may be possible to visualize both the female mite and nymphs.

17.7   Treatment

All clothing or bed linen in contact with the infested individual must be washed in hot water and dried in a hot setting. It is very important to treat all contacts at the same time to prevent "ping-pong" scabies. Elimite® cream contains 5% permethrin for topical application. The permethrin is a 1:3 mixture of *cis-* and *trans-*isomers of pyrethroid. Before treatment, the patient is requested to bathe or shower. After drying the skin, the cream is applied over the entire skin surface, skin folds, from the neck to the soles of the feet, and under the nails. It is applied only to the face and scalp when these sites are infested. The cream is removed after 10–12 h by bath or shower. Even though the package insert indicates one application is sufficient, a repeat treatment in 7 days is recommended. A clinical study with 5% permethrin cream reported a cure rate of 91% one month after a single treatment.[18]

Elimite may cause a temporary stinging sensation especially in excoriated skin. It is important to inform the patient that itching will not subside for 1–2 weeks after treatment. Itching is produced by the host's sensitization to the mite and its feces. Residual pruritis can be alleviated by topical antipruritic lotions or topical steroids after the scabicide has been washed off. Oral antihistamines are sometimes helpful, but oral steroids are usually not indicated. It is important to caution the patient not to use the scabicide other then as prescribed because that can produce irritation and pruritis.

Kwell® is a 1% gamma benzene hexachloride scabicide available both as a cream and lotion. It is applied the same as Elimite. Although they are approximately equally efficacious, Elmite is safer since it is less absorbed and more rapidly metabolized.

Eurax® is a scabicide available either as a cream or lotion. It is far less effective than either Elimite or Kwell.[18] It contains 10% synthetic crotamiton and is occasionally used for its antipruritic effect after treatment with either Elimite or Kwell.

Ivermectin, an antihelminthic agent, was used for treating both healthy and HIV scabies patients. A single oral dose of 200 μg/k of Ivermectin was administered to both groups. The results in this study indicated the Ivermectin demonstrated significant scabicide activity.[21] In patients less than 2 years of age, during pregnancy, and nursing mothers, use of either Elimite or Kwell is contraindicated. In these patients a 6% precipitated sulfur in petrolatum is applied nightly for 3 nights with washings between applications. Although this is messy and odoriferous, it is probably the safest treatment unless the patient is allergic to sulfur.[8]

HIV patients may require treatment with Elimite several times a week for multiple weeks. However, caution should be used to prevent excessive treatment which will produce irritation and itching.

A patient with crusted scabies may require removal of some of the thick crusts before treatment. Multiple treatments are required with the scabicide. Care must be taken not to introduce the scabicide into the mouth or eyes. Because of the large number of mites present on the patient, clothing, mattresses, bedding, chairs, and the surrounding area, decontamination is required to eliminate infestation.[22]

References

1. Parish, L.C. History of scabies, In: Orkin, M., Maibach, H.I. (ed): *Cutaneous Infestations and Insect Bites.* New York, Marcel Dekker, Inc. 3–8, 1985.
2. Renucci, S.F. These inaurale sur la decouverte de i'insecte qui produit la contagion de la gale du purigo et du phlyzacia. Paris, These No 83, 41, 1835. Cited in: Heilsen, B. Studies on Acarus Scabiei and Scabies. *Acta Derm. Vernereol. (Stockh.)* 26(Suppl. 14), 1–370, 1946.
3. Alexander, J.O. Scabies. In: *Arthropods and Human Skin:* Berlin, Springer-Verlag, 225–292, 1984.
4. Dagnew, M.B., Erwin, G. Epidemiology of common transmissible skin diseases among primary school children in north-west Ethiopia. *Trop. Geograph. Med.* 43, 152–5, 1991.
5. Srivastava, B.C., Chandra, R., Srivastava, V.K., et al. Epidemiological study of scabies and community control. *J. Commun. Dis.* 12, 134–8. 1980.
6. Stein, D.H. Scabies and pediculosis. *Curr. Opin. Pediatr.* 3, 660–6,1991.

7. Menking, T.L., Taplin, D. Advances in pediculosis, scabies, and other mite infestations. *Adv. Dermatol.* 5, 131–52, 1990.
8. Rasmussen, J.E. Scabies. *Pediatr. Rev.* 15, 110–14, 1994.
9. Paules, S.J., Levisohn, D., Heffron, W. Peristent scabies in nursing home patients. *J. Fam. Pract.* 37(1), 82–6, 1993.
10. Fain, A. Epidemiological problems in scabies. *Int. J. Dermatol.* 17, 20–30, 1980.
11. Arlan, L.G., Estes, S.A., Vyszenski-Moher, D.L. Prevalence of *Sarcoptes acabiei* in homes and nursing homes of scabietic patients. *J. Am. Acad. Dermatol.* 19, 806–11, 1988.
12. Forsman, K.E. Pediculosis and scabies. What to look for in patients who are crawling with clues. *Postgrad. Med.* 38, 89–100, 1995.
13. Estes, S.A., Estes, J. Scabies research: another diminsion. *Semin. Dermatol.* 12(1), 34–8, 1993.
14. *Lice and Scabies: From Infestation To Disinfectation.* Reed and Carnick, Kenilworth, NJ, 11–15, 1976.
15. Oliver, R.P. Norwegian scabies. *Central Afr. J. Med.* 23, 105–6, 1977.
16. Burns, D.A., Lampe, R.M., Hansen, G.H. Neonatal scabies. *Am. J. Dis. Child.* 133, 131–134, 1979.
17. Denam, S.T. A review of pruritus. *J. Ann. Acad. Dermatol.* 14, 375–392, 1986.
18. Taplin, D., Menking, T.L. Scabies, lice, and fungal infections. *Prim. Care, Clinics Office Pact.* 16(3), 551–76, 1989.
19. Nicholls, P.H. When your resident has scabies. *Geriatr. Nurs.* 15(5), 271–3,1994.
20. Donabedian, H., Khazan, U. Norwegian scabies in a patient with AIDS. *Clin. Inf. Dis.* 14(1), 162–4, 1992.
21. Menking, T.L., Taplin, D., Hermida, J.L., et al. The treatment of scabies with ivermectin. *N. Eng. J. Med.* 333, 26–30, 1995.
22. Haag, M.L. Brozena, S.J., Fenske, N.A. Attack of the scabies: What to do when an outbreak occurs. *Geriatrics.* 48, 45–53, 1993.

chapter eighteen

Lice

Kenneth A. Borchardt, Axel W. Hoke, Nino Maida, and Michael Z. Zhang

18.1   Introduction...323
18.2   Head lice...324
    18.2.1   Epidemiology...324
    18.2.2   Clinical disease 324
        18.2.2.1   *Pediculus humanus capitis*.....................................324
    18.2.3   Diagnosis 324
    18.2.4   Treatment...324
18.3   Body lice 326
    18.3.1   Epidemiology...326
    18.3.2   Clinical disease 328
        18.3.2.1   *Pediculus humanus corporis* 328
    18.3.3   Diagnosis 329
        18.3.3.1   *Pediculus humanus corporis* 329
    18.3.4   Treatment...329
18.4   Pubic lice...329
    18.4.1   Epidemiology...329
    18.4.2   Clinical disease 329
        18.4.2.1   *Phthirus pubis*...329
    18.4.3   Diagnosis 329
        18.4.3.1   *Phthirus pubis*...329
    18.4.4   Treatment...329
References..331

18.1   Introduction

Lice are wingless, blood-sucking insects that infest both mammals and birds. They are classified as ectoparasites because their life cycle occurs on the host. Human lice are classified into: *Pediculus humanus capitis*, the head louse; *Pediculus humanus corporis*, the body louse; and *Phthirus pubis*, the pubic or crab louse. Only *P. corporis* can transmit disease. Because the head and body lice are morphologically similar and may interbreed, it is theorized that the body louse evolved from the head louse. Lice feed by employing a stylet in their mouth parts to penetrate the skin. Saliva is introduced to prevent clotting while the louse seeks a blood vessel.[1]

18.2   Head lice

18.2.1   Epidemiology

Head lice have been plaquing humans for thousands of years. Lice were prevalent in both Central and South America in the pre-Columbian era.[2] From 1970 to 1987 pediculosis infestations in the U.S. had a prevalence rate in schools that ranged from approximately 10–40%.[3] A higher rate was demonstrated in the U.K. in industrialized cities then in less populated areas.[4]

Females and children have more infestations than males. Perhaps this is related to their longer hair and the proclivity of women and children to be physically closer to one another. Men rarely have head lice after the age of 20. Adult males have more hair follicles which are empty and resting than either women or children. This results in a less dense hair which is not necessarily ideal for infestation. It has been hypothesized that male hormones may affect egg fertility of head lice.[5]

The incidence of head lice among blacks in the U.S. is extremely low. Their tightly curled, oval hair prevents the head louse from firmly grasping the hair shaft. Head lice in Africa are capable of infestation because there claws are more curved enabling them firm attachment to hair.[6]

18.2.2   Clinical disease

18.2.2.1   Pediculus humanus capitis

Hygiene does not significantly prevent head lice infestations. The most susceptible hosts are children, usually, between the ages of 3–10. Although direct contact with an infested individual is the usual method of transmission, hats, combs, and brushes may be vehicles for transmission.[1] The infestation does not produce an immune response.

18.2.3   Diagnosis

The female head louse is between 3–4 mm long, with a diamond-shaped head, and claws on its legs to grasp scalp hair. During its life span of approximately 40 days, it produces between 7–10 nits (eggs) per day. Nits have a lid or operculum covering the free end[1] (Figure 1).

Diagnosis may be established by examining the patient for the presence of nits, lice, and the distribution of lesions. One can suspect head lice being present on a patient's scalp or the nape of the neck when impetigious, crusted, or weepy areas are present, often accompanied with lympadenopathy. Lice are frequently present in the warmer sites covered by long hair, such as at the nape of the neck and retroauricular area. The nits are attached by the adult female to the base of the hair shaft where it is warmest. Therefore, one can estimate the duration of the infestation by the nits' location on the hair shaft. Nits may be differentiated from scales of dandruff or hair casts. Sehorrhic dermatitis is often misdiagnosed as *Pediculus capitis* (Figure 2–4).

18.2.4   Treatment

It is recommended that in treatment the pediculicide be used twice, 7–10 days apart. This eliminates any nymphs that may have survived the initial treatment and hatched. Removal of nits from scalp hair is often difficult even with the use of a special fine toothed comb in the over-the-counter pediculicides.

NIX® is a 1% permethrin cream rinse shampoo with significant residual ovicidal activity. It is formulated with a hair conditioner that enables the hair to be easily combed. A double-blind clinical study evaluated 263 patients treated with NIX and only 5(2%)

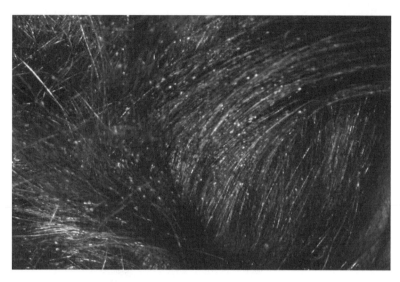

Figure 1 A psychotic patient with a significant infestation. (Photo courtesy of A.W. Hoke, M.D.)

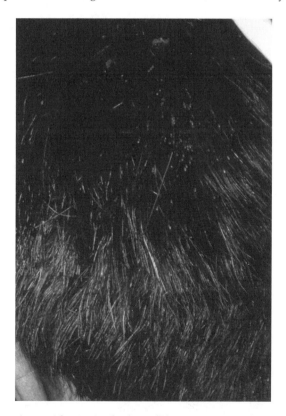

Figure 2 A patient with nits in the hair. (Photo courtesy of A.W. Hoke, M.D.)

were treatment failures. Of the 172 treated with lindande shampoo (Kwell®), 52 (30%) were treatment failures.[7-9]

RID® is a liquid pedicullicide for treatment of head lice, which contains 0.33% pyrethrins and piperonyl butoxide. Pyrethrin acts as a contact poison and piperonyl butoxide reacts synergistically increasing the effectiveness of the pyrethrin. The recommended application time is 20 min with subsequent washings with warm water, soap, or shampoo. A clinical

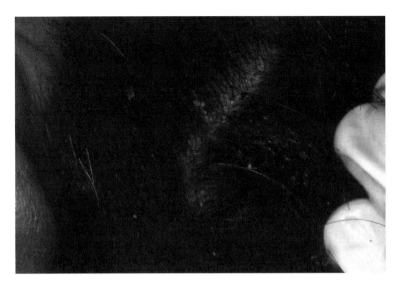

Figure 3   This patient has evidence of both lice and nits. (Photo courtesy of A.W. Hoke, M.D.)

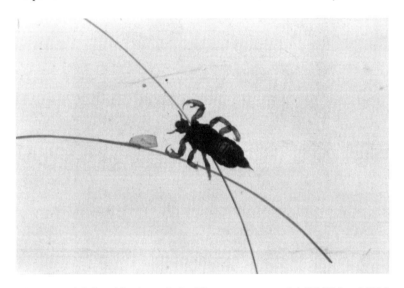

Figure 4   Adult with nit on hair. (Photo courtesy of A.W. Hoke, M.D.)

evaluation comparing RID with NIX demonstrated that after one week of treatment with NIX, 205 (98%) of the patients were lice free compared to 164 (85%) treated with RID.[10]

A-200® is a pediculicide shampoo for head lice which contains 0.30% pyrethrins and 3.0% piperonyl butoxide. Warm water, soap, or shampoo may be used to remove the pediculicide after 10 min. A-200 is not an effective ovicide because 30% of viable eggs have been observed to hatch after being immersed in an undiluted solution.[11]

18.3   Body lice

18.3.1   Epidemiology

Morphologically the body louse resembles the head louse but it is larger. The body louse completes its entire life cycle, eggs through mating, in the seams of the host's clothing.

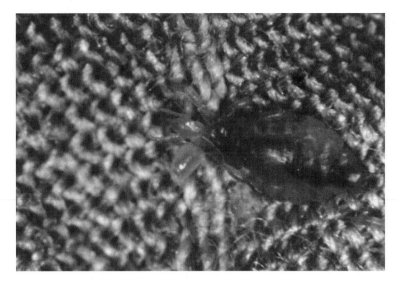

Figure 5   Adult with eggs. (Photo courtesy of A.W. Hoke, M.D.)

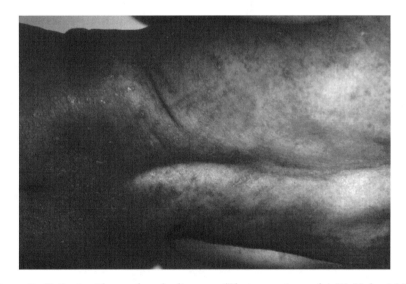

Figure 6   Patient with vagabonds diseases. (Photo courtesy of A.W. Hoke, M.D.)

This may be reflected in the phrase, "the seamy side of life." It prefers an adult male host rather then either a female or child. Eggs are attached to the seams of inner clothing both for their protection and the hosts body heat. The body louse has a particular preference for certain types of clothing. Body lice have been found in necklaces when little clothing was worn.[12] Wool and natural fibers are preferred to either cotton or synthetics (Figures 5 and 6). A human odor in the clothing is preferable to its absence. When cloth is unavailable for attachment, the louse will not attach any eggs to body hair but indiscriminately release their eggs. The population of lice may increase to several thousand, and a patient may experience a thousand bites each day. Louse saliva produces a local sensitization 3–4 weeks after infestation. The bite site becomes a red elevated papule 2–4 mm in diameter. Wheals occur at the bite site for excoriations and are commonly observed in the scapular area, flanks, and abdomen. In chronic cases the skin of the axillae, groin, and upper inner thighs are diffusely pigmented with a bronze

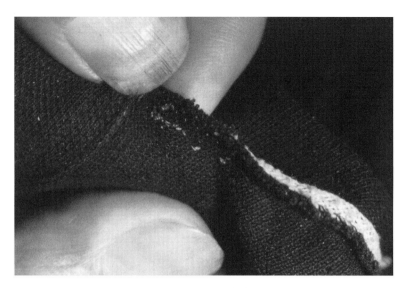

Figure 7   Adult with eggs in seam of clothing. (Photo courtesy of A.W. Hoke, M.D.)

hue. The skin may become lichenfied, a syndrome identified as vagabond's disease[13] (Figure 7). A subsequent infection with body lice may produce a slight increase in temperature and muscular aches both in the legs and feet. A transient rash occurs resembling German measles concomitantly with a feeling of apathy and irritation. This may be the derivation of the phrase "feeling lousy."

The body louse abandons the host when the blood pressure drops.[14] Body lice may be maintained on rabbits.[13]

18.3.2   Clinical disease

18.3.2.1   *Pediculus humanus corporis*

Historically, *P. humanus corporis* has been the major insect vector of diseases in third world countries. Body lice transmit classic typhus fever (*Rickettsia prowazekii*), trench fever (*Rochalliamea quintana*), murine typhus (*Rickettsia typhi*), and epidemic relapsing fever (*Borrelia recurrentis*).

R. prowazekii transmits classical typhus fever to the host through a scratch contaminated with rickettsia in the louse feces. The rickettsia may produce the infection through the conjuctiva or lung when the dried, powdery feces contaminate the eye or are inhaled. Clinically one sees fever, chills, headache, rash, and myalgia. Typhus is frequently fatal when not diagnosed and treated promptly.[5]

Trench fever is similar to typhus but less severe. Transmission occurs via rat feces. Although this was a significant infection in World War I, it was not significant in World War II, and presently occurs infrequently.[5] The usual host for murine typhus is the brown rat, *Rattus norvegicus*. Transmission to humans occurs when contaminated rat feces enter the host through scratched skin. Transmission to another host occurs via infected lice. Murine typhus is not as severe as classic typhus.[5]

The etiologic agent for louse borne relapsing fever is the spirochete *B. recurrentis*. This blood-borne spirochete enters the host when an infected body louse is crushed releasing infectious hemolymph on to either intact or scratched skin. The infection is characterized by recurrent fever. The louse carries the spirochetes in its circulating fluid transmitting the organism.[15]

18.3.3   Diagnosis

18.3.3.1   Pediculus humanis corporis

P. corporis should be suspected in any patient with severe itching at body sites in close contact with clothing, such as the axillae, waist, and crotch. It is more important to examine the patient's clothing rather than the patient, especially the seams at the waist, collar, and crotch. The homeless, street people, and drug addicts are frequently infested with body lice. Viable lice are easily seen without magnification.

18.3.4   Treatment

Treatment is necessary to control an epidemic.[1] To prevent reinfestation, all personal clothing and bed linens should be laundered in hot water. Carpets, mattresses, and upholstered chairs should be thoroughly vacuumed.

A 1% lindane cream or lotion (Kwell) requires application from the chin to the toes for appropriate louse eradication. The medication should remain on the skin for a minimum of 12 h before removal by shower or bath. Lice resistant to 1% lindane have been reported in other countries, but not in the U.S.[7]

Appropriate application of 5% permethrin requires only a single treatment.

18.4   Pubic lice

18.4.1   Epidemiology

Pubic lice infestations have increased significantly in recent years. Sexual contact is one of the most common modes for transmission, particularly between the ages of 15–40.[1] The infestation is equal in both heterosexual and homosexual persons. One STD clinic reported that 38% of patients with pubic lice had been infected with other STD diseases.[16] An evaluation of male homosexuals reported that 67% had head or pubic lice at least once.[17] The French have named it "pallons d' amour," which translates as butterflies of love.

18.4.2   Clinical disease

18.4.2.1   Phthirus pubis

The pubic louse is 3–4 mm in size and has a shape similar to a crab with legs that have hook shaped claws to grasp hair (Figure 8). Any hirsute part of the body may be infested with pubic lice, including the eyelashes, but rarely the scalp. These lice prefer hairs that are widely spaced, such as in the pubic area, thighs, abdomen, and axillae[18] (Figures 9–11).

18.4.3   Diagnosis

18.4.3.1   Phthirus pubis

As has often been stated "moles that move should always raise suspicion." Frequently the patient establishes the diagnosis of infestation by bringing a louse to the clinician for identification. The louse is readily seen by using a well-lighted magnifying lens, appearing as a small brownish-red speck. After feeding, it is more easily identifiable.

18.4.4   Treatment

Both 1% lindane shampoo (Kwell) and pyrethrins (A-200) require a second treatment 7–10 days after the initial one.

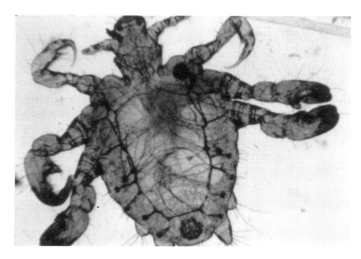

Figure 8   Adult *Phthirus pubis* (Photo courtesy of A.W. Hoke, M.D.)

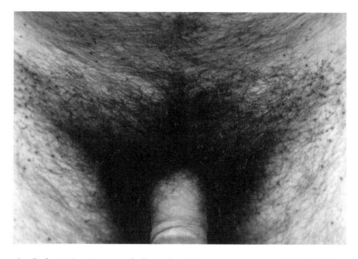

Figure 9   Infestation in an adult male. (Photo courtesy of A.W. Hoke, M.D.)

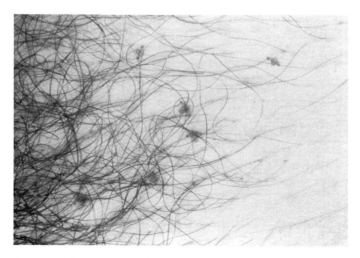

Figure 10   Magnification to demonstrate adults on pubic hairs. (Photo courtesy of A.W. Hoke, M.D.)

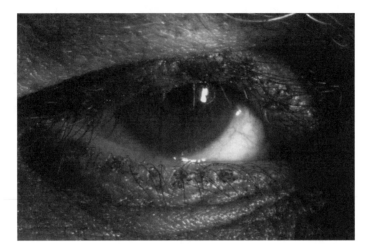

Figure 11 Palebra pediculosis. (Photo courtesy of A.W. Hoke, M.D.)

Eyelash infestation may be treated by either careful manual removal of the nits with a serrated forceps, or by application of ophthalmic ointment daily for one week and removal of the nits with serrated forceps.

References

1. Forsman, K.E. Pediculosis and scabies. What to look for in patients who are crawling with clues. *Postgrad. Med.* 98(6), 89–100, 1995.
2. Horne, R.T., Kawaski, S.Q. The prince of El Plomo. A paleopathological study. *Bull. N.Y. Acad. Med.* 60(9), 925–931, 1984.
3. Taplin, D., Menking, T.L. Infestations. In: Schnachner, L.A., Hansen, R.C. (Eds.) *Pediatric Dermatology*, New York, Churchill Livingstone, 1465–1515, 1988.
4. Donaldson, R.J. The head louse in England; prevalence amongst school children. *Health Educ. Council Rep.*, 1975.
5. Maunder, J.W. The appreciation of lice. *Proc. R. Inst. Great Britain* 55, 1–55, 1983.
6. Taplin, D., Meinking, T.L. Scabies, lice, and fungal infections. *Prim. Care Clin. Office Prac.* 16(3), 551–76, 1989.
7. Taplin, D., Meinking, T.L., Castillero, P.M., et al. Permithin 1% creme rinse (NIX) for treatment of *Pediculus humanus.* var. *capitis* infestation. *Pediatr. Dermatol.* 3, 344–48, 1986.
8. Bowerman, J.G., Gomez, M.P., Austin, R.D., et al. Comparative study of permithin 1% creme rinse and lindane shampoo for the treatment of head lice. *Pediatr. Infect. Dis.* 6, 252–55, 1987.
9. Bradenburg, K., Deinard, A.S., DiNapoli, J., et al. 1% Permethrin cream rinse vs. 1% lindane shampoo in treating *pediculosis capitis. Am. J. Dis. Child* 140, 894–6, 1986.
10. DiNapoli, J.B., Austin, R.D., Englander, S.J., et al. Eradication of head lice with a single treatment. *Am. J. Public Health* 78, 978–80, 1988.
11. Menking, T.L., Taplin, D. Advances in pediculosis, scabies, and other mite infestations. *Adv. Dermatol.* 5, 131–52, 1990.
12. Elgart, M.L. Scabies. *Dermatol. Clinics* 8(2), 258–63, 1990.
13. Alexander, J.O. *Arthropods and Human Skin.* Berlin, Springer-Verlag, 225, 1984.
14. Cole, M.M. Body Lice: In: Smith C.N., (Ed.) *Insect Colonization and Mass Production*, New York, Academic Press, 15–24, 1966.
15. Burgdorfer, W. The relapsing fevers. In: *Tropical Medicine*. Philadelphia, W.B. Saunders, 137–40, 1976.
16. Judson, F.N., Penley, K.A., Robinson, M.A., Smith, K. Comparative prevalence rates of sexually transmitted diseases in heterosexual and homosexual men. *Am. J. Epidemiol.* 112, 836–43, 1980.
17. Darrow, W.W., Barrett, D., Jay, K., et al. The gay report on sexually transmitted diseases. *Am. J. Public Health* 71, 1004–11, 1981.
18. Lane, A.T. Scabies and head lice. *Pediatr. Ann.* 16, 51–4, 1987.

Index

A

A-200, 326, 329
Abortions, 11, 13, 15–16, 84, 138
AccuProbe, 91
Acid-fast staining, 182–183, 197–198, 200
Acidolin, 5
Acinetobacter, 76
Acquired immune deficiency syndrome (AIDS).
    See also Human
immunodeficiency virus
    amebiasis and, 172
    candidiasis and, 155, 157
    cryptosporidiosis and, 190–191, 193, 197, 200,
        202
    gay bowel syndrome and, 300, 303–304
    herpesviruses and, 231–234, 238, 240
    human papilloma viruses and, 273
    molluscum contagiosum and, 285–288
    overview of, 131, 246
    scabies and, 318
Acyclovir
    gay bowel syndrome and, 303, 306
    herpesviruses and, 219, 230, 232, 235–236, 238
    interferon-α, 219, 238
ADC (AIDS dementia complex), 252
Adefovir, 263
Adenitis, 117
Adenopathy, 119, 121, 140, 227, 304
Adhesin, 172
Affirm VP III Microbial Identification Test, 25
Africa
    cryptosporidiosis in, 193
    Donovanosis in, 106
    herpesviruses in, 237, 239
    human immunodeficiency virus in, 246
    lice in, 324
    scabies in, 315
African-Americans
    bacterial vaginosis in, 6, 9
    chancroid in, 63
    gonorrhea in, 78
    herpesviruses in, 226
    lice in, 324
    vaginal pH of, 6
AFST (antifungal susceptibility tests), 158–159
Age and STDs, 78
Agglutination tests, 91, 136, 181, 209, 230
AIDS. *See* Acquired immune deficiency
        syndrome
AIDS dementia complex (ADC), 252
AIDS-Related Complex (ARC), 247–248
Albendazole, 306–307
Alcoholism, 171
Algae, 201

Allergies, 251
Alopecia, 144
Alprazolam, 262
Althaun. See Lymphogranuloma venereum
Alysiella, 76
Amebiasis. *See also Entamoeba histolytica*
    clinical manifestations of, 168–169, 175–179
    diagnosis of, 179–185
    epidemiology of, 171–172
    hepatic, 170, 175, 178–179, 181, 184
    immunology and, 169–171
    inflammatory bowel disease (IBD) and, 185
    intestinal, 184
    microbiology of, 172–173
    overview of, 167–168
    transmission of, 174–175
    treatment of, 172, 185–186
Amebic colitis, 169, 171
Amikacin, 306
Amino acid metabolism, 6
Aminoglycosides, 61
Amiodarone, 261
Amniotic fluids, 15, 19, 137
Amoxicillin, 70, 111
Amphotericin B, 159
Ampicillin, 27, 111, 306–307
Ampicillin digoxigenin conjugate, 133
Amsel's diagnostic criteria, 4, 19–20
Androscopy, 276
Anemia, 233, 255, 259, 261
Anilingus, 172, 192, 296–297, 301
Anorexia, 121, 197, 227
Antabuse, 262
Antifungal susceptibility tests (AFST), 158–159
Antigen detection, 47–48, 69
Antimony, 110
Antisense constructs, 238
Anus
    anal carcinoma, 252, 298, 305
    candidiasis and the, 151
    chancroid and the, 67
    condyloma acuminata and the, 273–274, 281
    Donovanosis and the, 107, 111–112
    lymphogranuloma venereum and the, 119
    syphilis and the, 140–141
Apicomplexa, 194
Appendicitis, 178
ARC (AIDS-Related Complex), 247–248
Arinine, 82
ART (Automated Reagin Test), 135
Arthritis, 83, 85, 118, 237
Asia, 78, 193
Asian-Americans, 9
Astemizole, 261
Asthma, 252

Ataxia, 138
Augmentin, 27
Auramine rhodamine staining, 200
Australia, 9, 43, 106, 193
Autoimmune diseases, 236. *See also* Acquired
    immune deficiency syndrome; Human
    immunodeficiency virus
Automated Reagin Test (ART), 135
Autoradiography, 152
Auxotyping, 81–82
Axenic culture methods, 168–169
Azithromycin, 70–71, 95, 111, 256, 306–307
Azothioprene, 236
AZT (zidovudine), 256, 258–263

B

Bacteremia, 97
Bacterial vaginosis (BV)
    diagnosis of, 4, 7, 19–25
    endometritis and, 11–13, 16
    epidemiology of, 7–11
    microbiology of, 5–7
    overview of, 4–5, 29
    pelvic inflammatory disease (PID) and, 11–13,
      17
    pregnancy and, 8–11, 15–19, 27–29
    treatment of, 10–11, 17–19, 25–29
Bacteroides, 5, 9, 11, 19, 67
Bacteroides bivius, 12
Balanitis, 119, 156
Balanoposthitis, 119, 208
Barium enema, 185
Bartholinitis, 83
Bartholins gland, 83–84
bcl-2, 226
Bcl-2, 236
Benign suppurative inguinal paradenitis. *See*
    Lymphogranuloma venereum
Benzathine penicillin, 71, 138
Bepridil, 261
BHRF1, 236
Biaxin, 262
Blacks. *See* African-Americans
Bladder, 107, 274
Blastocystis hominis, 171, 301, 307
BL (Burkitt's lymphoma), 219, 225, 236–237
Blindness, 84, 233
Bone marrow, 237–238, 277
Boric acid, 158
Borrelia burgdoferi, 136
Borrelia recurrentis, 328
Bowel disease, inflammatory (IBD), 185, 304
Bowenoid papulosis (BP), 274
Brachyspira aalborgii, 299, 302
Breasts, 228, 318

Bright-field microscopy, 198
Burkitt's lymphoma (BL), 219, 225, 236–237
Butoconazole, 156–157
Butyrate, 6
BV. *See* Bacterial vaginosis

C

Cachexia, 250
Caco-2 cell monolayers, 190
Cadaverine, 6
Calcofluor white staining, 201
Calmodulin, 80
Calves, cryptosporidiosis in, 189, 192, 195, 200
Calymmatobacterium granulomatis, 103–105,
    109–110. *See also* Donovanosis
Campylobacter, 302–306
Campylobacter cinaedi, 300
Campylobacter fenneliae, 300
Campylobacter fetus, 300
Campylobacter jejuni, 300, 303
Canada, 9, 43, 82
Candida, 64, 252
Candida albicans, 83, 149–152, 154–155, 157, 159,
    209
Candida glabrata, 149–151, 155, 157
Candida guilliermondii, 151, 155
Candida kefyr, 151
Candida krusei, 151, 155
Candida lusitaniae, 155
Candida parapsilosis, 150–151, 155
Candida rugosa, 155
Candida tropicalis, 150–151, 155
Candida vulvovaginitis (CVV), 150, 152
Candidiasis
    antibiotic use and, 155
    clinical manifestations of, 155–156, 160
    diagnosis of, 154–155
    epidemiology of, 149–154
    human immunodeficiency virus and, 64, 155,
      158, 160, 247
    oropharyngeal, 159
    treatment of, 156–160
    vulvovaginal (thrush), 249–251, 264
Candidiemia, 152
Cantharidin, 287
Carbohydrate utilization tests, 91
Carbolic acid, 287
Cat-scratch disease, 122
Cattle, 205
CD (Crohn's disease), 185
CDC (Centers for Disease Control), 171, 193,
    211, 246–249, 273, 277
CD4+ T lymphocytes
    AIDS and, 246–247, 249–250, 252–258, 260
    amebiasis and, 170

cryptosporidiosis and, 197, 201–202
herpesviruses and, 231, 238
Cecum, 178
Cefixime, 92, 95, 306
Cefmetazole, 95
Cefotetan, 95
Cefoxitin, 93
Ceftriaxone, 70–71, 92–93, 95, 306–307
Cefuroxime, 95
Cell-mediated immunity, 170, 207, 285–286
Cellulitis, cuff, 11, 13
Centers for Disease Control (CDC), 171, 193,
    211, 246–249, 273, 277
Central America, 171, 193, 324
Central nervous system (CNS), 232
Cephalosporins, 92, 95–96
Cerebrospinal fluids (CSF), 137, 228, 230, 263
Cervical cancer, 13–14, 247, 249, 274–275, 298
Cervical intraepithelial neoplasia (CIN), 11, 14,
    274
Cervicitis, 83–84, 92, 207–208
Cervix, 42, 107, 205, 208, 227, 273
Chancroid. *See also Haemophilus ducreyi*
    diagnosis of, 64, 68–70
    epidemiology of, 62–64, 119
    HIV-1 and, 63–64, 68, 71
    overview of, 59–62
    pathogenesis of, 65–70
    syphilis and, 64, 68, 71
    treatment of, 70–72
CHEF (contour clamp homogeneous field gel
    electrophoresis), 152
Chemiluminescence, 133
Chemotherapy, 191, 197, 277
Chickenpox, 219, 237–238
Chickens, 205
Child sexual abuse, 9–10, 85, 106, 275
China, 106
Chlamydia pneumoniae, 48
Chlamydia psittaci, 48, 118
Chlamydia trachomatis. See also
    Lymphogranuloma venereum
    bacterial vaginosis and, 11–12, 19
    culture of, 46
    diagnosis of, 44–49, 90
    epidemiology of, 42–44, 76
    gay bowel syndrome, and, 299, 302–307
    microbiology of, 118
    Neisseria gonorrhoeae and, 83, 92
    papilloma viruses and, 272
    treatment of, 49–50, 91
    urethritis from, 42, 45, 82
Chloramphenicol, 61, 111
Chloroquine, 185
Cholecystitis, 178, 197
Chorioamnionitis, 84

Chromatin, 177, 224
Chronic venereum ulcer. *See* Donovanosis
Cidofovir, 306–307
CIN (cervical intraepithelial neoplasia), 11, 14,
    274
Ciprofloxacin, 61–62, 70, 92, 96, 306
Circumcision, 63, 65, 68
Cirrhosis, 136
Cisapride, 261
Citrulline, 82
Clarithromycin, 256, 262, 306–307
Clavulonic acid, 70, 95
Clearview Chlamydia assay, 47–48
Cleocin Vaginal Cream, 26
Climatic bubo. *See* Lymphogranuloma
    venereum
Clindamycin cream, 10, 17–18, 26–28
Clorazepate, 262
Clostridium sporogenes, 29
Clotrimazole, 156–158, 211
Clozapine, 262
Clue cells, 10, 14, 20–22
CMRNG (chromosomally mediated resistant
    Neisseria gonorrhoeae), 92–96
CMV. *See* Cytomegalovirus
CNS (central nervous system), 232
Coagglutination tests, 91
Coccidiodes immitis, 251
Coccidioidomycosis, 247
Coliform bacteria, 194
Colitis
    amebic, 169, 171
    Crohn's, 304
    enterocolitis, 234, 304
    proctocolitis, 296–297, 300, 302–304, 307
    ulcerative (UC), 185
Colon, 178, 232
Colon adenocarcinoma, 190
Colonic neoplasia, 13
Colonoscopy, 185
Colpitis, anaerobic, 4
Complement activation, 169–170
Complement fixation, 48, 123, 230, 286
Con A (concanavalin A), 170
Concanavalin A (Con A), 170
Condyloma acuminata
    cancer and, 275
    clinical manifestations of, 66, 273–275,
        279–281
    diagnosis of, 275–276
    epidemiology of, 272–273
    exophytic, 273–274
    gay bowel syndrome and, 298, 303, 305
    overview of, 272
    treatment of, 276–279
Condyloma latum, 141–142

Conjunctivitis, 83–84, 118, 121, 219, 286
Constipation, 28, 83, 121, 197, 228, 303
Contagious granuloma. *See* Donovanosis
Contour clamp homogeneous field gel
  electrophoresis (CHEF), 152
Contraceptives and STDs, 9, 12
Coproantigens, 200
Coprophagy, 296
Corynebacterium diphiteriae, 105
Corynebacterium vaginalis, 4
Crack cocaine usage and STDs, 63
Crixivan (indinavir), 256, 258–260, 262–263
Crohn's colitis, 304
Crohn's disease (CD), 185
Cryotherapy, 277, 287
Cryptococcosis, 247, 250, 287
Cryptococcus neoformans, 159, 287
Cryptosporidiosis
  clinical manifestations of, 190–191, 197
  diagnosis of, 198–202
  epidemiology of, 191–194
  gay bowel syndrome and, 301, 304–307
  human immunodeficiency virus and,
    190–191, 193–194, 247, 250
  overview of, 189–190
  prevention and treatment of, 193, 202
  respiratory, 191, 200
  transmission of, 192–194
Cryptosporidium
  detection of, 198, 201
  gay bowel syndrome and, 302, 305–306
  in history, 189–190
  microbiology of, 192, 194–197
  treatment of, 202
Cryptosporidium parvum, 172, 182–183, 191,
    193–197, 199–200
Cryptosporidium serpentis, 195
CSF (cerebrospinal fluids), 137, 228, 230, 263
Curatek (Metro-Gel Vaginal), 26, 28
CVV (candida vulvovaginitis), 150, 152
Cyclospora cayetanensis, 182–183, 201
Cyclosporin A, 236
Cysteine proteases, 207
Cystitis, 45, 83
Cytobrushes, 45
Cytokines, 225, 236
Cytomegalic inclusion disease, 219
Cytomegalovirus (CMV)
  clinical manifestation of, 233
  diagnosis of, 224, 234–235
  epidemiology of, 233
  gay bowel syndrome and, 298, 302, 304–307
  human immunodeficiency virus and,
    233–235, 247, 250, 252, 256
  overview of, 218
  treatment of, 235

D

Dapsone, 256
Darkfield microscopy, 62, 69, 133, 135, 305
ddC (zalcitabine), 256, 258–261
ddI (didanosine), 256, 258–261
Dehydroemetine, 185
Delavirdine (DLV), 257–259, 262–263
D'emblé bubo. *See* Lymphogranuloma
  venereum
Dementia, 248, 252
Denmark, 8–9
Deoxyuridine triphosphatase, 223
Desciclovir, 236
DFA. *See* Direct fluorescent antibody testing
DGI (disseminated gonococcal infection), 83,
  85–87
Diabetes mellitus, 155, 160
Diamines, 24
Diamonds culturing, 209–211
Diarrhea, 28, 189–191, 197, 248, 303
Diazepam, 262
Didanosine (ddI), 256, 258–261
Dientamoeba fragilis, 171, 301
Diloxanide furoate, 185
Dinitrochlorobenzene (DNCB), 278
Direct fluorescent antibody (DFA) testing
  for *Chlamydia trachomatis,* 44, 47
  for cryptosporidiosis, 197, 200
  for *Haemophilus ducreyi,* 64, 69
  for trichomoniasis, 209–210
Disseminated gonococcal infection (DGI), 83,
  85–87
Disulfiram, 262
Diverticulitis, 178
DLV (delavirdine), 257–259, 262–263
DMP-266, 263
bDNA assay, 253
DNA hybridization, 136, 276
DNA polymerases, 223, 235
DNA probes, 48, 64, 90, 152, 180, 209
DNCB (dinitrochlorobenzene), 278
Döderlein's lactobacillus, 4, 28
Donovanosis
  chancroid and, 68–69
  clinical manifestation of, 107–108,
    111–115
  diagnosis of, 108–110
  epidemiology of, 106, 119
  overview of, 103–105
  systemic, 107
  treatment of, 110–115
Doves, 205
Doxycycline, 92, 111, 124, 138, 306–307
Drug usage and STDs, 63, 77, 132
Dysentery, amebic. *See* Amebiasis

Dyspareunia, 207
Dysuria, 82, 207, 227

E

EBERs (Epstein-Barr encoded small
  nonpolyadenylated RNAs), 225–226
EBNAs (Epstein-Barr nuclear antigens),
  225–226
EBV. *See* Epstein-Barr virus
Eczema, 119, 252, 318
EIA. *See* Enzyme immunoassay
Eikenella, 76
Electron microscopy, 198
Electrophoresis, 49, 152, 168, 284
Electrophoretic karyotyping, 152–153
Elephantiasis of the genitals, 121–122,
  124
Elimite, 321
ELISA (enzyme-linked immunosorbent assay),
  48, 124, 137–138, 230
Encainide, 261
Encephalitis, 219–220, 228, 234, 237
Encephalitozoon, 301
Encephalitozoon intestinalis, 172
Endocarditis, 83, 85, 249
Endolimax nana, 171
Endometritis, 11–13, 16, 19, 29, 83
Endoscopy, 305
Endotoxin, 5–6
Enoxacin, 70
Entamoeba coli, 168, 171, 174, 177, 180, 301
Entamoeba dispar, 168–169, 174, 177, 180
Entamoeba hartmanni, 174, 177, 180, 301
Entamoeba histolytica. See also Amebiasis
  detection of, 179–184
  distribution of, 171
  gay bowel syndrome and, 301–307
  immunology of, 169–171
  microbiology of, 170–177
  overview of, 167–168
  transmission of, 171–172, 179
  treatment of, 185
Entamoeba nana, 301
Enteritis, 296–297, 302, 304
Enterobius vermicularis, 301
Enterococcus, 18, 26, 29
Enterocolitis, 234, 304
Enterocytozoon bieneusi, 172, 301
env, 94
Enzyme immunoassay (EIA)
  Chlamydia trachomatis and, 42, 45–48
  cryptosporidiosis and, 198, 200
  Entamoeba histolytica and, 181–183
  Neisseria gonorrhoeae and, 89
  trichomoniasis and, 209

Enzyme-linked immunosorbent assay (ELISA),
  48, 124, 137–138, 230
Epidemic inguinal lymphadenopathy. *See*
  Lymphogranuloma venereum
Epidermodysplasia verruciformis, 275, 285
Epididymitis, 42, 83, 108, 208, 304
Epivir (lamivudine), 256, 258–261, 263
Epstein-Barr encoded small nonpolyadenylated
  RNAs (EBERs), 225–226
Epstein-Barr nuclear antigens (EBNAs),
  225–226
Epstein-Barr virus (EBV)
  cancers and, 225–226, 237
  clinical manifestations of, 236–237
  epidemiology of, 236
  gay bowel syndrome and, 298
  human immunodeficiency virus and, 236–237
  overview of, 218
  pathology from, 224–226
Erythema nodosum, 121
Erythromycin
  bacterial vaginosis and, 17–18, 27
  chancroid and, 70–71
  cryptosporidiosis and, 202
  Donovanosis and, 111
  gay bowel syndrome and, 306
  gonorrhea and, 95
  lymphogranuloma venereum and, 124
  syphilis and, 132
Escherichia coli, 18, 26, 80, 95, 133
Esophagus, 205, 232, 247
Estazolam, 262
Ethambutol, 306–307
Ethidium bromide staining, 152
Eurax, 321
Exanthum subitum, 219
Eyes
  Chlamydia trachomatis and, 50
  Donovanosis and, 107
  gonorrhea and, 96
  herpesviruses and, 228
  Kaposi's, 265
  lice and, 331
  molluscum contagiosum and, 288
  syphilis and, 145

F

FA (fluorescent antibody) techniques, 91,
  181–183, 198, 286
Fallopian tubes, 79, 84, 108
Famciclovir, 306
Feces, 151, 296
Fellatio, 296
Field inversion gel electrophoresis (FIGE), 152
Finland, 9

Fitz-Hugh-Curtis syndrome, 84
Flagyl. *See* Metronidazole
Flecainide, 261
Fleroxacin, 70
Flow cytometry, 200
Fluconazole, 152, 156, 158–159
5-Fluocytosine, 159
Fluorescent antibody (FA) techniques, 91,
    181–183, 198, 286. *See also* Direct fluorescent
    antibody testing
Fluorescent treponemal antibody absorption
    test (FTA-ABS), 136
5-Fluorouracil (5-FU), 277, 306
Flurazepam, 262
Focal epithelial hyperplasia, 275
Foreskin. *See* Penis
Foscarnet, 219, 233, 235, 238, 306–307
France, 8
Frei's test, 123–124
FTA-ABS (fluorescent treponemal antibody
    absorption test), 136
5-FU (5-fluorouracil), 277, 306
Fusobacterium, 67

G

Gallbladder, 200
Ganciclovir, 219, 235, 238, 306–307
Gardnerella, 23
Gardnerella vaginalis
    bacterial vaginosis and, 4–6, 9, 11, 15, 19, 26
    detection of, 20–21, 23–25, 209
Gas liquid chromatography (GLC), 9, 15, 19
Gastritis, 234
Gastroenteritis, 192
Gay bowel syndrome
    clinical features of, 301–304
    diagnosis of, 304–306
    epidemiology of, 172, 296
    microorganisms associated with, 297–301
    treatment of, 306–307
GC-Lect medium, 87
Gel agar diffusion techniques, 286
Gel electrophoresis, 49, 152, 168, 284
Gene amplification techniques, 48
Genital herpes, 68–69, 119, 219, 226–232, 256. *See*
    also Herpes simplex viruses
Genital ulcer disease, 62–64
Genital warts. *See* Condyloma acuminata
Gentamicin, 111, 306
Gentian violet, 110
Germ tube test, 155
Giardia, 194, 201
Giardia lamblia, 171, 200, 300, 302, 304–307
Giemsa staining, 104, 109, 197, 230, 286
Gingivitis, 6

Gingivostomatitis, 219
GISP (Gonococcal Isolate Surveillance Project),
    92–93
GLC (gas liquid chromatography), 9, 15, 19
Glomerulonephritis, 237
Glucophosphate isomerase (GPI), 168
Glucose metabolism, 5
Gonococcal Isolate Surveillance Project (GISP),
    92–93
Gonococcemia, 97
Gonorrhea. *See Neisseria gonorrhoeae*
Gonostat, 90
Gonozyme, 89–90
Gout, 261
GPI (glucophosphate isomerase), 168
Gram stains
    bacterial vaginosis and, 9–11, 14, 16, 19–25
    chancroid and, 60–61, 69
    Chlamydia trachomatis infections and, 42
    gay bowel syndrome and, 305
    gonorrhea and, 88–91
    molluscum contagiosum and, 286
Granuloma donovani. *See* Donovanosis
Granuloma inguinale. *See* Donovanosis
Great Britain, 193
Griseofulvin, 287
Guillain-Barré syndrome, 233
Guinea pig, Hartley, 225

H

Haemophilus, 95
Haemophilus ducreyi. *See also* Chancroid
    biology of, 60–62
    identification of, 122
    overview of, 59–60
    treatment of, 70–72
Haemophilus influenzae, 252
Haemophilus vaginalis, 4
Halofuginone, 202
HCT-8 (human ileocecal adenocarcinoma), 202
Headache, 28, 121, 227–228, 261
Heat shock protein, 49
Helicobacter, 300, 302, 306
Hemagglutination tests, 136, 181, 230
Hematoxylin and eosin (H&E) staining, 182,
    201, 286, 305
Heme, 81
Hemophiliacs, 262
Heparin, 118, 222
Hepatitis
    cryptosporidiosis and, 197
    cytomegalovirus and, 237–238
    gay bowel syndrome and, 297–298
    human immunodeficiency virus and, 251, 256
    tests for, 135

Hepatosplenomegaly, 138, 233, 238, 304
Herpesviruses. *See also* Herpes simplex viruses; Herpes simplex virus type 1; Herpes simplex virus type 2
   alphaherpesvirinae. *See* Herpes simplex virus type 1; Herpes simplex virus type 2
   betaherpesvirinae. *See* Cytomegalovirus (CMV)
   cell transformation by, 225–226
   clinical manifestations of, 226–229, 231–232, 237, 239–242
   cytopathology from, 224, 229
   gammaherpesvirinae. *See* Epstein-Barr virus (EBV)
   gene expression in, 222–224
   human immunodeficiency virus and, 228, 231–240, 251
   latency of, 224–225
   overview of, 218
   structure and replication of, 218–222
Herpes simplex viruses (HSV). *See also* Herpes simplex virus type 2; Herpes simplex virus type 1; Herpesviruses
   clinical manifestations of, 226–228
   cutaneous lesions and, 232
   diagnosis of, 229–230
   epidemiology of, 226
   gay bowel syndrome and, 298, 302, 304–306
   genital herpes, 68–69, 119, 219, 226–232, 256
   Haemophilus ducreyi and, 62, 69
   human immunodeficiency virus and, 228, 231–233, 247, 250, 252
   Neisseria gonorrhoeae and, 83
   treatment of, 230
   Trichomonas vaginalis and, 206
Herpes simplex virus type 1 (HSV-1)
   clinical manifestations of, 232
   cytopathology from, 224, 229
   gay bowel syndrome and, 302, 306
   human immunodeficiency virus and, 228
   latency of, 225
   overview of, 218
Herpes simplex virus type 2 (HSV-2)
   clinical manifestations of, 227, 232
   cytopathology from, 224
   epidemiology of, 226
   gay bowel syndrome and, 302–303, 306
   human immunodeficiency virus and, 228
   latency of, 225
   overview of, 218
Herpes zoster (shingles), 249–250, 252
Hexokinase (HK), 168
HHV-1 (human herpesvirus-1). *See* Herpes simplex virus type 1
HHV-2 (human herpesvirus-2). *See* Herpes simplex virus type 2

HHV-3 (human herpesvirus-3). *See* Varicella-zoster virus
HHV-4 (human herpesvirus-4). *See* Epstein-Barr virus
HHV-5 (human herpesvirus-5). *See* Cytomegalovirus
HHV-6 (human herpesvirus-6), 224, 238
HHV-7 (human herpesvirus-7), 218–219, 238
HHV-8 (human herpesvirus-8). *See* Kaposi's sarcoma
Hispanics, 63, 78
Histoplasma capsulatum, 251
Histoplasmosis, 109
HIV. *See* Human immunodeficiency virus
Hivid (zalcitabine), 256, 258–261
HK (hexokinase), 168
Hodgkin's disease, 122, 286
Hollander's culturing, 209–210
Homosexual males
   amebiasis in, 171–172
   cryptosporidiosis in, 192
   Donovanosis in, 106
   gay bowel syndrome in, 296–301, 306–307
   herpesviruses in, 231, 239
   lymphogranuloma venereum in, 118–119
HPV. *See* Human papilloma viruses
HSIG (human serum immunoglobulin), 202
HSV-1. *See* Herpes simplex virus type 1
HSV-2. *See* Herpes simplex virus type 2
Human B-lymphotropic virus (HHV-6), 219, 224, 238
Human herpesvirus-1 (HHV-1). *See* Herpes simplex virus type 1
Human herpesvirus-2 (HHV-2). *See* Herpes simplex virus type 2
Human herpesvirus-3 (HHV-3). *See* Varicella-zoster virus
Human herpesvirus-4 (HHV-4). *See* Epstein-Barr virus
Human herpesvirus-5 (HHV-5). *See* Cytomegalovirus
Human herpesvirus-6 (HHV-6), 219, 224, 238
Human herpesvirus-7 (HHV-7), 218–219, 238
Human herpesvirus-8 (HHV-8). *See* Kaposi's sarcoma
Human ileocecal adenocarcinoma (HCT-8), 202
Human immunodeficiency virus (HIV). *See also* Acquired immune deficiency syndrome
   amebiasis and, 172
   antiretroviral therapy and, 256–263
   bacterial vaginosis and, 7, 11, 14–15
   candidiasis and, 64, 155, 158, 160
   chancroid and, 63–64, 68, 71
   in children, 248
   Chlamydia trachomatis and, 64
   classification of, 246–250

cryptosporidiosis and, 190–191, 193–194
disease progression of, 251–255
Donovanosis and, 107–108
gay bowel syndrome and, 297–307
gonorrhea and, 85, 96
herpesviruses and, 228, 231–240, 279
Kaposi's sarcoma (KS) and, 238–240, 247–248, 250, 252, 264–266
laboratory investigations of, 255
lymphogranuloma venereum and, 119
molluscum contagiosum and, 283, 285, 287
pet ownership and, 193
prevention and treatment for, 256
scabies and, 318, 321
syphilis and, 132–133, 138
Trichomonas infection and, 64, 207
vaginal pH and, 7, 14
Human papilloma viruses (HPV). *See also*
    Condyloma acuminata
    bacterial vaginosis and, 13
    cancer and, 275
    clinical manifestations of, 273–275, 279–281
    diagnosis of, 275–276
    epidemiology of, 272–273
    gay bowel syndrome and, 298, 302, 306
    human immunodeficiency virus and, 252
    treatment of, 276–279
    types of, 272
Human serum immunoglobulin (HSIG), 202
Hybridization techniques, 48, 136, 152–153, 276
Hydrogen peroxide production, 5–6, 11
Hyperglobulinemia, 124
Hypogammaglobulinemia, 191
Hypoxanthine, 82
Hysterectomies, 11–13, 29, 84

I

IBD (inflammatory bowel disease), 185, 304
IDV (indinavir), 256, 258–260, 262–263
IFN (interferons), 191, 225, 236, 278
IgA, 7, 14, 169, 207
IgE, 169
IgG, 169, 207, 256
IgM, 207, 234, 285
Immunocompromised individuals. *See also*
    Acquired immune deficiency syndrome;
    Human immunodeficiency virus; Organ
    transplant recipients
    cryptosporidiosis and, 191, 193, 197, 200, 202
    herpesviruses and, 228, 233, 236, 238
    molluscum contagiosum in, 285–287
    scabies and, 316
Immunofluorescent detection methods, 192, 230, 234–235
Immunoglobulins

heavy chain locus, 237
IgA, 7, 14, 169, 207
IgE, 169
IgG, 169, 207, 256
IgM, 207, 234, 285
Immunoperoxidase (IP)-labeling, 234
Imodium, 307
India, 106
Indinavir (IDV), 256, 258–260, 262–263
Indirect fluorescent antibody (FA) tests, 181–183
Indirect hemagglutination tests, 181
Indirect immunoperoxidase assay, 48
Indonesia, 9–10
Infertility, 42, 49, 76, 208
Inflammatory bowel disease (IBD), 185, 304
Inguinal granuloma. *See* Donovanosis
Inguinal lymphogranuloma. *See*
    Lymphogranuloma venereum
InPouch TV, 209–210, 212
in situ hybridization, 236, 276
Interferons (IFN), 191, 225, 236, 278
Interleukins, 5, 191
Intertrigo, 119
Intestines, 178, 191, 201, 205
Intrauterine devices, 9
Invirase (saquinavir), 256, 258–259, 261, 263
Iodamoeba butschlii, 301
Iodoquinol, 185–186, 306–307
IP (immunoperoxidase) labeling, 234
Iritis, 138
Iron, 81
Iron hematoxylin staining, 200
Isoenzyme analysis, 152, 168
Isoleucine, 82
Isoniazid, 256
Isospora, 304–305
Isospora belli, 172, 182–183, 194–195, 201, 301–302
Isosporiasis, 247, 250, 301
Israel, 43
Itraconazole, 156–157
Ivermectin, 321

J

Japan, 43
Jaundice, 178

K

Kaposi's sarcoma (KS)
    gay bowel syndrome and, 298, 304–305
    human immunodeficiency virus and, 231, 238–240, 247–248, 250, 252, 264–266
    overview of, 219
Keratoconjunctivitis, 121, 219
Ketoconazole, 156–159

Kidney stones, 259
Kingella, 76
Kingella denitrificans, 91
Kinyoun's staining method, 197
Kissing disease, 236
Klebsiella granulomatis, 105
Klebsiella rhinocleromatis, 105
KS. *See* Kaposi's sarcoma
Kwell, 321, 329

L

Labia, 107, 119, 139, 142
Lactacin G, 5
β-Lactams, 61, 93–95
Lactobacilli, 4–5, 11, 20, 22–23, 25–26, 28
Lactobacillus acidophilus, 5, 29
Lactobacillus crispatus, 5
Lactobacillus fermentum, 5
Lactobacillus gasseri, 5
Lactobacillus jensenii, 5
Lactoferrin, 81
Lambs, cryptosporidiosis and, 192
Lamivudine (3TC), 256, 258–261, 263
Lanosterol, 156
Larynx, 274–275
Latency associated transcript (LAT), 225, 236
Latency membrane proteins (LMPs), 225–226, 236
Latex agglutination, 209
LE (leukocyte esterase) test, 45
Leishmania, 110
Leishmaniosis, 109
Lesbians, 9, 208, 297
Letrazuril, 202
Leukemia, 237, 246, 285
Leukocyte esterase (LE) test, 45
Leukorrhoea, 4, 21, 28
Levamisole, 278
LGV. *See* Lymphogranuloma venereum
Lice
    body, 326–329
    head, 324–326
    overview of, 323
    pubic, 329–331
Ligase chain assay, 44, 48, 90
Lincomycin, 111
Lindande shampoo, 325
Lindane cream, 329
LIP (lymphoid interstitial pneumonitis), 247
Lipooligosaccharides (LOS), 79–81
Listeriosis, 249
Lithium thyomalate, 110
Liver
    abcess of, 170, 175, 178–179, 181, 184, 186

hepatic disease, 138, 178–179, 184, 186, 233, 238
LMPs (latency membrane proteins), 225–226, 236
Lobucavir, 263
Lomotil, 307
Long terminal repeat (LTR), 238
LOS (lipooligosaccharides), 79–81
Loviride (LOV), 257–259, 262–263
Lugol's iodine stain, 126
Lymphadenopathy
    Chlamydia trachomatis, 117
    Haemophilus ducreyi, 59, 67
    lice and, 324
    lymphogranuloma venereum and, 120
    persistent generalized (PGL), 249–250
    syphilis and, 138
Lymphocytosis, 233
Lymphogranuloma venereum (LGV). *See also*
        Chlamydia trachomatis
    clinical manifestations of, 119–123, 125–126
    diagnosis of, 122–124
    epidemiology of, 118–119
    overview of, 117–118
    treatment of, 124
Lymphoid interstitial pneumonitis (LIP), 247
Lymphomas, 247–248, 250

M

MAC (membrane attack complex), 81
Macrophage migration-inhibition assays, 170
MAI *(Mycobacterium avium intracellulare)*
        infection, 300, 302, 304, 306–307
Major outer membrane (MOMP) antigens, 48
Malaria, 237
Malate dehydrogenase (ME), 168
Malaysia, 106
MC. *See* Molluscum contagiosum
McCoy cells, 46–47
MCV *(Molluscum contagiosum* virus), 283–284
ME (malate dehydrogenase), 168
Megacolon, 304
Meingasser's method, 211
Membrane attack complex (MAC), 81
Men
    Chlamydia trachomatis in, 42
    condyloma acuminata in, 273
    lice in, 324
    Neisseria gonorrhoeae in, 82–83, 86
    scabies in, 315
    Trichomonas vaginalis in, 208
Meningitis
    gonorrhea and, 83, 85
    herpesviruses and, 219, 228, 238
    human immunodeficiency virus and, 249

lymphogranuloma venereum and, 121
  syphilis and, 138
Meningococci, 88
Meningoencephalitis, 121, 233
Menopause, 13
Mental institutions, 171
Meperidine, 261
Methionine, 82
Methotrexate, 285
Metro-Gel Vaginal (Curatek), 26, 28
Metronidazole
  for amebiasis, 185–186
  for bacterial vaginosis, 10, 12–13, 17–18, 26–28
  for gay bowel syndrome, 306–307
  for trichomoniasis, 210–212
Metrorrhagia, 12
Mexico, 171
MHA-TP (*Treponema pallidum*
  microhemagglutination test), 136
Miconazole, 156–157
Microimmunofluorescence (MIF), 48
Microscopy, 62, 69, 133, 135, 198, 305
Microsporidia, 201, 301–302, 304–306
Midazolam, 262
Mobiluncus, 5, 9, 12, 20–21, 23, 25
Modified Thayer-Martin (MTM) medium, 87
Molecular typing methods, 152–153
Molluscum contagiosum (MC)
  clinical manifestations of, 285–286, 288–289
  condyloma acuminata and, 275
  diagnosis of, 286–287
  epidemiology of, 284–285
  overview of, 283–284
  treatment of, 287
Molluscum contagiosum virus (MCV), 283–284.
    See also Molluscum contagiosum
MOMP (major outer membrane) antigens, 48
Mongolism and scabies, 316
Monkeys, 197
Monoclonal antibodies
  Chlamydia trachomatis and, 49, 118, 124
  cryptosporidiosis and, 200
  Entamoeba histolytica and, 180
  Haemophilus ducreyi and, 64
  herpesviruses and, 230
Mononucleosis, 135, 219, 233, 236, 251
Moraxella, 76
Mouth
  candidiasis and the, 151
  Donovanosis and the, 108
  herpesviruses and the, 228, 236–237
  human immunodeficiency virus and the, 259
  Kaposi's, 264
  lymphogranuloma venereum and the, 119
  papilloma viruses and the, 275, 279
  syphilis and the, 140–141

trichomoniasis and the, 205
MTM (modified Thayer-Martin) medium, 87
mtr, 94
Mucinase, 7
Multilocus enzyme electrophoresis, 152
Murine typhus, 328
c-*myc*, 237
Mycobacterium avium, 247, 252, 256, 307
Mycobacterium avium intracellulare (MAI)
    infection, 300, 302, 304, 306–307
Mycobacterium kansasii, 247
Mycobacterium tuberculosis, 122, 247, 249
Mycobutin (rifabutin), 256, 261–262, 306–307
Mycoplasma, 5, 135
Mycoplasma hominis, 5, 9, 11–14, 19, 26
Myelopathy, 234, 248
Myeloperoxidase, 6
Myocarditis, 83, 233
Myositis, 259, 261

N

Nasopharyngeal carcinoma, 219, 225
National Institutes of Health (NIH), 193
National Sanitation Foundation (NSF), 194
Native Americans, 78
Nausea, 28, 121, 197, 261
Neisseria, 95
Neisseria elongata, 76
Neisseria gonorrhoeae
  antimicrobial resistance by, 91–98
  bacterial vaginosis and, 11–12, 14, 19
  Chlamydia trachomatis and, 42
  chromosomally mediated resistant
    (CMRNG), 92–96
  clinical manifestations of, 82–85, 96–98
  culture media for, 87–88, 90
  diagnosis of, 85–91, 98
  epidemiology of, 76–79, 297
  gay bowel syndrome and, 299, 302, 305–306
  HIV infection and, 85
  papilloma viruses and, 272
  pathogenesis of, 79–82
  penicillin-producing (PPNG), 84, 92–96
  tetracycline resistant strains (TRNG),
    92–94
  treatment and prevention of, 76, 91–92
Neisseria lactamica, 91
Nelfinavir, 258, 263
Neonates, 83, 86, 118, 219
Neopterin, 254
Nerve growth factor (NGF), 225
Neuropathy, peripheral, 248–249
Nevirapine (NVP), 257–259, 262–263
New Guinea, 106, 108, 284
NGU (nongonococcal urethritis), 82

Nicolas-Favre-Durand disease. *See* Lymphogranuloma venereum
NIH (National Institutes of Health), 193
Ninorazole, 210
NIX, 324, 326
Nocardiosis, 249
Non-nucleoside reverse transcriptase inhibitors (NNRTIs), 257, 259, 262–263
Nonoxynol-9, 9
Norvir (ritonavir), 256, 258–263
Nosema, 301
NSF (National Sanitation Foundation), 194
Nucleic acid probes, 25, 48
NVP (nevirapine), 257–259, 262–263
NYC medium, 87

O

Octreotide, 202
OFAGE (orthogonal-field alternation gel electrophoresis), 152
Ofloxacin, 27, 61–62, 70, 92, 96, 306
OHL (oral hairy leukoplakia), 219, 236–237, 249–250, 252, 304
Onychomycosis, 264
Oocysts, 190–198, 202
Oophoritis, 83
Opacity proteins, 80
Ophthalmic infection. *See* Eyes
Optic atrophy, 138
Oral contraceptives, 9, 12
Oral hairy leukoplakia (OHL), 219, 236–237, 249–250, 252, 304
Organ transplant recipients, 236, 238–239, 285
Ornidazole, 210
Ornithosis, 118
Oropharyngeal infection, 83, 232
Orthogonal-field alternation gel electrophoresis (OFAGE), 152
Ovaries, 108
Oxidase test, 90

P

Pace 2, 90
Pacific Islanders, 78
PAGE (polyacrylamide gel electrophoresis), 152, 284
Pallons d'amour, 329
PAM (penicillin aluminum monostearate), 138
Pancreatitis, 197, 259, 261
Papanicolaou smears
    bacterial vaginosis and, 9, 14, 21–22
    condyloma acuminata and, 273, 276
    Donovanosis and, 114
    herpes simplex viruses and, 230

human immunodeficiency virus and, 252
    trichomoniasis and, 209
Papilloma viruses. *See* Human papilloma viruses
Parametritis, 83
Paromomycin, 185, 190, 202, 306–307
PAS (periodic acid-Schiff), 182
Passive hemagglutination, 230
PBMC (peripheral blood mononuclear cells), 191, 240
PCP (*Pneumocystis carinii* pneumonia), 248, 250, 256
PCR. *See* Polymerase chain reaction
Pediculus humanus capitis, 323–324, 328–329. *See also* Lice
Pediculus humanus corporis, 323. *See also* Lice
Pelvic inflammatory disease (PID), 11–13, 17, 42, 76, 83–84, 249
pen, 95
Penicillin
    Donovanosis and, 110
    Haemophilus ducreyi and, 62, 71
    Neisseria gonorrhoeae and, 82–85, 92–93
    syphilis and, 132, 137–138
Penicillin aluminum monostearate (PAM), 138
Penis
    cancer of the, 110, 115
    candidiasis in the, 151
    chancroid of the, 66, 68–69
    condyloma acuminata of the, 66, 273, 279
    Donovanosis of the, 107–108, 112–113
    elephantiasis of the, 121–122
    herpesviruses and the, 227
    molluscum contagiosum of the, 288
    saxophone, 121–122
    scabies of the, 317, 320
    syphilis and the, 139–140
    trichomoniasis of the, 205
Pentamidine, 256
Pentatrichomonas hominis, 205
Peptostreptococcus, 5, 9, 11, 19, 26
Periappendicitis, 42, 83
Peridontal disease, 6
Perihepatitis, 42, 83–84
Perineal lesions, 112–113
Periodic acid-Schiff (PAS), 182
Peripheral blood mononuclear cells (PBMC), 191, 240
Perisplenitis, 83
Peritonitis, 6, 11, 42, 83
Permanent stained smears, 179–183, 199
Permethrin, 321, 324
Pets, cryptosporidiosis and, 193
PGL (persistent generalized lymphadenopathy), 249–250
PGM (phosphoglucomutase), 168

pH, vaginal, 6–7, 9–10, 14, 20, 27
PHA (phytohemagglutinin), 170
Pharyngitis, 82–84
Phimosis, 119
Phosphoglucomutase (PGM), 168
Phospholipases, 7, 13
Phthirus pubis, 323, 329–330. *See also* Lice
Phytohemagglutinin (PHA), 170
PID (pelvic inflammatory disease), 11–13, 17, 42, 76, 83–84, 249
Pigeons, 205
pil, 80
Pilin, 79
Pimozide, 262
Pinta, 132
Piperonyl butoxide, 325–326
Piroxicam, 261
Pleistophora, 301
PLH (pulmonary lymphoid hyperplasia), 247
PML (progressive multifocal leukoencephalopathy), 247, 250, 252
PMNs (polymorphonuclear leukocytes), 42, 45, 79–80, 170, 235
Pneumocystis, 234
Pneumocystis carinii, 247–248, 250, 252, 256
Pneumonia
    herpesviruses and, 237
    human immunodeficiency virus and, 247, 250
    lymphogranuloma venereum and, 121
    Pneumocystis carinii (PCP), 248, 250, 256
Pneumonitis, 233, 237–238
Podophyllin, 277, 281, 287, 306
Podophyllin emodi, 277
Podophyllin peltatum, 277
Poliovirus, 50
Polyacrylamide gel electrophoresis (PAGE), 152, 284
Polymerase chain reaction (PCR)
    Chlamydia trachomatis and, 42, 46, 48
    condylomata acuminata and, 276
    Cryptosporidium and, 201–202
    cytomegaloviruses and, 235
    Haemophilus ducreyi and, 64, 70
    herpesviruses and, 230, 238–240
    RT, 253
    syphilis and, 136–137
Polymorphonuclear leukocytes (PMNs), 42, 45, 79–80, 170, 235
Porphomonas, 5
Por protein, 80
PPNG (penicillin-producing *Neisseria gonorrhoeae*), 84, 92–96
pPROM (preterm premature rupture of membranes), 15–17, 29
Prednisolone, 236
Prednisone, 285

Pregnancy
    bacterial vaginosis during, 8–11, 15–19, 27–29
    candidiasis during, 155–156
    condyloma acuminata during, 272–274, 277
    ectopic, 76
    gonorrhea during, 84
    herpesviruses during, 228
    syphilis during, 132, 138
    trichomoniasis during, 207–208, 211
    tubal, 42
Preterm birth, 4, 7, 15–19, 29
Preterm labor (PTL), 16–17, 29
Preterm premature rupture of membranes (pPROM), 15–17, 29
Prevotella, 5, 11, 23, 25–26
Prevotella bivius, 19
Probenecid, 95, 307
Procaine penicillin G, 138
Proctitis
    gay bowel syndrome and, 296–297, 299, 302–304, 306–307
    gonorrhea and, 82–84, 92
    herpesviruses and, 231
    lymphogranuloma venereum and, 119
Proctocolitis, 296–297, 300, 302–304, 307
Progressive multifocal leukoencephalopathy (PML), 247, 250, 252
Proline, 82
Proline amniopeptidase, 24
Propafenone, 261
Propoxyphene, 261
Prostaglandins, 5, 7
Prostatitis, 42, 208
Prostitution and STDs, 63, 118
Protozoal infections, 135
Pruritis, 207, 318, 321
Pseudomonas, 95
Psittacosis, 118
PTL (preterm labor), 16–17, 29
Pudendi tropicum granuloma. *See* Donovanosis
Pulmonary lymphoid hyperplasia (PLH), 247
Pulsed-field gel electrophoresis, 49
Putrescine, 6, 20
Pyrethrins, 321, 325–326, 329
Pyridoxine, 256
Pyruvic acid, 6
Pyuria, sterile, 42

Q

Quinacrine, 306
Quinidine, 261
Quinolones, 92–93, 95–96

R

Radiculopathy, 234, 303
Random amplified polymorphic DNA (RAPD), 195
Rapid Plasma Reagin (RPR) test, 135–136, 306
Rattus norvegicus, 328
Rectal cancer, 123
Rectitis, 121
Rectum, 83, 119, 121, 151
Reiter's syndrome, 42, 118, 136
Relapsing fever, 328
Renal allograft recipients, 236, 238
Rescriptor (delavirdine), 257–259, 262–263
Respiratory disease, 191, 197, 200
Restriction enzyme analysis, 49, 82, 284
Retinitis, 233–235, 247, 256, 307
Retrovir (zidovudine), 256, 258–263
RFLP, 152
Rhinoscleroma, 105, 109
Ribonucleotide reductase, 223
Ribotyping, 49, 64
Ribozymes, 238
Rickettsia prowazekii, 328
Rickettsia typhi, 328
RID, 325–326
Rifabutin (Mycobutin), 256, 261–262, 306–307
Ritonavir (RTV), 256, 258–263
Rochalliamea quintana, 328
Rosaxcin, 70
Roseola infantum, 219, 238
RPR (Rapid Plasma Reagin) test, 135–136, 306
RTV (ritonavir), 256, 258–263

S

Sabouraud dextrose agar (Sab), 154
Saline wet mounts, 209–210
Salmonella, 95, 302, 304–306
Salmonella septicemia, 247, 250, 300
Salpingitis, 11–12, 29, 42, 50, 83–84
Saquinavir (SQV), 256, 258–259, 261, 263
Sarcocystis, 194
Sarcoidosis, 285–286
Sarcoptes scabiei hominis, 315
Scabies, 315–321
Scarlatiniform eruption, 121
Sclerosing granuloma. *See* Donovanosis
Scotland, 284
Scrofuloderma, 122
Scrofulous bubo. *See* Lymphogranuloma venereum
Scrotum, 107, 121, 317
SDS-PAGE, 284
Secnidazole, 210
Seminal vesiculitis, 83

Septata intestinalis, 301
Serology, 48–49, 135–136, 155, 169, 230, 305–306
Serotyping, 81–82, 94
Serpiginous ulcer. *See* Donovanosis
Sexual abuse in children, 9–10, 85, 106, 275
Sexual behavior and transmission, 9–10, 44–45, 71–72, 78, 118, 172
Sexually transmitted disease (STD) clinics, 7–8, 12, 43, 85, 88
Sheather's sugar solution, 198
Shigella, 95, 302–303, 305–306
Shigella flexneri, 300
Shigella sonniae, 300
Shingles, 249–250, 252
Sialic acid, 81
Sialidase, 7, 14
Sigmoidoscopy, 179, 185, 231, 303–305
Simonsiella, 76
Sixth disease, 219, 238
Skene's gland, 84
Skin, 143, 151, 233–234, 252
Smoking and STDs, 14
Snakes, 195
Sodium polyanetholsulfonate, 87
South Africa, 69, 71
South America, 171, 193, 324
Southern blot hybridization, 48, 152–153, 276
Spectinomycin, 92–93, 95
Spiramycin, 202
Spirochetes. *See* Syphilis; *Treponema pallidum*
Spirochetosis, intestinal, 299–300, 305–306
Sporogony, 195
Sporozoites, 196–197
Sputum, 201
Squamous cell carcinoma, 109, 274–275
SQV (saquinavir), 256, 258–259, 261, 263
Sri Lanka, 106
Staphylococcus epidermidis, 5
Starch gel electrophoresis, 168
Stavudine (d4T), 256, 258–259, 261, 263
STD (sexually transmitted disease) clinics, 7–8, 12, 43, 85, 88
Stevens Johnson's syndrome, 262
Streptococcus pneumoniae, 252, 256
Streptomycin, 111
Strongyloides stercoralis, 301–302
Strongyloidiasis, 250, 301
Struma. *See* Lymphogranuloma venereum
Subacute inguinal lymphogranulomatosis. *See* Lymphogranuloma venereum
Succinic acid, 6
Sulbactam, 95
Sulfadiazine, 124
Sulfa drugs, 110
Sulfametoxazole, 111
Sulfisoxazole, 124

Sulfonamides, 61
Surgery and STDs, 124
Susceptibility testing, 158–159
Sweden, 8–10, 14, 43
Swimming pools, cryptosporidiosis and, 194
Syphilis. *See also Treponema pallidum*
    clinical manifestations of, 139–145, 304
    congenital, 132, 136, 145
    diagnosis of, 135–136
    elephantiasis and, 121
    epidemiology of, 119, 132–133
    HIV infection and, 132–133, 138, 251, 298
    meningeal, 138
    neurosyphilis, 136–138
    overview of, 131–132
    papilloma viruses and, 272
    pathology of, 134–135, 137
    treatment of, 134, 138

T

Tarter emetic, 110
T-cell lymphomas, 237
Tenesmus, 83, 121, 231, 303
Tenosynovitis, 83, 98
Terconazole, 156–157
Terfenadine, 262
Tetracyclines
    Donovanosis and, 111
    Haemophilus ducreyi and, 61
    lymphogranuloma venereum and, 124
    Neisseria gonorrhoeae and, 92–93, 95
    syphilis and, 132, 138
Thiamine, 82
Thrombocytopenia, 233, 238, 249, 255
Thrush, 249–251, 264, 304
Tianfenicol, 111, 124
αTIF (α-*trans*-inducing factor), 220–222, 225
Tinidazole, 210, 306
Tioconazole, 156–157
Tissue culture neutralization, 286
TK, 223, 230, 232
TMP-SMX, 306
TNF (tumor necrosis factor), 236
Toxoplasma gondii, 194
Toxoplasmosis, 247, 250, 252, 256
TPI (*Treponema pallidum* immobilization) test, 136
Trachoma, 118
trans-activating transcription factors, 238
Transferrin, 81
α-*trans*-inducing factor (αTIF), 220–222, 225
Trench fever, 328
Treponema carateum, 132
Treponema pallidum, 122. *See also* Syphilis
    detection of, 64, 136–137

dormant phase of, 135
epidemiology of, 297
gay bowel syndrome and, 299, 302–303, 306
microbiology of, 132–134
pathology of, 134
Treponema pallidum immobilization test (TPI), 136
Treponema pallidum microhemagglutination test (MHA-TP), 136
Treponema paralius-cunniculi, 133
Treponema pertenue, 132, 136
Tretinoin, 287
Triazolam, 262
Trichloroacetic acid, 277, 287
Trichomonas, 64
Trichomonas foetus, 205–206
Trichomonas gallinae, 205–206
Trichomonas tenax, 205
Trichomonas vaginalis, 14, 19, 82–83, 205–212
Trichomoniasis
    clinical manifestations of, 207–209
    diagnosis of, 209–210
    epidemiology of, 205–207
    gonorrhea and, 82–83
    papilloma viruses and, 272
    treatment of, 210–212
    urogenital, 209
    vaginal pH and, 6
Trichosel culturing, 209–211
Trichrome staining, 182–183, 197, 200–201
Trichuris, 301
Trimethalamine, 6
Trimethoprim, 61–62, 70, 256
Triple sulfa cream, 27
TRNG (tetracycline resistant *Neisseria gonorrhoeae*), 92–94
Trophozoites, 173–176, 179–182, 186, 205, 305
Tropical bubo. *See* Lymphogranuloma venereum
Tropical disease. *See* Donovanosis
Tropicum granuloma. *See* Donovanosis
Tuberculosis
    elephantiasis and, 121
    human immunodeficiency virus and, 247, 249–252, 256
    lymphogranuloma venereum and, 117–118, 122
    pulmonary, 108
Tumor necrosis factor (TNF), 236
Typhus, 328

U

UC (ulcerative colitis), 185
Ulcerating granuloma. *See* Donovanosis
Ulcerative colitis (UC), 185

United Kingdom, 8–9
United States
    amebiasis in, 171
    bacterial vaginosis in, 8–9
    Chlamydia trachomatis in, 43
    cryptosporidiosis in, 192–193
    herpesviruses in, 226, 233
    Neisseria gonorrhoeae in, 82
    syphilis in, 132–133
Uracil, 82
Ureaplasma, 64
Ureaplasma urealyticum, 5, 12, 82
Urethra, 82, 89, 208, 273–274
Urethritis
    Candida and, 82
    Chlamydia trachomatis and, 42, 45, 82, 118
    gay bowel syndrome and, 304
    Haemophilus ducreyi, 68
    herpes simplex and, 82
    lymphogranuloma venereum and, 119
    Neisseria gonorrhoeae and, 82–84, 92, 96
    nongonococcal (NGU), 82
    Trichomonas vaginalis, 82, 208
    Ureaplasma urealyticum and, 82
Urine testing procedures, 45–46
Uterus, 11–12, 84, 205

V

Vaccines, 50, 134, 138, 172, 256, 279
Vagabond's disease, 327–328
Vagina
    candidiasis in the, 151
    chancroid infections of the, 66–67
    condyloma acuminata of the, 273, 280
    discharge from the, 4–5, 42, 83, 207–208, 227, 273
    Donovanosis of the, 107
    fluid composition in the, 5, 20–21
    herpesviruses and the, 227
    trichomoniasis in the, 205, 208
Vaginal bacteriosis. *See* Bacterial vaginosis
Vaginitis
    anaerobic, 4
    candida vulvovaginitis (CVV), 150, 155–158
    Gardnerella, 4
    Haemophilus vaginalis, 4
    nonspecific, 4, 8
    trichomoniasis and, 207
Valacyclovir, 306
Valium, 262
Vancomycin, 87–88
Varicella-zoster virus (VZV), 219, 232, 237–238
Venereal Disease Research Laboratory (VDRL), 135–136
Venereal warts. *See* Condyloma acuminata

Venereum granuloma. *See* Donovanosis
Verruca vulgaris, 275
VHS (virion host shut off) protein, 220, 224
Vidarabine, 238
Videx (didanosine), 256, 258–261
VIN (vulvar intraepithelial neoplasia), 274
Viramune (nevirapine), 257–259, 262–263
Virion host shut off (VHS) protein, 220, 224
Vitamin A acid, 287
Vitamin B-12 absorption, 190
Vulva, 107, 121, 227, 273
Vulvar carcinoma *in situ,* 275
Vulvar intraepithelial neoplasia (VIN), 274
Vulvovaginitis, 119
VZV (varicella-zoster virus), 219, 232, 237–238

W

Wasserman antibodies, 135
Water contamination and cryptosporidiosis, 192–194, 201–202
Western immunoblot technique, 136
Whites, 78
WHO (World Health Organization), 246, 248–250
Women
    Chlamydia trachomatis in, 42
    condyloma acuminata in, 272
    gonorrhea in, 83–84, 86
    herpesviruses in, 226–227
    lice in, 324
    scabies in, 315
    trichomoniasis in, 207
World Health Organization (WHO), 246, 248–250
Wright staining, 109, 230, 286

X

D-Xylose test, 190

Y

Yaws, 132, 136
Yeast vaginitis, 28. *See also* Candidiasis
Yogurt, 29

Z

Zalcitabine (ddC), 256, 258–261
Zidovudine (AZT, ZDV), 256, 258–263
Zolpidem, 262
Zoonosis, 189
Zoster, 219
Zymodemes, 168–169, 185